PHARMACEUTICALS

-A LAYPERSONS GUIDE TO SUPPLEMENTS-

FOR WRITERS AND FILM MAKERS

COMPLIED BY THE MYSTERIOUS SIMON VON WOLFIE

TLS

ISBN13: 978-1-959350-08-8

Set in, Fries & Ketchup 29/72pt, Georgia 11pt

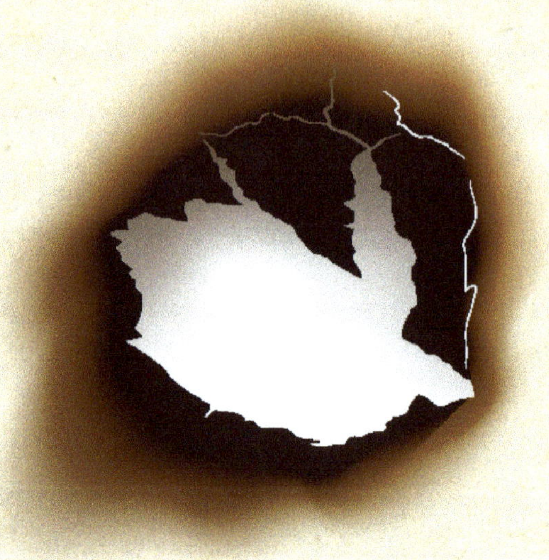

The following document is not meant as a medical guidebook.

It is not advised that anyone use this book as such.

It is meant as a resource guide for writers of screenplays and books so that when they write of drugs, medicines, antibiotics or herbals they do so armed with accurate information.

Contents

An Introduction

The purpose of the works in this collection is to provide a realistic guide for authors writing about survival after the downfall of civilization as we know it. This has nearly become a genre in its own right, spreading to encompass every form of speculative fiction from realistic projection to the fantastic. One thing that is often a major issue is the question of medication access after current pharmaceuticals have run out (or when they just aren't available). The obvious answer is that the surviving characters will go back to herbalism. But the commonly known- and used-herbs are not necessarily going to help in a number of situations – extreme pain, severe congestive heart failure, anaphylactic shock. And, in order to have characters using the dangerous plants which could help in such situations in a believable manner, the author, too, has to have some idea of what sort of dosage and preparation they might be using, how the character learned how to do this (a little hint: it's called Mrs. M. Grieve's Modern Herbal, and every post-apocalyptic character needs a copy) – and what could happen if they get the dosage wrong.

The only herb I discuss at any length here which is not potentially deadly, or even measurably toxic, is cannabis. I include it because it has been the topic of so much social prejudice, is now showing so well as a potential medicine in a great multiplicity of studies, and is probably the most vital herb any small band of survivors could possibly cultivate. This is not intended to be a complete herbal or medical guide to the post-Catastrophe author (or prepper): there are many plants native, for instance, to the Americas which could be classed as "extreme herbs".

I am focusing mainly on those which, having a long place in Western tradition and usually roles in the real-life pharmaceutical industry, are best-known in the West. With the exception of cannabis (still illegal where I live at the time of writing) I have grown the vast majority of these as ornamentals and historical display plants, though thankfully, having access to modern medicine, I have never had any need to use them. The information on use and dosage is drawn variously from older herbals, recent pharmaceutical guides and medical protocols, recent scientific studies, and occasionally professional modern herbalists. Measurements are generally given (with the exception of dosages for many medicines, since both the US and the rest of the world use metric for these) in rough equivalents of both metric and Imperial, because stories with American or older Irish/British protagonists will probably have their characters working/chiefly familiar with Imperial (or the American version, in which 1 pint = 16 rather than 20 oz...a pint is not "a pound the world 'round"!) measurements.

Also for the benefit of US writers who are not familiar with the metric system, to avoid the sort of terrible howlers that riddle John Ringo's otherwise entertaining and imaginative far-future twist on the Catastrophe, his Council Wars series (worst example in There Will Be Dragons: a character who is described as a metre and a half tall – four foot eleven – and sturdy, but not notably massively muscled or gifted with an adamantium skeleton, says of a female character on his work crew that she may have lacked the mass to do as well as he did at a physically demanding job...the female character in question having been described as 2 metres tall – a whisker under 6'7" – and "built like a male bodybuilder"). Ringo should beat his editor about the head and shoulders for having allowed him to embarrass himself in public by letting this and many other gross errors in metric understanding get through to publication stage; but he also should be slapped a little himself for not having bothered either to use a simple conversion chart or to accurately visualize his characters from one page to the next.

Another Authorial Knowledge Fail in the same series, which actually helped inspire me to write the first section of this book: at one point, a health-care-professional character grudgingly prescribes 5 mg of codeine for a man in agony from a severe injury.

Why not just give the poor guy a single aspirin or tell him to "offer up his suffering to God"?

This isn't a commonly quoted law of writing, but it should be: "When thou knowest not thine arse from thine elbow, LOOK IT UP, idiot!" Or carefully gloss it over without giving any specifics at all. The moment you (and by "you" in this instance I mean the author, not the fictional character) cite a number or a technique in any detail, you had better get it right, or at least a fair percentage of your readers will promptly lose their belief in the rest of your story.

There is a phrase to the effect that, "The secret of realism is to describe the thumb so well, the reader thinks he has seen the whole hand". This is true – but it only works if you don't then make the hand work like a foot without a really, really good explanation. Throughout these works, I shall use "they", "their", and "themself" to refer to people of non-specified gender. For many years, s/he, his/her, etc., seemed to be generally preferred and the redefinition of formerly plural forms was resisted. That formulation is, however, clunky (and some people are non-binary or gender-identity-fluid in any case).

Most Western doctors are dubious about herbalism for one basic reason. Medicine is, ultimately, based on playing the percentages – betting health against illness, and life against death. Figures are usually available for the effectiveness, safety, dosage, and metabolism of single-component, pharmaceutically pure, clinically-tested drugs – and for the risks and consequences involved in any given condition.

With tested pharmaceutical drugs, it is also possible to minimize risks by, for instance, choosing something else if the patient is in a population group likely to make them more sensitive to the negative effects; or by preparation.

For instance, the cephalosporin antibiotics (such as ceftriaxone, the first line in bacterial meningitis) have a 10% chance of cross-reactivity in a patient with a known penicillin allergy. Depending on the circumstances, the drug might be given anyway – but with preparations already on hand to enact at the first sign of an allergic reaction.

A natural plant product contains hundreds of components, and the percentage of the known active one or ones still have to be lab-tested in order to establish a precise dosage – for every batch. In addition: clinical studies are expensive, and generally pharmaceutical companies are not motivated to spend a great deal of money on something which is unlikely to benefit them, such as testing whole plants that anyone can grow or buy over the counter.

In general, the Western approach is geared towards an optimum combination of safety and efficacy. However, that only works as long as pharmaceutical products are available – hence this book, much of which deals with possible survival improvisations when the current basic pharmaceutical tools of medicine are no longer available.

Previous attempts to neologize non-gender pronouns (hir, xey, SHe) are even clunkier and more distracting; Lois McMaster Bujold's brave effort to redefine "it" as a non-perjorative in a culture with a significant hermaphrodite minority (her Miles Vorkosigan series; Baen, 1986 ff.) only works for characters of hers from that particular world, and even those characters have to lecture outsiders on why that usage is acceptable. In the immortal words of K.J. Charles, expressing in simple terms the essence of courtesy regarding the gender spectrum, "Call people what they want to be called, and treat them as they want to be treated" (An Unsuitable Heir; Penguin Random House, ebook, 2017). This should offend no one of any decency or courtesy.

My personal toxicity scale for herbal use. Note that, with the exception of hemp, essential oils should be considered as at least one level higher than the plant they come from. Essential oils are extremely concentrated (very high dosage), and do not necessarily have the same chemical profile as the raw plant material: some, in particular wintergreen, thyme, and the artemisias (mugwort, wormwood, southernwood, rue), may contain a higher percentage-per-dose of compounds that, while usually inoffensive at low to moderate whole-plant dosages, are toxic in concentration. One is unlikely to suffer harm from drinking a cup or two of wintergreen tea, but wintergreen essential oil, if not very highly diluted or if taken internally, is likely to be harmful or even fatal. The safety regarding oral use of essential oils is debated, but the evidence so far is that low-level oral dosage (1-3 drops/day – a drop is ca. 1/20 ml) is likely to be safe for the vast majority of oils. Topical use is considerably more common, as essential oils are readily absorbed through the skin and into the circulation. A famous test involved shaving a patch of fur on a rabbit, applying topical lavender oil, and then dissecting the rabbit: its liver had a distinct aroma of lavender oil.

0 – No herbs can properly be listed here, because there are no plants on this Earth to which someone might not be severely, even fatally, allergic. Some people can probably be allergic to fake flowers made from the wrong material. Even the two least toxic herbs on the planet, chamomile and cannabis, carry this risk. If a patient has not used an herb before, it would be ideal to do three specific allergy tests (topical patch test) before using freely. This may, of course, not be an option in a crisis. To be honest, I've never even heard of anyone in the health-care field doing it with any pharmaceutical medication either, even though the allergy concerns are similar; though with things like the infusion of biologicals such as are used for some auto-immune diseases, we usually do have someone standing by ready to act in case of incipient anaphylaxis.

0.5 – Cannabis and German chamomile. No direct toxicity even in the highest doses imaginable. As there has never yet been a case of death by cannabis overdose, we do not know what the LD50 for humans is, though estimates based on animal studies suggest somewhere in the region of 135 mg/kg, or ca. 8.5 kg (17.7 lbs) of pure THC in a single dose to kill an average-sized human. An extremely strong cannabis strain might contain as much as 25% THC; even the most powerful concentrated extracts seldom top 80%.

Even with purified THC, I am quite certain that if you were to inject 8.5 kg of anything into an otherwise healthy human body in one bolus, that person would not survive the injection (sometimes with severe haemorrhage, a patient might end up getting as much or more in continuous blood replacement; but the key-word there is replacement...and the prognosis is not good; one urban trauma centre evaluation of people receiving 20 units [ca. 10 kg] or more of blood had a survival rate of 30.5% and a death rate of 69.5%, although other risk factors such as aortic cross-clamping, prolonged hypotension, and the need for inotrope support seem to be more relevant to the odds of survival than the amount of blood given).

LD50 is the lethal dose in 50% of test subjects, usually rats and/or rabbits. It may vary significantly by species: for instance, the absence of certain liver enzymes in the cat mean that menthol is 3-4 times more toxic to cats than to rats. However, rodent LD50 values are generally taken as the starting point in determining toxicity.

The LD50 for oral German chamomile essential oil is > 5 grams/kg; German and Roman chamomile oils, along with lavender, are among the very, very few which are safe for infants and nursing mothers (in fact, chamomile essential oil is a splendid treatment for "cradle cap" and diaper rash). Note that a patient with ragweed allergy may have a cross-reaction to the chamomiles and other plants in the same family: if a known allergy is related to a potential herbal treatment, you really should do that triple patch test.

But even cannabis may present hazards to patients with certain pre-existing conditions, notably cardiovascular; the full safety profile regarding conception and pregnancy is not properly determined; there are some concerns about possible neurological effects in genetically-vulnerable children and adolescents; and, as mentioned above, individuals can be allergic to pretty much anything. Essential oil processed from either medicinal or fibre-only hemp is similarly safe: you have to have a toxin present in the first place in order to concentrate a toxin!

One caution about fibre-hemp products in the real world: the cannabis plant is excellent at drawing heavy metals and a number of other toxins from the ground, making industrial hemp an increasingly attractive and popular option for reclaiming chemically poisoned earth...and a bit of a concern as a source for CBD oil if specific standards are not demonstrably met by the producer.

1 – Most common kitchen herbs, lavender, etc. No toxicity in normal dosages as used for tea, cooking, or medicine. Extremely high doses of these herbs may be toxic; unless the essential oil is specifically known to be safe to use undiluted as a topical, it should generally only be used topically in a 3-5% dilution or in minute oral doses. The essential oils of chamomile and lavender are safe to use as undiluted topicals; in fact, pure lavender essential oil is one of the best possible immediate treatments for burns (along with aloe vera gel, separately or together – many people keep lavender oil and an aloe vera plant in their kitchens for just that reason). On the other hand, cinnamon is usually quite safe to eat in normal quantities, but cinnamon essential oil can actually directly burn the skin of a sensitive person.

2 - Some kitchen herbs and most "home medicinals". Mugwort, rue, tansy, pennyroyal, and wormwood are among the best-known in this class. Toxic in larger doses or to the sensitive or vulnerable individual, and may have serious acute consequences in some circumstances even at low to normal whole plant doses: e.g., the abortifacient nature of tansy, pennyroyal, and rue. Using the essential oils (one danger level higher) of these plants, topically or orally, is strongly dis advised.

3 – This is the level at which "extreme herbalism" properly begins. Except in the most desperate circumstances, these herbs should not be used for any purpose other than as garden ornamentals by anyone who is not a medically-trained herbalist. Some of these herbs are still either the direct source of or the original molecule for many real-life pharmaceuticals, but no doctor in the world would suggest that using the (unknown potency) raw herb is in any way an option when it is possible to administer pharmaceutical doses which can be judged, if necessary, down to the microgram. Henbane, deadly nightshade, woody nightshade, datura, mandrake, Chinese ephedra, opium poppies. Note that deadly nightshade, in particular, should not be grown anywhere that children might access it, as the deep purple berries are very sweet...and very poisonous!

4 – Herbs that probably should not be attempted for any medical purposes by anyone who is not a fictional character named Brother Cadfael (Monk's Hood, Edith Pargeter); and that are really too dangerous to grow even as garden ornamentals unless you can effectively fence out children and animals. Hemlock, aconite (a.k.a. monkshood, wolfbane). If growing a display garden of ancient medicinal plants, avoid touching these plants without gloves on, and be careful to bag and remove the flowers the moment they start to fade in order to avoid accidental self-seeding.

Part I: Papaver Somniferum

Introduction

Many speculative authors ask questions regarding availability of major pain medication in the event of a complete breakdown of society, after which there will be no pharmaceutical industries to supply purified and strength-quantified medications, nor doctors readily available to prescribe them and properly oversee their use. Time-travel into the past by someone with modern medical knowledge also comes up, but I think Diana Gabaldon's Outlander series and S.M. Stirling's Nantucket trilogy pretty much covered that one between them. Hence, an obvious question is whether home cultivation of the opium poppy (Papaver somniferum) might offer an alternative to the lucky survivors, assuming they are actually lucky to have survived and are not living in the equivalent of Nevil Shute's On The Beach, in which latter case they probably won't live long enough to cultivate their own poppies.

This section is written primarily as a reference for authors of fiction writing about life after a society-destroying catastrophe who wish to maximize the realism of their descriptions. It does include some details relevant to current times: e.g., pain control principles as understood in modern medical practice, the dangers of opiates/opioids in general and home-made poppy drugs in particular, and, for my fellow enthusiastic gardeners who live where it is legal to grow this beautiful flower among one's ornamentals, some cultivation, species, and sourcing details for what I consider to be some of the most attractive cultivars. Otherwise, the "you" addressed is, unless otherwise stated, specifically the fictional character preparing ahead in case of and/or living after the Catastrophe.

I emphasize, and shall continue to do so, that the non-prescription use (with the exception of low-dose over-the-counter codeine in Britain and Ireland) and/or personal production of opiates are currently illegal almost everywhere in the world. I hope that the safety issues I discuss here will help clarify why that is so. I do not advocate, recommend, or otherwise encourage the illegal production or consumption of any form of opium-related drug. In real life as we know it now, these substances should only be used under the guidance of a qualified medical practitioner.

It should be noted that, in the US, which probably has the harshest laws in this regard in the West: it is legal to sell and possess seeds of Papaver somniferum. Growing small amounts in one's garden as an ornamental is technically illegal: very seldom if ever prosecuted in normal flower-garden quantities, as shown by the vast number of garden centres that do sell these seeds (and presumably do so and continue to do so because a lot of people are buying and growing them for purely decorative purposes), but legally prosecutable under the exacting US narcotics laws. In the US, technically the presence of a live P. somniferum plant = the possession of opium.

While enforcement of this upon the home gardener growing for ornamental purposes is rare if not effectively nonexistent, certainly if anyone were to grow poppies as a garden flower and then slit the green pods for opium or get caught doing anything other than seed collection or flower arranging with the dry pods - in the US or, indeed, pretty much anywhere in the West or most of the world - the DEA or other country's equivalent will absolutely lock that person up and eat the key. So don't do it. However, even in the US, you can legally own and store your seeds against the day when you might need them (replace ca. every 2 years, they don't last forever).

Then you can plant them when either there is no longer any government or law to prevent you, or your local council is desperately grateful that some serious painkillers might still be available, as per the awesomely brilliant post-Catastrophic writings of S.M. Stirling (the Nantucket trilogy and Emberverse series), in which ornamental poppies, presumably with a lot of help from local chemistry teachers, become the source of injectable morphine in the altered world.

I will refer to the hypothetical breakdown as "the Catastrophe" without specification. There are many potential ways by which such a breakdown could occur – war, plague, massive social or geological upheaval, alien invasion, a change in the laws of the universe, causes yet unimagined. My concern here is purely: what might fictional survivors be able to do in terms of major pain control when there is no longer a pharmaceutical industry to provide products of known strength and purity, nor, necessarily, trained health-care personnel available to oversee their prescription and administration? And how could those hypothetical survivors minimize the risks associated with home production and administration of a potentially extremely hazardous drug while maintaining its efficacy when it is truly needed?

I. Pain Evaluation and Appropriate Levels of Medication

Before prescribing, providing, recommending, or using any pain medication, it is crucial for both the real-world doctor and the fictional character who is or must, after the Catastrophe, become an health-care provider to have a framework for evaluation regarding the appropriate strength and character of the same. The standard for medication choice in the Western world in real life (and hence presumably for Westerners who survive the Catastrophe) is the WHO (World Health Organization) Pain Pyramid. The WHO Pain Pyramid is defined by levels as follows:

1) Acetaminophen, most non-steroidal anti-inflammatory drugs (NSAIDs...aspirin, ibuprofen), caffeine often used as an adjunct. Most readily available herbal remedies will fall into this class.
2) Weak opiates or opioids (codeine, Tramadol), strong NSAIDs (diclofenac)
3) Strong opiates: morphine, various synthetic opioids (Oxycontin, Oxynorm)
4) Extremely strong opiates: heroin/"diamorphine" (used in the UK and some European countries for palliative care pain relief), fentanyl (generally used in time-release patches for major chronic pain management; 100x stronger than morphine. Evidence is increasingly showing that the rise in opioid ODs in both the prescription and abuser populations is due to the misuse of fentanyl, either by the patient in hopes of more relief or by the supplier of illegal opiates/opioids cutting various substances with fentanyl to deceive the consumer into believing they are actually getting what they paid for). Singers Prince and Tom Petty both died from accidental fentanyl overdoses in attempts to deal with severe chronic pain.

!

An opiate is an alkaloid or alkaloid-combination naturally produced by P. somniferum: opium, codeine, morphine. An opioid is a synthetic product based on a P. somniferum alkaloid, but which has had structural molecular alterations made in a laboratory to suit it for human use – e.g., thebaine, the main base for many opioid drugs; toxic and non-narcotic in the natural state, requiring considerable processing to make it into a human painkiller. Opium is the whole-plant extract, which includes all the natural alkaloids in the percentages present in the specific plant.

The phrase "opiate-naïve" refers to a patient who has never used opiates/opioids; has used them for only short periods of time in the past; or who has discontinued use long enough for their tolerance to return to its original level. It is considered the baseline state for establishing the likeliest safe dosage in any patient who does not have a well-established current tolerance.

Cannabis (hemp) should be considered, according to dosage/plant strain/ method of preparation, as falling into the 1-2 levels of pain control. Oral lipid-based extracts, which include all products made with cannabis-infused butter, are metabolized through the liver, altering delta-9-THC into 11-hydroxy-THC, and have a significantly more potent effect and much longer duration (ca. 8-10 hours vs. the 2-4 hours expected from normal levels of inhalation use), and should be considered more appropriate to WHO 2, whereas low to moderate quantities of inhaled hempflower are a closer equivalent to WHO 1.

This is based on reports from states and countries which have legalized cannabis for either medical or general usage. So far, while cannabis seems to be proving acceptable as a single drug or adjunct for WHO 1 and 2 pain treatment, and as an adjunct allowing reduction of opiate/opioid dose at WHO 3, the consensus appears to be that it will never replace the WHO 3 drugs in treatment of severe pain. Decreases in opiate/opioid prescription levels in recent "legalized states", do seem to indicate that hemp may potentially be a valuable tool in reducing opiate/opioid use and abuse, particularly in chronic pain.

Generally, when going up the WHO pain pyramid step by step (the usual process for chronic pain; in acute pain, of course, one may skip straight to level 3 if needed, plus lower-level adjuncts as appropriate), one does not cut out levels 1 or 2, but rather keeps them as adjuncts to minimize the dose of stronger pain control required. Take the hypothetical post-Catastrophe case of Grandma Annie, whose arthritis has been controlled effectively for a while by willow bark (NSAID...salicylic acid, level 1) and a dose of cannabis (levels 1-2) when required.

Since both osteoarthritis and rheumatoid arthritis are degenerative conditions, and since in the case of the latter, the drugs that have proved most effective in controlling the condition will no longer be available, Grandma Annie may reach the point where her herbal NSAID and hemp are no longer doing the job, or so much cannabis is required that she can no longer keep track of her rows and stitches while she knits, which has a significant negative impact on her self-image and quality of life.

Both an increase in herbal treatment (various topicals added to the willow bark and either a lower dose of cannabis or a switch to a higher CBD/lower THC strain if available, say) to reduce inflammation, and, if that doesn't work, a codeine-equivalent dosage of poppy product (1/10th the dose for oral morphine as per each individual batch) may be necessary to control pain and restore function. Grandma A. is now solidly up to WHO level 2, while keeping the WHO level 1 drugs which also have a direct effect on the causative condition.

If her condition becomes still worse (more likely if she had rheumatoid all along rather than osteo), the level of opiate may be slowly titrated up to WHO level 3 if necessary while maintaining or increasing the adjuncts at levels 1 and 2, trying to find the optimum balance for her between pain management and general function/ enjoyment of life. Your responsibility for Grandma Annie's treatment does not stop with evaluating her and producing her medications, either. Massaging her poor distorted, painful hands with anti-inflammatory oils on a regular basis in addition to her oral pain meds will probably also be a huge help to her, as will making sure that she has things to do that help her remember that she is still a valuable and contributing member of the community, such as teaching others how to perform the skills she can no longer carry out herself, or telling instructive stories to the children. And the latter, after the Catastrophe, will be far more than simple entertainment!

Unless the carer-character or someone in their survivor group is in a position to refine morphine to heroin, level 4 will not be possible to achieve after the Catastrophe. Upwards opium-extract titration and adjunct use will most likely be the only option in extremely severe palliative pain cases. More dubious substances like krokodil can allegedly be made more easily, but given the gruesome side effects, you might as well just take an axe to your patient's skull: it would achieve the same results in a cleaner and kinder manner. Establishing where on the WHO scale a patient may fall at any given time is a dodgy and difficult process, as pain is fundamentally subjective. An injury one person hardly notices may be agonizing for another; and only the patient truly knows how much pain they are feeling. The standard initial medical guide is the subjective (= patient's opinion) 0-10 Pain Scale...0 being "no pain", 10 being "worst pain imaginable".

However, that varies hugely from person to person, both in terms of intrinsic pain perception and in terms of...how accurately the scale is understood and the pain is reported. Some people will claim an 8 or 9...when they were sitting up in bed happily playing with their Internet device as the doctor entered. Some people will say, "Nah, not more than a 3", despite the fact that they have a compound fracture and their broken leg bone is sticking out into the open air. Duration of pain is also a relevant issue. A good punch in the nose may reach 6 to 7 for a few seconds to as much as half a minute, and a sharp blow to the gonads even higher for a little longer; but then the pain usually dulls down to a 3 or lower...easily tolerated by most people with no more than a WHO 1 drug at most, or even just a bit of ice.

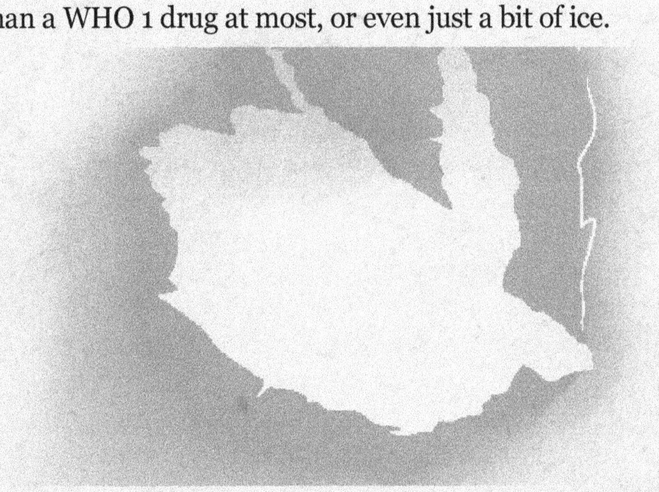

Ask any guy who's ever taken a good one in the meat-and-two-veg – the pain can be sometimes bad enough to cause vomiting initially, but seldom if ever requires as much as a low dose of codeine by the time the drug could be requested and supplied unless real structural damage were done. But if the degree of pain from the initial impact were steadily ongoing for hours, it would be difficult to endure and would definitely require major analgesia. Some unfortunate women, most often as a result of endometriosis, have the same pain level during the first day or two of menstruation as that Dreaded Nut Shot, if the blow in question were repeated every few minutes for several hours, and most certainly need WHO 2 plus smooth muscle relaxant adjuncts until their inner parts and possibly ectopic tissue quiet down. I myself once experienced a 10 during a medical procedure in a very sensitive region, but thankfully, it only lasted for a fraction of a second (just seemed like forever), and so nothing besides my already-ongoing post-surgical analgesia -WHO 2 at the time - was required. Whereas a constant, unremitting 5 that doesn't respond to WHO 2 may eventually become unbearable without titrating up towards WHO 3.

My personal observational pain scale - note that this does not necessarily refer to chronic pain patients or patients who have undergone repeated or prolonged experiences of major pain in the past, many of whom have learned by necessity to function and appear relatively normal in spite of considerable suffering! Also recall that some people really are just bloody stoic, whereas others really do have pain thresholds that are more like pain gutters. If in doubt, check your patient's chart and history, and consider their physical situation.

1-3...patient may appear somewhat annoyed/unhappy. Needs aspirin/ ibuprofen/ acetaminophen or herbal equivalent (WHO level 1).

4-5...patient is rubbing the spot (if there is a particular spot and if they can bear to touch it), moving carefully, and may start looking a bit pale or flushed. If a WHO 1 drug has already been administered and failed to work, patient probably needs a low to medium dose of codeine (ca. 8-30 mg); minute/diluted poppy extract equivalent for codeine; or – post-Catastrophe or where medically available and recommended for this purpose - a solid dose of cannabis (WHO level 2; roughly estimated at 20-30 mg THC for the cannabis-naïve or occasional user; the cannabis-experienced can estimate their own dosage without risk). Many or most patients may still be able to distract themselves to a greater or lesser degree with activities or mental pain control, though mild to moderate analgesia is recommended unless refused.

6-7...patient is short of words; disinclined to move unnecessarily or do anything that might be mildly pleasurable. Definitely not chatting cheerfully with their mates on the phone or playing games on their device, or whatever the post-Catastrophe equivalent may be (knitting, whittling, whatever). Patient needs something from a solid dose of codeine (60 mg, equivalent to 6 mg oral morphine) to, if absolutely necessary, a low starter dose of morphine (oral 10 mg) or post-Catastrophe poppy-drug equivalent (WHO upper 2 to low 3).

8-9...patient can't do much beside lie there, moan, and if they're one of the "I am so tough" people, may grit out, "I'm fine, it's no more than a 3 or 4" between their teeth. Patient definitely needs something comparable to an oral 20 mg or IV/IM 10 mg dose of morphine. More may be required if that is ineffective. WHO pain pyramid 3 (IV/IM morphine 10 mg, oral 20-30 mg; strong opioid such as Oxycontin or Oxynorm). However, if they refuse any particular suggested analgesia, they have the right to do so and you cannot ethically administer it. Check every 15 minutes or so until either they are hurting less or change their mind.

10...patient is lying there screaming, if they have the strength, or just sort of moaning incoherently in agony. Patient should get at least 10 mg of morphine IV/IM if possible or 20-30 mg oral/equivalent at once, with the option of titrating up carefully if needed. Observe carefully and titrate up with care until relief is obtained. Remember that oral analgesics take longer than IV or IM analgesics to absorb, so treat appropriately. If it looks as though you may need to titrate up, do not pump a new oral dose into them before they have had a full hour for the plasma levels of the last one to peak. WHO pain pyramid a solid 3, and if the pain continues at that level on an ongoing basis without responding to maximum tolerable levels of WHO 3 plus adjuncts, it may even be time to consider moving to WHO 4 if you can. This sort of thing is why we developed fentanyl patches in real life.

10+...allegedly reported from some severe jellyfish stings in Australia and some particularly disastrous large-body-area burns. Not even on the subjective scale: patient has been rendered apparently unconscious by a large dose of morphine, and is still writhing and screaming in their state of incomprehensible agony. Good luck to you and the patient, you'll both need it. Not sure if even WHO pain pyramid 4 would do the job, were it available to you, which it may or may not be in a modern hospital context (fentanyl generally is, but due to its extreme strength...ca. 100x morphine, remember!...it is not often, actually never to my knowledge, used in emergency situations, given the incredible ease of overdose), and certainly won't be after the Castastrophe, unless you actually cleaned out the hospital pharmacy before fleeing to the hills. Fortunately, unless you live in Australia or are dealing with the aftermath of a major fire incident, you will probably never see a 10+. If you're religious, pray you never do.

Negative values (again, may not be relevant to the chronic pain or pain-experienced patient, who can often fake normalcy surprisingly well):

» Patient's colour is good, showing little signs of suffering, sitting up in bed, and lively, and then they go, "Argh, it's at least an 8". While it is not ethically acceptable to whack such a patient on the head, no matter how tempted you may be, it most certainly is ethically acceptable and maybe ethically required to offer them only the appropriate drug for their apparent level of pain, which is most probably WHO 1.

Some hospital health-care personnel, especially those in ER practice who have seen more than their share of drug-seekers, have more elaborate equations regarding subtractions for things like, "I have a really high pain threshold, but this is...", or "I can't take any synthetic drugs, I have to have real codeine/morphine". Sometimes actually true, but not nearly as often as claimed. Check chart and history. If patient does have a history of violent nausea or other reaction after synthetic opioid administration, they're telling the truth...and I've seen that, too. Give them the opiate if their pain level appears to make it appropriate; the last thing a patient in pain needs is to start vomiting violently on top of the initial problem. Not that the latter will be a problem after the Catastrophe, since there won't be any synthetic opioids after the existing supply has run out.

II. Dangers and Concerns Associated with Opiate/Opioid Use; Recognizing and Treating Toxicity

a) Addiction: I hardly need to discuss the dangers of opiate/opioid addiction and the difficulties and agonies of withdrawal, as these are well-known. It only remains to say: if enough opiates can be extracted from any part of the poppy by any means, and are consumed with sufficient frequency, poppy seed tea can be just as addictive eventually (if not quite as swiftly, due to the slower uptake and lesser reward-rush in the brain) as shooting heroin. The crushed-pod product known as "doda" is, indeed, becoming an increasing problem in regards to abuse and addiction in the West as controls are tightened on pharmaceutical opiates. Just because it's natural doesn't mean it's safe: hemlock and Destroying Angel mushrooms are natural too.

b) Dosage control: This is the most immediate concern with any medication made directly from herbs in situations which do not allow a thorough assay of the medication's chemical constituents, especially herbs on which it is easy to go from "insufficient dose" to "fatal overdose" (low therapeutic index). It's true for digoxin (foxglove); it's true for atropine (deadly nightshade); and it's just as true for opiates (P. somniferum). This is a very significant reason why the vast majority of doctors prefer pharmaceutical products of proven potency to the herbs from which they are refined, and why no health-care professional today in real life, at least certainly not in the West (or anywhere else where a professional pharmaceutical alternative presents itself), would voluntarily make their own digoxin, atropine, or opiates.

Even the same strain of poppy, grown at the same times of year on the same land with the same fertilizers, etc., may vary considerably in active components for year to year due to weather. Therefore, the extract you make in year 8 ATC (After The Catastrophe) might prove to be twice as strong as the extract you made the year before, and using the same dosage levels without through and careful testing beforehand could kill you or a loved one with an overdose, because naloxone is not something you can make in your post-Catastrophe kitchen. Or it could be half as strong, and the same dosage would not suffice for appropriate analgesia.

Each batch of any herbal product which could so readily become fatal would have to be tested individually, starting with a minute account and titrating successively upwards until the desired strength is reached (see below under "Extraction" for some general estimates and hypothetical trial dosage levels). The ideal tester for poppy products would be a healthy adult who has experienced prescribed opiates in the past (for instance, post-surgical/emergency injury morphine followed by codeine), but has not done so for some time, returning them to an opiate-naïve level of sensitivity. Such a person is likely to be able to compare dosage strength to pharmaceutical opiates of known potency, but will not underestimate efficacy at normal minimal doses as, for instance, a chronic pain patient who is still accustomed to necessary pharmaceutical opiates might do.

However, the latter might well be able to give an experienced opinion on strength of a given dose as compared to their normal known pharmaceutical dosage, so their advice should not be ignored. If you are a time-traveler into the past, the need for you to see to your own testing of poppy products will vary according to when you are. At any time prior to the sixteenth century, when Paracelsus created the first known recipe for laudanum, poppy preparations were not even slightly standardized. Even if your colleague was a student of Hippocrates or Avicenna (ibn Sina), or trained in Alexandria, the dosages he (most likely) recommends for his own poppy concoctions should probably be taken as a general guideline from which to formulate your own test for each batch, rather than a final evaluation.

With the introduction of standardized recipes and concurrent dosage recommendations for laudanum, the reliability of pre-testing increases, but is not conclusive. Laudanum was generally a tincture made with whole opium (plus various flavorings, apparently opium by itself is nasty bitter); and the potency of the opium crop in India, for instance, might have been well over the odds one year, and absolute crap the year following, with a matching increase or decrease in the potency of laudanum made to the same recipe each year. If you are going back no further than the American Civil War (1860-65), purified injectable morphine will be available, with the corresponding increase in dosage reliability. You will probably be quite shocked by how freely your colleagues administer any poppy product from paregoric to injected morphine (try to hide your shock, it's not normal for the era and could get you in trouble – and trouble, even as late as the 19th century, could mean a lot worse than people looking at you funny), and by their common failure to wean patients off morphine long after the original injury has healed. But at least you can rely to a reasonable degree on measurements of the drug itself.

In the contexts of either time travel or post-Catastrophe surgery: one should note that Galen didn't believe in surgical analgesia at all, probably because he had seen it kill as many patients as the original condition or the surgery. Galen was also able to perform the most complex and dangerous operations...some of which, like a hemipericardectomy when an infection of the sternum proved to have spread, would be challenging to a modern surgeon under optimal conditions...at roughly the speed of light. Unless you have Galen's insane level of surgical skill, which is like saying, "unless you can lift heavier rocks than Hercules or Grettir the Strong", he should be admired, but not considered a practical example. I refer to the nineteenth-century surgeon Dr. Robert Liston, who tried to match Galen for speed, and was, to be fair, very good at what was a necessary skill in his time to avoid just losing the patient from shock...but is also famed and shamed for being the only surgeon ever to perform an operation that achieved a 300% mortality rate. That's not a typo or bad math. 300%.

The patient died of a post-surgical infection; so did Liston's assistant, whose fingers Liston managed to amputate in the process of the operation; and one spectator was so terrified when Liston's scalpel slashed his coat that he dropped dead from "fright". I'd be very nervous about consulting any student of Galen's for any purpose, though if I needed a major operation in his era, he'd be the only surgeon I'd even consider would give me a fair chance of survival...and if I were writing a novel with a super-surgeon as the hero/ine, I would absolutely use Galen as the model, allowing me to express a well-documented "neener neener" to any critic who suggested that the surgical feats were impossible.

I refer to Susan P. Mattern's: The Prince of Medicine: Galen in the Roman Empire (Oxford University Press, 2013) for any post-Catastrophe or time-travel author who wants to know what is theoretically, and at least proven once in practice, possible for the most extremely gifted surgeon. And I don't doubt that Galen, in whatever afterlife the huge amount of good he did in his life is almost certainly allowing him to enjoy, is smirking right now as I stroke his stereotypical surgeon ego, which he certainly did not lack.

With proper attention to dosage safety, even if one does not have the capabilities (or the nerve, given its explosive character and lower safety profile compared to current real-life anaesthetics) to make ether, a reasonable middle ground should be attainable when there is no option outside of invasive surgery. High levels of opiates as the primary anaesthetic may well be more dangerous than ether, but at least they are preferable to alcohol, which has been the usual Western alternative. Cannabis may safely be combined with either, but while it is a fair adjunct, it won't do much for a major surgery patient on its own.

The desired initial single-dose strength, for opiate-naïve adults in severe pain, is generally accepted in medical practice as the equivalent of 10 mg morphine IV/IM or 20-30 mg morphine oral (absorption is less when administered orally; recommendations range from 2-3x the IV/IM dose. Intravenous takes effect more swiftly than intramuscular, but the potencies are comparable). This may be titrated upwards as necessary by effect, to a reasonable degree depending on the patient and the circumstances. Codeine is metabolized to morphine in the human liver, but the potency is much weaker in comparison to the original dose (1/10 the strength of oral morphine), and the onset is slower. That severely injured John Ringo patient-character I mentioned earlier should have gotten at least 5 mg, and more likely 10 mg, of IV/IM morphine, not 5 mg of codeine!

Codeine phosphate can be administered intramuscularly or subcutaneously, but I have never seen nor directly heard of this being done and was never so much as taught that it was an option. I had to check the Internet to find out if it was even possible. Usually codeine is only given orally; presumably the injections are reserved for patients who do not require morphine, but do require codeine, and are vomiting too badly to get pills down. Codeine makes up a much lesser part of the alkaloid content of P. somniferum, but is generally not present to a degree which would make a significant difference, for help or harm, in a whole-opium extract. Pharmaceutical codeine is normally synthesized from morphine, as, being a much milder and thus relatively safer drug, it is far more commonly administered and prescribed than its chemical predecessor.

Therefore, much larger quantities are required worldwide than could be directly extracted from poppies. It is crucial to be aware that an oral dose of 100-200 mg morphine (= 50-100 mg IV/IM morphine) is often fatal in opiate-naïve adults. However, a patient in palliative care, or a long-term chronic pain patient, may eventually require rather more than that on a regular basis due to both increasing tolerance and increasing pain. I have personally seen palliative-care cancer patients whose pain was barely or even inadequately controlled by a dosage that would undoubtedly kill an opiate-naïve person.

The question of the morality of prescribing, to a terminal patient in severe pain, a high enough level of opiates that their life may be further shortened (but its quality improved) thereby is the subject of much debate. However, it is commonly accepted throughout the Western medical profession that, in a terminal patient who is nearing a potentially agonizing end, quality of life trumps quantity of life. Addiction is obviously not a matter of concern in someone who is extremely unlikely to live long enough for drug weaning/withdrawal to ever be a concern. This is why the UK, for instance, still uses pharmaceutical heroin when necessary in the latter stages of palliative care. Although they call it diamorphine, not least to avoid distressing the patient/their family with the social-stigma implications..."My God, you're giving Grandpa HEROIN! Like a JUNKIE!" In addition to yearly variability, all strains of P. somniferum are not created equal in terms of alkaloid content.

The morphine content of dry ornamental cultivar capsules has been shown to range from as low as 50 mg/100 grams of dry deseeded capsule (.5 mg morphine/gram) to over 700 mg/100 grams of dry deseeded capsule (7 mg of morphine/gram), with pods of even the same cultivar in the same trial varying by as much as +/- 70 mg/100 grams, for a total variance of 1.4 mg morphine/gram, or a light morphine IV shot's difference between two single 4 gram pods of the same cultivar grown at the same time in the same field.

A moderately large ornamental 4 gr. capsule, depending on its cultivar of origin (and assuming the exact same growing conditions), could theoretically provide anything from 2 mg to 28 mg of oral morphine – or from the equivalent of slightly less than 2 over-the-counter low-codeine pills (25 mg codeine is the maximum dosage for OTC codeine in Ireland/UK), to nearly the maximum possible recommendation for initiating oral morphine. Varieties used for pharmaceutical cultivation, many of which are also grown as ornamentals, can have even higher concentrations. The same source cited the "Buddha" strain as 1640 mg morphine/100 g dry poppy capsule, that is, 1.6% morphine content, or 64 mg/4 gr. capsule (slightly over two maximum oral morphine doses for the opiate-naïve), and noted that generally the minimum content for pharmaceutical-cultivation varieties is ca. 800 mg/100 grams (32 mg morphine, the maximum oral dose plus the equivalent of 20 mg codeine extra, from that hypothetical 4 gram capsule). These figures, however, are based on using modern techniques to assay morphine content.

It is extremely improbable that, however hard the post-Catastrophe survivor tries, they will be able to extract 100% of that content with the methods available to them. However, until proven otherwise by careful testing of each batch, the higher contents must be assumed. It is better to delay full relief by cautious observation and slow titration than to cause an overdose. The former is unpleasant and certainly not ideal; but the latter may well be fatal.Different patients also metabolize opiates at different rates, so even a dose of pharmaceutically-assayed potency may prove problematical in some people with no obvious indications for concern, as any quick survey of adverse events associated with opiate treatment will show.

As with any drug that has not been used on that particular patient before: the rule is "start low, go slow" until individual tolerance under the specific circumstances is ascertained. Even if the Catastrophe caught you by surprise, do not just bung pods into your grinder, make a tea, and drink it yourself or feed anyone else the whole thing, as some people writing on the Internet today are wont to do. First, the majority of said people are not exactly opiate-naïve – some are long-term addicts to a frightening degree - and so are at less risk of overdose from any given preparation than someone who does not commonly use opiates, due to increased (sometimes vastly increased) tolerance.

Second, they are often working with pods grown for crafting purposes, most commonly the "Giganteum" strain preferred for decorative flower arrangements, which is comparatively low-morphine for ornamental strains (the previously-cited study evaluated Giganteum as running around 200 mg/100 grams, or a maximum of 8 mg from that hypothetical 4 gram pod – still more than a maximum post-surgical 60 mg dose of codeine!). Extraction inefficiency and tolerance levels lead to the common Internet tea-user suggestion of 3-4 pods/dose as a starter. But if an opiate-naïve person got hold of some stronger pods and used the same dosage, it would very probably be fatal. Third, making up one batch with pods of untested potency and consuming the whole thing in one go is likely to be either dangerous or ineffective.

As P.J. O'Rourke observed in Republican Party Reptile (Grove, 1987), more or less: recreational drugs come in only two dosages: not enough and way too much. This can also be true when working with untested medications of any sort, except for cannabis; the only practical way to kill someone with cannabis is to shove their head into a bale and suffocate them with it, or drop a tightly compressed 20-lb. brick on their head from a great height. And even cannabis, now that proper studies can be done, is showing indications that it may well be hazardous to those with uncontrolled high blood pressure, cardiac issues, or stroke history/high stroke risk.

If these indications prove to be correct, and so far they seem quite solid, I would expect to see cannabis at least relatively contraindicated in such patients. Opiates, and to a lesser degree pretty much everything else that grows in your garden, including common kitchen herbs such as thyme and rosemary, have a much, much lower therapeutic index (the difference between "dose needed to be effective" and "dose that has a fair chance of causing seriously undesirable consequences, like killing the patient"). So, Catastrophe survivor, if you want to keep surviving: be very very careful with your testing, measurements, and dosage. Do not play Russian roulette with single batches of pod tea.

This goes ten, or perhaps an hundred, times over for poppy seed tea, the dosage of which is far harder to estimate even on a preliminary basis, because there is literally no way to guess how much powdered opiate-containing poppy detritus got caught on the seeds' coats in any given batch, even if they come from the same source every time. Poppy seed tea isn't just Russian roulette; it's Russian roulette where the player doesn't even know how many chambers are loaded and how many are empty. So if you were hoarding unwashed poppy seeds in bulk as the most obviously legal way in the US to have a stash of opiates available in case the world falls apart suddenly...don't.

Just don't. Wash those seeds, toast them, grind them, and bake with them once they are safely deopiated. Or, instead of being the surviving protagonist of your story, you could well end up as "poor bugger who survived the Catastrophe, then accidentally killed themself by doing something stupid". Of which there will no doubt be quite a few. It is true that some people have succeeded in growing poppies from bakery seeds thrown into their backyard. The beautiful and comparatively strong (for an ornamental) cultivar "Lauren's Grape" is said to be descended from seeds planted off a bagel by Colorado garden notable Lauren Springer. Apparently she saw the rich purple flowers produced by one of these seeds and decided to propagate it, producing one of the most popular ornamental varieties today.

But since it is legal to own and store poppy seeds everywhere in the West, it's probably a better idea to just order some from a garden centre and tuck them away. Then at least, when you need to sprout them after the Catastrophe, you have the beginnings of a clue about what you might be getting. Children and the elderly, as well as patients with liver disease, metabolize opiates more slowly than healthy adults. As a consequence, not only is overdose more likely, but it may well be delayed past the point where a young/healthy adult in great pain might be needing another dose. With these patients, start very low and go very slow; and always make sure that, if opiate treatment is necessary for a vulnerable patient, someone is monitoring them for at least 12 hours after the most recent dose.

Paediatric pharmacokinetics, in particular, are often not the same as adult pharmacokinetics. One cannot assume a safe dose of any drug for a child simply by calculating by weight percentage unless the specific pharmacokinetics for that drug in children are known! Having said that: after the Catastrophe, it is possible that you, by using a minute dose of poppy, could save the life of an infant or small child with extreme diarrhoea...they can dehydrate with shocking speed!...but careful observation to make sure that the cure isn't as deadly as the disease is necessary. If the diarrhoea is caused by poisoning, opiate should not be administered until the toxin has been cleared from the body. Modern pharmaceutical paregoric, at a strength of 2 mg morphine/5 ml liquid (1/25th the strength of opium tincture in the modern pharmacoepia, which is 10 mg/ml), is given to paediatric patients at a dosage of 0.1-0.2 ml/kg (0.04 – 0.08 mg morphine/kg), no more frequently than an absolute maximum of every 4 hours, with a dose spacing of 6 hours being the more usual maximum.

Children have died because a prescriber carelessly abbreviated "diluted tincture of opium" (paregoric) as DTO, and someone read that as "deodorized tincture of opium" (full-strength morphine-wise, but with the unpleasant odour and emesis-promoting poppy alkaloid noscapine removed), thus giving the child 25 times as much of the drug as they ought to have had – like giving an opiate-naive adult 250-500 mg of oral morphine instead of 10-20 mg.

I repeat myself again, because this is crucial. It is always best to start at the minimum possible effective dose of an opiate (or, indeed, any drug). If necessary, titrate up slowly and carefully; and reduce the dose/cease the medication whenever it is possible to do so without causing your patient needless suffering.

c) Signs of opiate toxicity:

Confusion, delirium, visible intoxication (may appear superficially similar to alcoholic intoxication)

--Cold, clammy skin

--Muscular limpness

--Vomiting. Actually one of the best things the patient can do if the dose was oral. If they are unconscious or their consciousness is significantly compromised, ensure that they do not aspirate the vomit and choke or develop aspiration pneumonia later by turning them on their side in "recovery position" (described below) and keeping a close watch on their airway status.

-- Miosis (the characteristic "pinpoint pupils" of opiate intoxication)

--Extreme sleepiness/loss of consciousness; the patient cannot be awakened.

--Intermittent loss of consciousness ("nodding off")

--Slow, irregular, difficult breathing (opiates/opioids depress the breathing reflex), which may proceed to complete cessation of breathing and major brain damage or death if intervention does not occur swiftly.

--Peripheral and central cyanosis (blueness of finger- and toetips, lips, and tongue), a sign of dangerously lowered oxygen levels. Also seen in general with severe lung and/or heart conditions, both of which can be provoked acutely by opiate overdose. Cyanosis, particularly central (lips and tongue), is always a worrying sign; but when the state of hypoxaemia has taken a while to develop, the body makes some adjustments (this is why giving high-percentage O_2 can actually be quite hazardous in patients with chronic low oxygen/high carbon-dioxide respiratory issues, who have come to rely on drops in their O_2 level rather than raised CO_2 levels to activate their drive to breathe). When cyanosis manifests within a very short period of time, as is the case when opiate overdose is the cause, it is a sign of serious and immediate danger.

--Pulmonary oedema (fluid filling the lungs)

--Death.

D) Treating an overdose

The most effective treatment for opiate/opioid overdose is an injection of naloxone. You can't make this in your kitchen, post-Catastrophe or otherwise, although if you start out as a prepper before the Catastrophe, you definitely want to stock up on it. One very positive result of the "opioid crisis recognition" is that, in the interest of harm reduction, naloxone is becoming much more commonly available, particularly to first responders. Some states are now permitting everything from "prescription to family/friends of opiate patients or abusers" to "over-the-counter". So the character preparing for disaster before the Catastrophe may not need to be a professional health-care provider themself at that time in order to obtain and stock up on this crucial drug.

Any US physician may prescribe naloxone without the legal concerns now associated with prescription of even necessary opiates. Naloxone is probably the most valuable single method of acute harm reduction in the context of opiate/opioid abuse. You, the survivor, will want to know about expired naloxone. If you're lucky and careful, it could be a long time after the Catastrophe when you have to use your stash, and it might well be out of date by then (total shelf life at full potency is between 18 and 24 months, expiration date is required to be at least 12 months from the time of purchase).

Naloxone will diminish in potency after its expiration date, but will not become toxic. If outdated naloxone is all you have, then use it! More of the expired stuff may be needed than if it were still in-date, but even a weakened dose will give your OD patient a better chance. There is, of course, every chance that you may have to use your naloxone hoard within quite a short period of the Catastrophe to head off one or more suicide attempts.

Herbal Laxatives

If giving stimulant herbal laxatives which stimulate a little too much for comfort, make sure the patient stays hydrated and administer tea made with a high-potassium herb such as dried chervil at ca. 83 mg per tablespoon. Poppy seeds are also quite high in potassium (63 mg/tablespoon). Diarrhoea notably causes potassium loss, and severely low potassium causes fatal heart complications (singer Karen Carpenter died of this, secondary to her anorexia).

The recommended daily dose for potassium is 3.5 grams/day, supplied by a normal diet that includes fruit and vegetables. If the diarrhoea is severe, oral rehydration salts may be needed. Commercial ones contain potassium; homemade ones must have it added.

Do not use any stimulant herbal laxative longer than needed. They may impair the bowel's ability to function on its own after discontinuance. Cut dosages down to the lowest effective level, and be sure to give plenty of fibre/bulking agents.

Aloe Vera. The yellowish layer inside the skin, not the gel that fills the leaf. Very harsh: dosage is 1/32 teaspoon, 150 mg., or 2 1/3 grains (see "Weights and Measures" for apothecary equivalents).

This part of the aloe can be dried and preserved for future use. Save it for your most urgent cases. Aloe is also a notable topical medication for burns, and should be considered one of your most valuable post-Catastrophe herbs.

For real-life doctors, first responders, etc., there is now a major ethical, and indeed sometimes a legal, issue involved in whether or not one has the right to forcibly interfere with the suicide of a competent adult who refuses life-saving treatment. As matters in the medical profession stand now, it is held that a competent adult cannot be forced to accept even life-saving treatment against their will.

After the Catastrophe, the legal issues will no longer apply, but the moral issues will. Ultimately it will come down to your conscience...if you were a professional health-care provider before the Catastrophe, your internalization of medical ethics, which very much do include the patient's right of autonomy, may lead you in a very different direction than if you are a Catholic priest.

At least I assume so: I do not actually know what the current position of the Catholic Church is in regards to individual autonomy in such matters. In any case, I think my point about differences in training and ideology determining different behaviours in such circumstances stands (and, for your author, opens up some interesting possibilities).

The chief risk of naloxone is the provocation of withdrawal in patients who are addicted to opiates. Otherwise, there is no risk known to any patient. Naloxone works purely as an opiate antagonist; you cannot kill your patient with it, although if they are addicted to opiates/opioids you can briefly make them quite unhappy by chucking them straight into withdrawal.

Since time is crucial in treating an overdose, naloxone dosing is always empirical (a.k.a. "best guess when we don't have time to run any tests or they aren't back yet"), often starting with 0.5 mg and increasing the dose every 3 to 4 minutes if there is no response (2 mg...4 mg...10 mg). Details of dosage may vary between areas, but this is a fairly common version and a good basic guide...remembering, again, that you just can't kill someone with naloxone.

!

To make activated charcoal:

Build a medium-sized fire outdoors. Fill a large metal pot with small pieces of hardwood (nutshells can also be used, as can bone). The pot should have a lid with a vent hole in it.

Cook the wood for 3-5 hours on your open fire until no more smoke or gas is escaping from the vent. At this time, it should have been rendered down into pure charcoal.

Allow to cool. When cool, rinse off all ash and debris with clean water.

Crush or grind the charcoal to powder and allow to completely air-dry.

If you have calcium chloride, combine it with water in a ratio of 1 part calcium chloride to 3 parts water. If not, lemon juice (or other acid solution such as vinegar) or bleach (or other strong base) can be used undiluted.

Mix the liquid and charcoal powder into a paste. Cover and allow to sit for 24 hours, then drain. Rinse thoroughly with sterilized water to remove traces of activating chemicals.

Cook (covered; at least the boiling temperature of water, 212 F/100 C) for three hours longer. The activated charcoal is now ready for use.

If there is no response after 15 mg (unexpired, full-strength), then there may be a problem other than the opiate. Hopefully you or another character did not, in your post-Catastrophe desperation, try to compound one of those ancient surgical anaesthesia remedies in which opiates are combined with henbane, mandrake, and deadly nightshade or similar.

Significant alcohol intoxication also potentiates the depressive effects of opiates, and while naloxone might deal with the opiate part of alcohol intoxication + poppy, it won't do a thing for the effects of the alcohol.

High cannabis dosage + poppy does not increase the risk unless the patient also had a pre-existing cardiovascular condition. If they did or might have done, you should be worried about cardiac issues and stroke, and take such measures as are available to you.

Otherwise, sufficient amounts of cannabis, particularly orally administered, may keep the fundamentally healthy patient unconscious even after the opiates have been blocked.

If there is no response to naloxone after you have given 15 mg of full-strength in-date, or somewhat more of possibly weakened expired, naloxone, offer supportive treatment as described below and keep a close eye on vital signs.

Note that naloxone may be shorter-lived than a large dose of opiates, and is definitely shorter-lived than the long-lasting pharmaceutical opioids (especially important to know if your patient got hold of some pre-Catastrophe Oxycontin or similar). Observe patient closely for at least 12 hours and repeat dosage if necessary.

Opium was used effectively to treat cholera in the 18th and 19th centuries. Fortunately, we now know that if a cholera patient is supplied with constant oral or IV re-hydration and electrolytes, they will survive and recover in a few days, no opiates required. However, in the absence of IVs and presence of the inability to tolerate the great volumes of oral re-hydration/electrolyte balance required (cholera can also cause vomiting), opium may still play a role in post-Catastrophe cholera outbreaks. When all the oral re-hydration salts packets have run out, the most adequate substitute would be:

--6 level teaspoons of honey or sugar (honey is preferred due to antibacterial activity, except in infants < 1 year, who are vulnerable to botulism spores in honey; give sugar or boil the honey with water at a rolling boil for at least half an hour.)

--½ level teaspoon salt

--Dissolved in 1 litre/5 cups water.

Potassium may be at least partially replaced by first making the water into a tea with 1-2 oz (28-56 grams) dried chervil, chamomile, nettle, alfalfa, parsley, spearmint, dill, or other high-potassium herb.

If the cholera patient is vomiting uncontrollably, inhalation of opium (together with continued efforts to administer anti-emetics such as cannabis, ginger, and mint) is likely to be the best option. Opium was traditionally taken from a specialized pipe, with a small metal bowl connected to the inhalation tube by an airhole; the paste was put around the rim of the hole or rolled into a ball on top of it. The reclining position was traditionally used; ideally the patient will already be reclining on a "cholera cot" (has a hole in the appropriate place above a bucket). The bowl would be inverted over a spirit lamp and the fumes swiftly inhaled through the tube. Peak plasma concentration is reached swiftly by this means, and the risk of overdose is diminished compared to IV or oral administration, while the option for further titration upwards if necessary is increased.

Other means of treatment involve:

--If possible, keep the patient awake and upright.

--Airway management (don't try intubation unless you are trained in it or have no choice – even most doctors in hospital generally call the airway management specialists when a patient needs intubation. You could rupture the patient's trachea and/or oesophagus if you make an error.

If you don't have a machine to basically breathe for them, which you most probably don't after the Catastrophe, intubation may not even do any good). Perform chin-lift and jaw-thrust as you would for any patient unconscious from uncertain causes where there is no risk that a cervical spine injury has been sustained, and make sure that the airway remains clear.

If the patient must be left at any time, put them in the "recovery position" (on side; upper elbow propped on lower elbow and upper hand under head, which helps keep the airway open and minimizes the risks of aspirating vomit; upper knee bent forward to prevent rolling onto stomach...the author should look up a picture of "recovery position" to make sure they can describe this with complete accuracy).

--Rescue breathing when the patient's breathing is visibly compromised. Note that the normal respiratory rate for an adult who is not consciously controlling their breath speed is 12-20 breaths/minute. A rate on either side of this (slower in the case of opiate overdose, assuming that the patient did not also take a major stimulant or other drug which might alter their breathing profile upwards) indicates that there is likely to be a significant problem. If the patient is conscious, take their wrist and tell them you're checking their pulse while surreptitiously counting their breaths.

People tend to change their breathing speed, deliberately or unconsciously, when they know you're counting. If the overdose is oral, administer activated charcoal to neutralize any remaining opiate in the stomach. If you didn't stockpile activated charcoal or ran out early...well, with a bit of luck, you shouldn't be running out. Activated charcoal is one thing you can make at home and should definitely keep a stock of (given the many post-Catastrophe options for one to poison oneself or another), assuming that you have both wood for charcoal production and calcium chloride, lemon juice, or bleach available.

Be aware that cardiac arrest may occur, and ready to use whatever treatments for same are available (chest compression +/- rescue breathing). Get at least one friend to help spell you if possible; chest compressions, with or without rescue breathing, can be exhausting. Assuming that you have been forethoughtful and lucky enough to equip yourself with the means of IV access and appropriate fluids, and know how to safely introduce an IV cannula into a peripheral vein, IV fluid support to maintain hydration and manage electrolyte and glucose balance (particularly if there has been significant vomiting) may be extremely useful.

Hypothermia may occur, so be sure to keep the patient warm. Although this may seem counter-intuitive, stimulants are not commonly used in treating real-life opioid overdoses. Naloxone is safer and far more effective in the first responder-to-hospital setting. However, they may play a role in post-Catastrophe emergency treatment, as a stimulant dose may help to counteract the respiratory and cardiac depression typical of opiate overdose.

E) Side Effects of Particular Concern:

Dry mouth (xerostomia). Though seldom a serious issue in and of itself, prolonged periods of dry mouth may lead to tooth decay and gum infections, which can be serious in the modern world if not promptly dealt with, and will be very serious and potentially fatal (in the long run if not the short, between infection and compromised nutritional intake) after the Catastrophe.

Some ways to mitigate this would be: sipping water regularly; chewing on a mint leaf or sour herb to stimulate saliva; and/or putting a pot of water by the head of the bed at night (or close enough to the stove or fireplace, if one is in the bedroom, to encourage evaporation without boiling the water, burning the pan, and starting a fire), or any other means of raising the humidity in the sleeping space that you can devise with the tools you have. A mixture of glycerine (you did stockpile some, didn't you?) and water may also serve as a saliva substitute, though go light on the glycerine, as it works by drawing water out of the surrounding tissues, and if used too freely may exacerbate the problem.

Nausea. Common (ca. 1/3 of patients), but generally self-limiting after ca. 1 week. Anti-nauseants such as peppermint, ginger if available, and cannabis may be useful for control.

Hallucinations – usually peripheral visual disturbances rather than the extreme and often distressing hallucinations caused by psychedelic drugs.

Nightmares – not actually harmful in nearly all cases today, but may be distressing to the patient. Personal therapy of some manner, according to the patient's own beliefs, may be of assistance. If they are religious, I would advise using counselling and appropriate forms of direct spiritual assistance from their own religion (prayer; partaking in the appropriate rites of cleansing and communion with the relevant deity or deities; and, if their religion encourages it, the use of amulets such as a cross, saint's medal, hamsa/Hand of Fatima, Thórr's Hammer, Medicine bag, or other physical focus of power and belief).

This is especially crucial if your post-Catastrophe environment includes significant supernatural activity. Nightmares under such conditions may threaten more than psychological stability, up to and including the suppression or dispossession of the patient's own spirit and full control of their body for malignant purposes by an invasive entity or force. The later books in S.M. Stirling's Emberverse series present a well-drawn picture of some of the possibilities in this regard; Samantha Nocera's Hellscape offers another plausible and highly entertaining perspective.

While it is unlikely that you will have the range of specialists to reproduce the real-life multi-disciplinary team (MDT) now considered optimal (and while some of the specialties, particularly imaging and most forms of lab work, will simply not be available), the inclusion of at least one spiritual or magical specialist on your MDT will be a matter of significant urgency. It is essential to match that specialist to the patient's own beliefs as closely as possible.

Their own beliefs may, specifically or generally, forbid either certain techniques from their religion in general (for instance, believers in some specific sects of Islam or Christianity may be unwilling or unable to work with a Qabalist, even one trained in the more modern iterations of that tradition which include a theoretically fully compatible theology) or calling on beings or powers from other faiths in specific (including a Wiccan, however skilled and virtuous, to carry out certain Christians' care in this regard would be actively counter-productive).

The same ethics hold for treatment involving spiritual and/or magical activity that are true for physical health care: however necessary a treatment may seem, if a patient refuses it, it cannot ethically be forced upon them. And in this situation, the risks of further weakening or injuring the patient by introducing a caregiver or treatment which they believe will endanger their intrinsic spiritual well-being may equal or exceed the risk of leaving the matter to the patient's own faith and their non-specialist co-religionists.

A note to the author: this is an article on maximizing the realism of pharmaceutical hypotheticals, not magico-religious ones. If you are considering writing about a faith or practice with which you are not closely personally familiar, I strongly suggest not only doing your research, as per the above-mentioned advice re ensuring the accuracy of your fictional presentation in those details on which you could and probably will be called out at least in the reader's mind, but consulting with a member or members of that faith or practice if available.

If the patient is not religious at all (and also if they are), regardless of the presence or absence of supernatural elements in your post-Catastrophe situation, talk therapy and working on the ability to direct their dreaming may be helpful. If that fails, and if the opiate dose cannot be reduced, making sure that there is someone close by at night who is able to awaken the patient if they display signs of distress in their sleep, or simply to be there and reassure them when they awake with the horrors, may be the only treatment.

The use of mild herbal calmatives such as chamomile and lavender, both physically applied as tea or an infused oil, and used to scent the sleeping room, may also be helpful. Do not use valerian or other strong herbal sedatives, including and especially cannabis, on this patient. This runs the risk of making awakening from the nightmare more difficult, and there is no reason to think it will relieve the nightmares; it may actually make them worse. Absolutely do not allow this patient to have any alcohol beyond the minute quantities needed to carry the opiate.

It should be added that anyone who has survived the Catastrophe ... whatever its nature or the character of the world which follows it...is probably going to be more prone to extreme nightmares, PTSD, adjustment disorders, and every psychological or psychiatric condition possible to someone who has gone through a great deal of stress and watched or at least heard about the deaths of a large percentage of the population around them, almost certainly including some of their friends and loved ones. These issues are going to be a massive epidemic: I would expect post-Catastrophe suicide rates to soar into the stratosphere.

Those who survive will probably all be more vulnerable to nightmares and night terrors. The wise pre-Catastrophe prepper character might consider taking a course in EMDR (Eye-Movement Desensitization and Reprocessing). Although this sounds appallingly New-Agey, there have just been too many studies showing its effectiveness, particularly in regards to PTSD, to dismiss it as the usual Newage b.s.; EMDR is presented as an option of great potential value to medical students on psychiatry rotations at orthodox universities now.

We still don't know exactly how or why it works, but evidence-based studies indicate that it does work. Hypnotherapy may also be of use, not only to the patient whose inner distress is brought out more strongly in nightmares by necessary opiate dosing, but to a great many others who are suffering from nightmares and other terrors due to what they lived through in surviving the Catastrophe. You may have all the food and bullets necessary to survive, but survival also entails keeping your sanity intact after living through horrors.

Which may be more difficult than simply training to fight, shoot, produce and store food, and practice skills such as textile production and herbal medicine. I could go on at far greater length here, but perhaps this should be a work of its own in the future. In the context of opiate side effects, one should expect that the likelihood of nightmares in general, and opiate-induced nightmares in particular, will be far more common and far more intense after the Catastrophe than as things currently stand in real life for most Westerners.

It would really suck to have saved your patient's life in the short run, only to have them take it themselves in the slightly longer run because they could not bear what they re-lived every night after falling asleep. Were that to happen because the necessary opiates you prescribed for their pain potentiated the existing risk, and you failed to realize how much of a problem that could be and did not do your best to mitigate it, that would be especially bad, and would place a good part of the blame right there on your shoulders.

Remember: a good doctor or nurse...or cunning-man, wise-woman, or just someone who actually cared enough to step up and shoulder part of the health-care burden after the Catastrophe...treats the whole patient, not just their obvious physical issues. In short, even with no supernatural elements as part of your life whatsoever: this opiate side-effect – generally considered minor in the current world - could easily be fatal to Catastrophe survivors.

Herbal Laxatives

If giving stimulant herbal laxatives which stimulate a little too much for comfort, make sure the patient stays hydrated and administer tea made with a high-potassium herb such as dried chervil at ca. 83 mg per tablespoon. Poppy seeds are also quite high in potassium (63 mg/tablespoon). Diarrhoea notably causes potassium loss, and severely low potassium causes fatal heart complications (singer Karen Carpenter died of this, secondary to her anorexia).

The recommended daily dose for potassium is 3.5 grams/day, supplied by a normal diet that includes fruit and vegetables. If the diarrhoea is severe, oral rehydration salts may be needed. Commercial ones contain potassium; homemade ones must have it added.

Do not use any stimulant herbal laxative longer than needed. They may impair the bowel's ability to function on its own after discontinuance. Cut dosages down to the lowest effective level, and be sure to give plenty of fibre/bulking agents.

Aloe Vera. The yellowish layer inside the skin, not the gel that fills the leaf. Very harsh: dosage is 1/32 teaspoon, 150 mg., or 2 1/3 grains (see "Weights and Measures" for apothecary equivalents).

This part of the aloe can be dried and preserved for future use. Save it for your most urgent cases. Aloe is also a notable topical medication for burns, and should be considered one of your most valuable post-Catastrophe herbs.

Myoclonic jerks, especially in overdose. Treat overdose if present and reduce overall opiate dose if possible. May be confused with epileptic seizures. This is not necessarily a disastrous misdiagnosis, as many of the drugs currently used to treat myoclonic jerking are the same that are used in epilepsy. Valerian appears to operate by the same mechanism as benzodiazepines (used for epilepsy and myoclonic jerks); high-CBD strains of cannabis are likely to be effective as well, as CBD has shown significant benefit in cases of intractable epilepsy. Although alcohol may be a muscle relaxant, it should not be prescribed in any quantity greater than the minimum required after the Catastrophe to preserve and carry the opiate, due to the increased risk of respiratory depression and loss of consciousness. Avoid stimulants, and I'm sorry for people from cultures that suck down coffee and tea all day (assuming you grow your own or stockpiled a huge amount, still have it available, and are still addicted), but no more than one cup in the morning to prevent withdrawal headaches, at maximum.

Pruritis (itching). Opiates promote histamine release, which can lead to generalized itching, often severe; and many of the drugs used to treat this condition in real life will not be available after the Catastrophe – the exception being NSAIDs, which fortunately are found in some herbs, chiefly in the form of salicylic acid, a predecessor to aspirin (acetylsalicylic acid, formed by reacting salicylic acid with acetic anhydride).

Treat with topical mild analgesics/anti-inflammatories such as lavender and chamomile; oral and/or topical willow bark, meadowsweet, or cannabis (your herbal NSAIDs); and reduce opiate dose if possible (always recommended with opiate treatment under any circumstances). In real life, switching to another opiate/opioid is often effective; but that is no longer an option for Catastrophe survivors.

Respiratory depression. Seldom seen whe gauged correctly to pain, but a significant an overdose (most common mechanism of OD reduced at the same rate as the patient is rec something that can just be left to run.

They must be reviewed regularly, and very acute condition, so that they can be decreased as the condition resolves. Paradoxically, opiates are not uncommonly used today to relieve the symptoms of dyspnoea (difficult/painful breathing), especially when caused by exercise, in COPD patients. I remember being shocked when a doctor I was shadowing prescribed morphine pills to one of his palliative COPD patients, because my knowledge at the time was limited to "causes respiratory depression", which I would have thought was the last thing one would want to risk in a patient with breathing issues.

He explained to me why it actually did help the patient's breathing. However, this may ultimately prove to be a quality of life vs quantity of life decision. Dyspnoea is a significant quality-of-life limiter; but there is also mounting evidence that opiates in such patients raise the risk of other respiratory problems and death.

In the post-Catastrophe world – less tobacco and industrial smoke, but far more smoky indoor fires with inadequate ventilation, the health-care provider who survives for two or three decades is increasingly likely to have to facilitate their patients in making that decision in an informed manner, as the palliative-care and respiratory specialists sometimes must do in real life.

Constipation. The downside of opiates' remarkable efficacy in controlling otherwise uncontrollable diarrhoea, for which purpose opium tincture and (generally paediatric) 1/25th strength tincture paregoric are still used today at need.

Treat the plants like children: pot in a 1:1 mix of sand and soil, and bring them into the warmest part of the house in winter. Do not water until the pot is completely dry down to the bottom. Aloes reproduce by "pupping" – sending out offshoots. When large enough, these can be removed with their portion of rootstock and replanted to increase your stock, give to friends, or use as trade goods.

Senna (Cascara sagrada, California buckthorn). A small tree native to the Pacific Northwest; the primary active ingredient in many pharmaceutical laxatives such as Senokot (first-line in hospitals for opioid constipation). Learn to recognise it in the wild; cultivate it if you can. A day's full dosage can be made with 2.5-5 grams of dried leaves or pods, the pods being less aggressive than the leaves. Divide the day's dose in two and administer one half of it every 12 hours.

Catnip (Nepeta cataria). A gentle herbal laxative; first choice as a prophylactic.

Coffee, if available, seems to have a mild laxative effect on ca. 30% of the population. This effect is not seen to any significant degree in caffeine pills, tea, or other caffeine sources.

Apples and other high-pectin fruits (quince, citrus, fresh plums, the Dreaded Prunes of Regularity) assist in softening the stool.

1 tablespoon of flax seed (yes, the exact same stuff that grows linen fibres), steeped in 1 cup (237 ml) water for 12 hours, produces a gel that is a notable stool softener.

Constipation is a common complaint of patients given opiates/opioids, even in the short run (post-surgical) and almost always in the long run. Opiate-type drugs slow down intestinal motility significantly. It is standard practice to prescribe mild prophylactic laxatives (a stool-softener plus a stimulant) together with higher doses of codeine (30-60 mg) or anything stronger over more than a day or two, especially if the patient is expected to require opiate/oid treatment for a while.

In real life, if a hospitalized patient hasn't moved their bowels today, they can pretty well count on getting a laxative to help them along. If that patient hasn't had a motion for a couple of days, they may get a lot of laxative, because doctors, especially surgeons, become very worried when a patient's internal functions are not manifestly functioning.

Making it through the ride home with clean trousers after being discharged is the patient's problem. For post-Catastrophe prophylactic use, it is best to begin with stool softeners and bulking agents such as flaxseed gel (described below), and save the powerful bowel stimulants for when and if a more serious problem begins to develop. Long-term constipation/motility diminishment has the potential to lead to consequences ranging from the need for enemas (no fun for the patient), to the need for manual disimpaction (no fun for patient or practitioner; hope you still have a few sets of disposable medical gloves in your stash), to megacolon (a very serious condition with the option of fatal ulceration, especially since you will no longer have the imaging to detect it with certainty, nor, in all probability, the OR facilities to operate if transit can't be restored), to, in extreme cases, complete intestinal paralysis, which can be fatal without swift treatment even in modern hospital conditions.

Appendicitis or diverticulitis due to impacted faeces are dangerous now, and will have a high chance of being fatal situations after the Catastrophe. So make sure that those bowels continue to function, particularly in your chronic pain patient! If the patient has been eating little, but is still passing gas normally and has normal bowel sounds, no distension or tenderness of the abdomen, and so forth, they are probably okay. Examine the abdomen, paying particular attention to bowel noises. Silence for more than one minute is worrying – more than five minutes is a very, very bad sign. A slow plop...plop...plop noise means that there is a nearly complete blockage in there.

In real life at this point, the patient is about to be scanned in great detail and may well be heading into surgery shortly thereafter. After the Catastrophe, if your strongest stimulating laxatives can't restore motility pretty quickly and you don't have surgical capability suitable for breaching the body cavity without the patient inevitably dying from infection...doom. Herbal laxatives may well be necessary post-Catastrophe for many reasons besides opiate use (diet, stress), but should be approached with some caution re strength and dosage. Stimulant herbal laxatives are generally quite harsh.

This is unlikely to kill your patient and may in some situations save them, so don't hold back too much when it seems necessary. However, after a night of cramps and squirting (especially since nice soft loo paper is also not likely to be in great supply after the Catastrophe), the patient may be ready to kill you when they finally get off the pot. Warn them first, and make sure they understand the gruesome alternatives. It's okay to get grossly graphic if necessary to communicate the extent of the risk to the patient. You're a doctor, or at least the closest thing to it that the post-Catastrophe world affords. In all cases of constipation, increase the patient's dietary fibre. Normal recommendations for fibre intake are 38 grams in men/25 grams in women. Dark green leafy vegetables are an excellent choice.

Poppy seeds also contain 2 grams of fibre per tablespoon (15 grams), making them useful for counteracting the constipating effects of the pod in which they grow.The seeds of Cannabis sativa (medicinal or purely fibre-production varieties) also provide good dietary fibre and many overall nutritional benefits; and no, regardless of the potency of the plant that it might produce, no C. sativa seed contains psycho-actives.

Make sure the patient stays well hydrated.

F) Injectable vs. Oral Opiates post-catastrophe

Producing a relatively safe injectable opiate requires more knowledge of practical chemistry than the average doctor has. An MD only means that you know how to prescribe and judge dosages and risks of purified pharmaceuticals of known potency, not that you know how to make any pharmaceutical at home.

They stopped teaching that kind of thing in medical school before the middle of the 20th century (in 1919, Harvard Medical school did teach how to make, for instance, your own digitalis-based drugs. The process involved killing three frogs in testing the potency).

Refining morphine may also call for the use of other purified substances such as ammonium chloride and hydrochloric acid, which may not be available in your post-Catastrophe kitchen or even lab.

No home-made poppy product should be used for injection except under extreme emergency conditions, unless you actually have chemistry experience and do know how to safely precipitate morphine from opium.

The process of precipitating morphine from opium is beyond the scope of this article, though a pre-Catastrophe survivalist character with some knowledge and experience of chemistry might do well to look into it in case it should ever become necessary – just as it is wise to learn how to recognise the penicillin mould and refine penicillin from it, or to refine insulin from animal pancreases for emergency use as was notably done by Eva Saxl during World War II when her own insulin supply ran out (she saved many lives, including her own, and no fatalities were reported from her homemade insulin).

All of these, like judging the strength of a batch of home-made digoxin (from foxglove) or estimating a probably-safe dosage of henbane or deadly nightshade, or making and using your own ether, are pieces of knowledge that you never wanted to have to use, but which might, in a post-Catastrophe situation, be less risky to a patient than not doing anything, assuming that "not doing anything" is clearly going to "= certain death". Diana Gabaldon's time-traveling doctor Claire Fraser does refine and use her own penicillin as best she can, and saves several lives with it – but loses one patient to graphically described anaphylactic shock, in a time when she can't just give said patient a swift jab of adrenaline. Her very crude penicillin is also probably a lot more effective than yours would be in a this-world-based future, since she was working in the late 18th century before bacteria even thought about developing penicillin-resistance.

On the other hand, due to a resurgence of interest in testing early historical medicines by modern means, we know more now about herbs such as plantain - surprisingly effective against Gram-positive bacteria, which include Staphylococcus, Streptococcus, and Clostridium (botulism, tetanus, gas gangrene) – than we did when Diana Gabaldon wrote most of the Outlander books. Otherwise, the alcohol in your home poppy extract is not necessarily a problem. Small amounts of ethanol (not methanol, it's poison!) can be injected IV or IM with relative safety. A burning pain at the site is usual, possibly with redness...and for an IV, careful observation is required to make sure you really got the IV into the vein and the redness is not a result of leakage into the surrounding tissues.

An IM alcohol injection that hits a myoneural junction may temporarily reduce a muscle's tone (and in real life, has been used specifically for that purpose in reducing cerebral palsy spasticity), but presents no lasting concerns. The effect of the alcohol in IV injection will be greater than that of oral consumption.

This should not be a concern if, for whatever reason, it were to become necessary to inject, say, 10 ml of a compounded extract as roughly a 10 mg. IV morphine equivalent; but could become much more of a problem at higher doses. Remember: oral morphine dosage should be 2-3x IV morphine dosage, and 10 mg is your standard starter for IV or IM.

While the alcohol is not an issue, opium or poppy pod extracts contain significant amounts of impurities at the best of times, and bacteria are a concern if the medium is not reasonably high-alcohol. These are of lesser relevance when taken orally (especially in an alcohol medium) or inhaled, but can cause everything from abscesses to total-body sepsis and anaphylactic shock when injected IV or IM. Even crude heroin analogues such as the Polish drug "kompot" contain these impurities and present significant dangers aside from the risks of overdose, unknown-substance additions, and the consequences of addiction. In the event that the patient is also vomiting severely and cannot keep an oral drug down, this might be time to find out how efficient inhaled opium (the dried sap of the pod) is for medical use; the risks are lower than those of injecting your homemade poppy extract with its inevitable impurities.

Probably the most likely reasons for injecting a homemade whole opium extract in a post-Catastrophe scenario would be situations where it is essential to either restore enough movement capability to a wounded comrade in order to get them out of a scene of deathly danger, and worry about other possible consequences later if there is a later, or to immediately ease a probably-soon-terminal patient's extreme pain. In the latter case, I decline to comment on the relative morality of "extreme palliative pain control" vs "the mercy stroke", as that is a decision which can only be made by the individual based on their personal beliefs and the situation with which they are confronted.

If the patient is conscious or has left a previous directive, however, their choice in such a matter ought, in my opinion, to take precedence. This may or may not be the opinion of the character(s) in the story. In general, oral use is likely to be the chief form of opiate medication after the Catastrophe, at least based on the history of Western medicine.

I do not know if any studies have been done on inhaled opium relevant to medical pain control, but the West has a long history of oral usage from ingested solid opium and poppy syrup, to laudanum, to our current morphine pills (long- and short-acting) used in palliative care and some chronic pain control, and the occasional use of liquid opiate extracts in, for instance, controlling intractable diarrhoea (which is still a life-threatener in many parts of the world, and would become one in the West again were a complete breakdown to occur).

In regards to intractable diarrhea: Clostridium difficile, a scourge of hospitals worldwide, is unlikely to be as much of a problem after the Catastrophe, since the most common cause of severe C. difficile infections is the scouring of normal intestinal flora by strong antibiotics, to most of which C. difficile is immune – and most of which will also not be readily available a few years after the Catastrophe. This scouring is not only the cause of normal antibiotic-caused bowel problems, but allows C. difficile to vastly over-grow its normal intestinal levels, which in turn results in serious and – even with modern hospital care – occasionally fatal diarrhoea. Standard antiseptic/antimicrobial solutions such as Betadine, chlorhexidine, and even alcohol do not kill C. difficile spores. Only soap does that. If there is any reason to suspect a C. difficile infection, always wash your hands thoroughly with soap, as per the basic initial scrub-in phase instructions given in a sidebar to Appendix III, section VII ("Menstrual Extraction").

Cholera treatment and rehydration salt recipe

Opium was used effectively to treat cholera in the 18th and 19th centuries. Fortunately, we now know that if a cholera patient is supplied with constant oral or IV rehydration and electrolytes, they will survive and recover in a few days, no opiates required. However, in the absence of IVs and presence of the inability to tolerate the great volumes of oral rehydration/electrolyte balance required (cholera can also cause vomiting), opium may still play a role in post-Catastrophe cholera outbreaks. When all the oral rehydration salts packets have run out, the most adequate substitute would be:

6 level teaspoons of honey or sugar (honey is preferred due to antibacterial activity, except in infants < 1 year, who are vulnerable to botulism spores in honey; give sugar or boil the honey with water at a rolling boil for at least half an hour.)

½ level teaspoon salt

Dissolved in 1 litre/5 cups water.

Potassium may be at least partially replaced by first making the water into a tea with 1-2 oz (28-56 grams) dried chervil, chamomile, nettle, alfalfa, parsley, spearmint, dill, or other high-potassium herb.

If the cholera patient is vomiting uncontrollably, inhalation of opium (together with continued efforts to administer anti-emetics such as cannabis, ginger, and mint) is likely to be the best option. Opium was traditionally taken from a specialized pipe, with a small metal bowl connected to the inhalation tube by an airhole; the paste was put around the rim of the hole or rolled into a ball on top of it. The reclining position was traditionally used; ideally the patient will already be reclining on a "cholera cot" (has a hole in the appropriate place above a bucket). The bowl would be inverted over a spirit lamp and the fumes swiftly inhaled through the tube. Peak plasma concentration is reached swiftly by this means, and the risk of overdose is diminished compared to IV or oral administration, while the option for further titration upwards if necessary is increased.

g) Combinations to Reduce Opiates While Maintaining Good Pain Control

It is always best to give the least possible opiate you can give while effectively controlling pain. Immensely useful as this drug is, it is also, as has been demonstrated, potentially immensely dangerous. And if even that doesn't get your attention, consider that, after the Catastrophe, you won't be able to just ring the hospital pharmacy and have them send up more when you run out.

Stimulants. While it is not common practice to prescribe stimulants together with opiates for pain control, it is effective and reduces the opiate quantity required while lessening the sedative and respiratory-depressive opiate effects.

In fact, those countries which make low-codeine content pills available over the counter sometimes combine the codeine (+ acetaminophen, aspirin, or ibuprofen) with caffeine for exactly the purpose of providing more pain relief with less opiate.

Some stronger prescription opiates also contain caffeine plus another adjunct: one tablet of Tylenol 3, for instance, contains 30 mg codeine, 300 mg acetaminophen, and 15 mg caffeine (a minute amount: a normal 8-oz cup of coffee contains ca. 95 mg caffeine, and a Midol tablet has 60 mg. Actual caffeine pills usually run between 100 and 200 mg). The combination of stimulants with opiates beyond low- to mid-level medications has probably been avoided in general prescribing for two main reasons.

One is the considerable potentiation of abuse risk (one might compare the street "speedball", a mixture of a strong illegal stimulant with a strong illegal opiate), but that is not going to be a concern in either opioid OD treatment or, really, for long-term pain relief in a patient who is not going to have any sort of life without some serious ongoing pain control. The second reason is that stimulants can mask opiate overdose symptoms (and vice versa), so if the OD'd drug is longer lasting than the counter-drug, the patient could quite suddenly have a very serious problem. These things make most doctors very cautious about prescribing strong stimulants together with strong opiates/opioids despite the potential benefits. Herbal options for stimulants are largely mild (peppermint; caffeine if you can get it). Ephedra sinica (Ma Huang) is a strong stimulant, and might be used for severe allergic and asthmatic attacks...but it is also potentially a very dangerous herb, as discussed in part III.

Analgesic adjuncts: It is common even in the modern post-surgical setting to provide a patient with a lower-level analgesic on an ongoing basis together with the minimum effective opioid dose. I have observed myself that acetaminophen is an effective trauma pain/post-surgical adjunct, though of lesser to no assistance in conditions where the pain is chiefly inflammatory. The chronic pain patient is extremely likely to benefit both in regards to pain control and function from anti-inflammatory treatment together with opiates, as many if not most chronic pain conditions are strongly associated with inflammation. Fortunately there are many readily available herbal anti-inflammatories such as willow bark and meadowsweet. Poppy seed oil, interestingly, is one of those anti-inflammatories, so, when ibuprofen and pharmaceutical opiates are no longer available, your poppies can help with pain two ways (as well as being a valuable nutritional source).

h)Veterinary Opiates

After the Catastrophe, you may not have a vet you can call when your cat or dog – beloved family member and/or valued member of your survival team – is injured or ill and suffering pain. Animals metabolize and react to many drugs differently than humans do. One standard human tablet of acetaminophen/paracetamol (Tylenol is the most common American brand name) will kill a cat; aspirin may be fatal to a cat or a dog.

The therapeutic index (range between "no appreciable effect" and "kills the patient") of ibuprofen is extremely low in both species. Even after the Catastrophe, it is not a risk to take with your companion's life. In real life, there are NSAIDs which are specifically formulated for animals, and which your vet will provide as appropriate. Do not dose cats or dogs with herbal painkillers which contain salicylic acid (willow bark, meadowsweet). They lack a necessary enzyme for metabolizing this substance. It is toxic to them. These herbs may, however, be used on horses, as may (and frequently is) aspirin (acetylsalicylic acid, metabolizes to salicylic acid, which is the effective form). Aspirin is often used as a mild analgesic and anti-inflammatory for horses (oral dosage: 0.01-0.1 mg/kg).

Horses commonly ingest salicylic acid-containing plants in their food, which has led to some controversy about the urine levels considered acceptable in competitive sports. Salicylic acid is also used topically for cows and horses. Fortunately for the post-Catastrophe dog who just had his belly ripped open by a feral pig (possibly while saving your life), or the post-Catastrophe cat who ran into the wrong feral dog or coyote, opiates are one of the few painkillers that, adjusting for body mass, are similar in effect and risk for dogs, cats, and humans.

The main difference is that neither dogs nor cats have any decent or reliable level of oral absorption of morphine, which means that the drug is probably best administered IM or SC (sub-cutaneous). IV can be used, but for someone who does not have veterinary training, IM or SC injection is easier for you and safer for the patient. Even if you know how to give humans an IV injection, the chances of going all the way through the tiny veins in a cat or the small veins in most dogs are vastly increased. Your human-sized large dog (somewhere between 45 and 100 kg, or 100-225 lbs), especially if in significant pain, is not necessarily going to cooperate with having a cannula put in unless they're sedated already, and if you had the means to do that, you probably wouldn't need to take the risks of giving them a homemade poppy injection.

There is also the warning that IV injection of a product with an alcohol base will affect the animal far more quickly and powerfully than either drinking alcohol or receiving an IM or SC injection. Absorption through oral membranes is possible, but the extreme bitterness makes the chances of being able to dose a cat or dog in this manner minimal. Cats, in particular, respond to bitter medications (such as some powdered antibiotics meant for oral intake) squirted forcibly into their mouths with what veterinary texts call "hypersalivation" and I call "frothing copiously at the mouth and gagging in a way that will make you think you just fatally poisoned your cat". Both dogs and cats may respond to a dose of morphine with immediate defecation and/or urination.

Be aware of this; prepare beforehand to minimize any chance of faeces contacting an open wound, and be ready to change the bedding and clean the animal immediately if it occurs. Poppy products, whether pharmaceutical or post-Catastrophe, should not be given to an animal wearing a vermin-control collar or being treated with an MAO inhibitor, as these drugs can interact with severe consequences. IM injections are generally given to animals in the large muscle of the upper hind leg. For SC injections in cats or dogs, common practice is to gently pinch up a skin fold at the back of the neck and inject into the fold. Veterinary dosage recommendations for morphine in animal species vary slightly. I present the most common values.

Remember, as always, that it is better to undermedicate and go up, than to overmedicate and hope your naloxone still works to a reasonable degree. Opiate-related respiratory depression is less often fatal in animals than in humans, but they can still die of overdoses. It is especially crucial to know the current weight of a cat or small dog when calculating an opiate dose. The smaller the patient, the lower the margin for error in administering any drug by weight. Start low, go slow! The feline dose for morphine ranges from 0.1 to 0.2 mg/kg (1 kg = roughly 2.2 lbs) by injection; the oral recommended dose, if it must be given orally, is 0.5 mg/kg, 4x/day. Minimum lethal dose (subcutaneous injection) is 40 mg/kg.

Thus, a five kilo (11 lb) cat in severe pain would receive an injected dose 0.5 ml (one tenth of a teaspoon) to 1.25 mg (one-quarter of a teaspoon) of an extraction which was judged to be of a strength roughly estimated at 1 mg morphine to 1 ml extract (5 ml, or one teaspoon, equalling roughly a post-surgical dose of codeine for an human). Excitation and "manic" behaviour has been reported as a result of giving higher doses of morphine to cats, but the frequency of this seems fairly rare: many studies remarked on its non-occurrence. Still, it should be watched for, as a cat with "opiate excitation" runs a risk of exacerbating its original injury.

Cannabis can safely be, and if available should be, used as an adjunct to decrease the dosage of opiates required in a cat. Catnip (Nepeta cataria) also has mild analgesic properties, and may be used as an adjunct as freely as the cat will take it. In dogs, catnip is a mild sedative; whether it has analgesic effects on them is not known. The canine dose for morphine is 0.5-1 mg/kg (oral), at a minimum interval of 4x/day (every 6 hours) or 0.3 to 1.5 mg/kg (injected), 4-6x/day. Minimum lethal dose is between 110-210 mg/kg by injection.

The effects of cannabis in dogs are less well-known than in cats (see Part II: Cannabis sativa), but preliminary evidence suggests that it can serve as an oral adjunct to opiates in dogs, and using cannabis plus a reduced opiate (especially homemade opiate) dosage in dogs is probably safer than using the higher dose of opiate alone. Horses are more sensitive to morphine than are either cats or dogs: the same pre-operative dose of morphine that suffices for a 30 kg (66 lb.) dog, 9-45 mg injected, is that which could be used for a 500 kg (1100 lbs) horse. The basic injection dose is 0.1 mg/kg (0.045 mg/lb). Injected doses of morphine have a short half-life in horses (1.5 hours), and may need to be given as often as every four hours for a horse in severe pain. Opiates are not given to horses orally because of the risk of bowel stoppage and colic.

The decreased intestinal motility which is a concern in other mammals receiving opiates presents a particular threat in horses; observe the animal closely and reduce or stop the dose if bowels are not moving normally. Poppy foliage, fresh or dry, should never be made available to horses. The vast majority will not usually eat it because of the extremely bitter taste; however, in matters of personal taste, there is always one outlier (the same horse that keeps trying to kill itself by going for fresh ragweed...and do not forget that dried ragweed loses its bitter flavour and is a serious danger to horses in the field or in fodder!), and serious hunger may also drive an animal to overlook flavour.

Horses can also become over-stimulated when receiving morphine by IV injection; the risk of this effect is much lower when the shot is given IM. Cannabis may be used as an adjunct to reduce opiate dosage in horses, although there do not seem to currently be any recommendation on dosage. Anecdotally, an oral (butter) cannabis preparation has been said to prove useful in reducing the pain and improving the quality of life for horses in chronic pain. CBD (see Part II) is often promoted for equine use, and may indeed function well and safely for that purpose, but not enough research has been done to establish optimum dosages.

Other adjuncts for horses include aspirin which is often used as a mild analgesic and anti-inflammatory to horses (oral dosage: 0.01-0.1 mg/kg), and the salicylic acid-containing herbal NSAIDs such as willow bark and meadowsweet. Horses commonly ingest salicylic acid-containing plants in their food, which has led to some controversy about the urine levels considered acceptable in competitive sports. Salicylic acid is also used topically for cows and horses. Naloxone may be administered in case of a suspected opiate overdose in all mammals, but may prevent further opiate-based pain control from being effective.

i) Opiates and Supernatural Beings

The relevance of this depends completely on your author and the post-Catastrophe environment they have created for you. Unfortunately, there have been no evidence-based studies published regarding the effects of opiates on various supernatural beings; Polish folklore (described in section III, 3, below) is our closest guide. There are, however, some tropes which are fairly common in novels dealing with beings which are, or might as well be, supernatural. Lycanthropes are generally considered to be more resistant to non-condition-specific toxins and drugs than standard humans. It has also been suggested (as in Laurell K. Hamilton's Anita Blake: Vampire Hunter series) that their increased metabolic rates may make the efficacious administration of analgesia difficult, requiring both higher and more frequent dosing. Until proper studies have been conducted and specific guidelines approved and published, this presents a challenge in terms of both achieving efficacy and maximizing safety.

When providing appropriate analgesia to a patient with lycanthropy, be mindful of the normal guidelines regarding caution in dosage and titration, and go slowly until you have determined the basic pharmacokinetics of the drug in that particular patient. In other words, treat under the same general principles you would use with a standard human, particularly one suspected or known to be an ultra-rapid metabolizer. In terms of general safety, however, it may sometimes be necessary to take a greater risk with the dosage if your patient is in too much pain to control themself, and is trying to shift shape with the apparent intention of eating your face. Zombies may be generated by supernatural means, physical toxins, diseases, or a combination of more than one element.

As George R.R. Martin's Dothraki (A Song of Ice and Fire series, 1996 ff.); would put it, "It is known" that the only effective way to sedate a standard zombie is via massive cranial trauma. Tossing out a piece of meat loaded with poppy extract is unlikely to do anything but encourage the zombie. The possibility exists that the dreaded "fast zombies", clearly possessing a higher level of neurological function than the slow-shambling "standard zombie", may be more vulnerable to drugs of this class. This has not, to my knowledge, been scientifically explored. Should you ever have the opportunity to test it, and survive that opportunity, please report your method and results for the benefit of others.

If the zombie or zombies with which you have a problem were created by the reported Haitian means of toxins-plus-ritual, it is highly inadvisable to treat them with opiates, as that runs the risk of interaction with whatever drugs they are already being given, and lowers your chances of eventually restoring the patient to life and sanity. Anecdotal reports concerning vampires tend towards the conclusion that, while they are less likely to be affected by the direct administration of opiates/opioids, these drugs and others, including alcohol, may be efficaciously given to them at second hand: that is, via the blood of someone who has ingested and absorbed the drug.

The second-hand ingestion trope appears in sources as diverse as Spider Robinson's short story "Pyotr's Tale" (in Callahan's Secret, Ace, 1986), Deborah Harkness' All Souls trilogy (Penguin: 2011-2014), and Cassandra Clare's Shadowhunter series (2007 ff.). This, of course, applies only to vampires of the classic Western type who subsist primarily or entirely on blood. It would not be relevant to, for instance, the life-energy absorbers of Jim Butcher's White Court (Dresden Files series; Roc, 2000 ff.); but vampires of that nature appear perfectly capable of taking their own medicinal (or recreational) drugs in the same manner as humans, with similar dosages and effects.

The effectiveness and safety of IV injections upon classic Western vampires is likely to depend on how recently the vampire has fed, as that will probably be the chief factor determining the efficiency of their circulation, rate of absorption, and overall capability to utilize medications delivered directly into their own bloodstream. However, as vampires appear to be largely immune to bacterial infections and are likely to be far less vulnerable to the harmful effects of impurities in an IV injection, the major cautions against injecting home-made poppy products into humans are unlikely to apply to them. Polish folklore regarding the capability of poppy seeds to keep the undead quiet and content in their graves (see below, section III, 3) suggests that, possibly regardless of actual morphine content, the spiritual effect of this plant on purely or primarily supernatural beings may be analogous to its physical effect on humans.

This is consistent with a general theme in folklore throughout the world: that the practical use of an herb can usually be taken as a guide to its magico-religious use. Thus plants with antibacterial capabilities and/or pleasing but penetrating odours, such as juniper, cedar, and sweetgrass, are not uncommonly seen functioning as supernatural protectives as well as assisting in the maintenance of household hygiene; the antibacterial properties of silver may also offer a hint towards its popularity as a means of defense against various otherworldly threats. This principle is likely to apply to all supernatural beings of a non-physical or largely non-physical nature. A dose of oral opioid is unlikely to directly affect a ghost or a witch on an extra-corporeal excursion; but the seeds of the source plant itself may do so.

III. Post-Catastrophe Opiate Production

Let us assume that, for whatever reason, national law no longer applies and moderate to major painkillers are no longer available through the currently legal, usual, and at least somewhat safety-moderated channels. So you, the fictional character, who happily have survived the Catastrophe and have some land, wish to be prepared to deal with medical situations involving urgent pain. Or maybe you fled to your grandmother's house, and she is suffering badly because she can't get her appropriate prescriptions for her dire rheumatoid arthritis any more.

A) Site, Soil, Sowing, and Major Pests (things real-life gardeners where P. somniferum is a legal ornamental may also want to know)

P. somniferum (or its sub-variant P. paeoniflorium) is the species you want for food and medicine. If you planned ahead, you ordered and preserved as seeds (or grew in your home garden STRICTLY AS AN ORNAMENTAL in those countries where it is permitted) one, or several, strains. It would be wiser to have available several strains, since disease/fungus/climate/pest resistance vary unpredictably. As we in Ireland know very well to our extreme historical cost, monoculture is Not Your Friend. Plus, the wide range of colours and shapes available just looks good and lends itself to all manner of attractive garden designing. And even (or maybe especially) after the Catastrophe, having that extra bit of beauty in your life can go a long way towards maintaining adequate mental health.

1) Site and Soil

Choosing the site: from halfway up a rise in the land to covering its top is very good. Anywhere that becomes even slightly squishy after a heavy rain, or catches runoff (unless you live in a very dry climate where your problem is getting enough water rather than getting too much), is very bad. Too wet = increased risk of fungus, and even modern gardeners can't do much about fungus. Poppies of nearly all species (except the Meconopsis species, which are of interest only aesthetically as garden plants) prefer full sun. Poppies like rich, but well-drained soil. Again: if you live in a dry spot, they will want irrigation, but not too much: they don't like having their feet wet.

If you live in an area with heavy clay or otherwise extreme soil, I recommend digging out the bed to at least 8" deep (if the soil is really problematic, you might want to go down to at least 1', assuming that you have a small household bed rather than trying to grow a field for a larger community) and replacing with a good compost blend - or the best equivalent you can manage, since there probably won't be a lot of garden centres with sacks of perfect soil after the Catastrophe. Your compost heaps and faithful livestock will be a great help here. Nitrogen and phosphorus seem to be the main fertilizer requirements for poppies; they don't actually seem to approve of too much potassium. Advice on post-Catastrophe (or real-life organic/homemade) fertilizer options is given in Appendix III: Fertilizing and Pest Control.

2) Sowing

In most temperate climates, it is recommended to sow in September to early October to give the plants a chance to root in before becoming dormant overwinter. Poppy seeds are tiny, and require light to germinate. They should be sown on top of the soil or just barely pressed in, watered in with a light sprinkler, then covered with a net if possible to keep the birds from eating them (see below, "Pests"). Cold stratification is sometimes recommended, but not necessary; I have grown ornamental poppies with an April sowing in Ireland.

But both Irish/UK and North American garden experts indicate that the early autumn sowing will give a better result, with stronger plants. And the plague of slugs is generally lessened in the UK/Ireland at this time. If you miss that period, sow in late March to early April...though some gardeners claim they just chuck their seeds out onto an inch of snow, and the seeds hit dirt and germinate when the snow melts. Thickness of sowing is debatable. One study (Tookey, Spencer, Grove, and Duke, 1975) indicated that the highest level of morphine was achieved with 6 cm (a bit over 2") between plants, ca. 1 foot between rows, double rows on ridges 1 metre (ca. 40") apart.

Other poppy advisors recommend no more than ca. 5 plants/square foot: still quite close for the size of the grown plant, but poppies seem to prefer clumping. This may be a "quality vs. quantity" issue: wider spacing tends to get bigger individual plants with more flowers, and is certainly best for ornamental purposes. In either case, it is recommended to sow more than you want and thin as appropriate...if the damned slugs don't do it for you first. If you live in an area with high winds, once the poppies start shooting up, you may want to stake them... tie a square foot's worth loosely together around the stake, just so they don't get knocked over.

Poppies resent transplanting after seedling stage. The only way you can do it is at seedling stage by hooking up the entire taproot and its dirt with a finger or small trowel, then setting it down in a hole, with no root disturbance. If you must have complete control over what goes where, and for a real-life ornamental garden with carefully-planned colours you may well want to, start them indoors in peat pots, which disintegrate on their own without disturbing roots, about a month or so before expected last frost. This also works for maize and other plants that resent transplanting. Poppies are, however, surprisingly frost-hardy, and not even intimidated by the winter's snow if they started in autumn.

Even poppy seedlings, roots and all, contain low levels of morphine. So if, after the Catastrophe, you oversow, it may be worthwhile putting young plants removed for thinning into an emergency tincture, particularly if you have a chronic pain patient who is out of their prescription meds. As the plant matures, the lower portions become increasingly alkaloid depleted: a poppy with pods will have virtually nothing you want in the roots, and little to nothing in the lower stem and leaves. Plough those parts back in for next year.

3) Major Pests

Birds - P. somniferum is also known as "birdseed plant" for a very good reason! How feasible netting is post-Catastrophe depends on the size of your plot. Unless your plots are quite small, or you live in a community where producing fishing nets is a major part of the winter's activities...or unless, early on, you totally cleaned out the bird-netting supply of a few garden centres...netting may be impractical.

Remember, however: the more people you're caring for, the more space you'll need...but the more help you should be getting. Netting a 10 x 10 plot, which is probably more medicinal poppy than two or three large families will need in a year (short of multiple disasters or chronic pain/palliative care patients), will likely still be quite possible. Netting a community-sized plot - especially given that the seeds and the oil should be as high or considerably higher on the priority list than the opiates, since with any luck you will only rarely need the opiates, but you need food and cooking oil pretty much daily - will not be, but a community should have no shortage of little kids to rotate in for bird-scaring duty. Especially after the birth-control devices run out and the contraceptive implants have all worn off.

Scarecrows are long-known, but of imperfect efficacy, even ones that are rigged to move with every gust of wind. Hint: if your main avian attackers are crows, carve up a mock shotgun or rifle to put in that scarecrow's arms! It has been exhaustively demonstrated that crows can recognise the silhouette of a human with a long gun, and know that such a monkey is best avoided. After the Catastrophe, you probably won't want to waste your valuable and possibly irreplaceable ammo on crows; but a shell or round fired once or twice at key times of year to keep them reminded of what that silhouette means is not going to be a waste. Other seed-eaters, sadly, are not nearly so bright.

Birds may become a problem again as the pods become ripe and begin to dry. They will peck through the pods to get at the seeds. Again, little kids plus scarecrows are probably your best defense.

Slugs and snails - Slugs and snails love poppy seedlings. The last time I grew an ornamental bed of poppies, I went out every day or so from first sprouting to hook up a few excess seedlings and move them to the bare spots where the slugs had been overnight. For control, see the "Fertilizing and Pest Control" chapter.

Small insects - Once poppies have formed the basic "rosette" or "cabbage" of leaves, they seem to be pretty much invulnerable to most macropests. Deer and the like tend to avoid them due to the extremely bitter taste of the latex. However, older poppies are still vulnerable to various small insects (beet leaf-miners, aphids, and so forth). In the absence of options that you can't produce yourself, tobacco extract plus soap in water, sprayed onto the leaves, is probably your best answer.

Fungi - sometimes a major problem, and not one that even modern gardeners, much less post-Catastrophe gardeners, can really treat directly. The wetter and warmer it is, the more of a problem fungi will be. Adjust your watering accordingly. Some varieties are more resistant to various fungi than others (Kykeon Plants recommend the purple Izmir Bush poppy, in particular, for its hardiness in cool damp conditions). Your choice of site will also have a significant impact on preventing fungal attacks: remember, well-drained!

b) Blooming Time/Preserving Varieties.

The one great curse of poppies is that their flowers don't last long, though many gardeners rhapsodize about the beauty of transience. Sounds like making a virtue out of necessity to me, but there you are. Other gardeners do a round of sowing every week for a month or so, in order to have some flowers for longer among the (attractive in themselves, but not so colourful) pods and foliage. Selecting one of the "bush" varieties of P. somniferum will also prolong your flowering period for any given plant.

Do not confuse these with the native Californian species called a "bush poppy", Dendromecon rigida. It is a member of the Papaveraceae family, and looks rather like a California poppy growing as a bush or small tree, but it does not produce opiate alkaloids or seeds. When growing poppies in real life, incidentally, a number of garden experts confirm that if you deadhead, poppies will produce more flowers. Cut the stalk just above the top leaf junction; the immature seeds are pretty useless, so just throw the pod in the rubbish bin, or burn it if concerned about accidentally poisoning any household pets who might have a propensity for bin-diving.

Of course, after the Catastrophe, you will be less concerned with how your garden looks and more with how it performs, and will want to leave that first main pod on the plant to make the various products you need. Poppy flowers start as bent-over buds, slowly straightening and finally bursting into bloom for a couple of days before the petals fall, leaving the pod to stand alone. One of Homer's finest poetic moments in the Iliad was his description of Prince Gorgythion's death: "As a garden poppy, burst into red blooms, bends, dropping its head to one side, weighed down by full seeds and a sudden spring shower, so Gorgythion's head fell limp over one shoulder, weighed down by his helmet".

The brief blood-red explosion of poppy flowers followed by the heavy-helmeted pod is extraordinarily evocative to anyone who has ever seen a corn poppy or a red P. somniferum going through the stages of its life, though it is...like the hero's death...a sad thing when the rains are heavy enough to actually cause a pod to flop over. They should stand straight up until harvested. If you want to keep your varieties pure (both for aesthetic purposes – they tend to revert to sort of muddy pink after crossbreeding randomly for a while – and for medicinal purposes, so you can at least kind of have a guess at where to begin estimating strength before you test a batch), this is the stage at which you want to cover them with a fine-mesh bag, tied carefully around the stem – tight enough to keep insects out, not tight enough to crush the stem.

The vast majority of poppy pollination is done by insects, so if you can keep the insects out, you are likely to keep a pretty pure strain. This is also a good way to isolate the first producers, best flowers (bag them all and leave the bags on the most attractive ones), largest pods, usw., for next year's generation. Because poppies are insect-pollinated, even planting plots of different strains at a good distance (some people recommend 250') from each other will not guarantee next year's purity. Poppies are self-fertile. Once the bagged poppy has bloomed, in order to achieve maximal seed production, you may want to hand-pollinate from either the same plant or a different one of the same strain with a fine paintbrush, replacing the bag immediately afterwards. Or you may want to deliberately cross different strains for visual or medicinal effect, growth habit, and so forth. Same process, only choose the pollen daddy as your source for hand pollination rather than the same plant's flower.

As your pods approach ripeness, birds may start pecking through them for the seeds. You are now back to the same netting/scarecrow/little kids method(s) which you used to protect the fresh-sown seeds. However, the most dangerous macropest that may invade your post-Catastrophe poppy plot or community field from the time the pods are showing, though it also goes on two legs, does not have wings, and won't stop with pecking through the outer pods to steal the seeds.

Nor can it readily be hand-collected and squished or frightened away by small children. In terms of attraction to raiders of all descriptions (assuming that one member of the band, nearby warlord's retinue, etc., can recognise a poppy pod or is aware that you/your community are able to produce poppy-based analgesia), this is more or less a field of gold – possibly worth a good deal more than gold in a post-Catastrophe environment, certainly until a non-survival-based economy has re-established itself.

Hopefully, having survived long enough to plant and grow your plot already, you know what to do about this particular species of vermin and are capable of doing it. The remains may gainfully be used for next year's fertilizer, unless you have severe religious objections.

A) The Harvest

1)Harvesting Seeds

For poppy seed harvest, which is the only legal poppy harvest (in places where you can grow P. somniferum at all) while our current civilization lasts - at least, without serious alterations to home opiate laws, which are unlikely in our lifetimes - leave the pod on the plant until it is dry, brown, and rattles when you shake it. Kykeon Plants, in the wetter climate of Northern England, recommend harvesting as soon as the pod turns yellow and the seeds start to rattle, as if it is left too long in a damp climate, the seeds will sort of turn to mush, or else start germinating inside the pod, neither of which is desirable.

Some varieties such as Elka are specifically bred not to open the vents in the top of the pod. Most vent and self-seed readily when mature, and therefore, in regards to harvesting seed, it is a good idea (if you can) to tie at least a paper or cloth bag loosely around the pod once it starts to dry so that there is minimal loss (this may also help with the bird problem). If you have a community-sized field, this is obviously impractical; but hopefully you are growing enough to offset the first self-seeding losses. Cut the pod off; pop the top and shake the seeds into a bag; and there you are.

If saving for future years, keep seeds in the fridge or at least a cool dark place in paper bags (if you have them; tight-woven linen or cotton if you don't; remember to label carefully) inside a sealed jar with, if possible, a good quantity of desiccant. Powdered milk is reputed to do the job if no commercial desiccants are available, as is dry rice. I cannot either disprove or vouch for this. Remember that commercial desiccant can usually be re-used indefinitely by gently heating it to dry it back out every so often. Otherwise, sow again in late summer/early autumn after you have tilled and refertilized the plot. The same storage principles hold true for poppy seeds stored as food: cool, dark, airtight, and dry.

The one downside of their high oil content is that, if exposed to too much air and moisture, they can go rancid quite easily. Remember to rodent-proof any area where poppy (or any other) seeds, in whatever quantity, are stored! If using seeds for food, toast gently in your dehydrator if it's still running, on the warming pan of your solid-fuel stove, or something similar. Central and Eastern European dishes relying on huge amounts of poppy-seed paste do this, then grind at the time of use. You'll want to have a hand-operated poppy-seed grinder – they do exist for this specific purpose, and are common, cheap, and easy to purchase. I wouldn't use my hand-operated grain mill; poppy seeds have a very high oil content as well as being extremely fine, and can gum a grain mill up like nobody's business.

Both toasting and grinding are noted for bringing out the characteristic flavour of these seeds, and the ground white seeds are commonly used as a thickening agent in Indian cuisine. Blue/black seeds would also serve well as a thickening agent, but white is preferred because of its neutral colour. It should be noted that if your varieties are high-alkaloid, whether grown as ornamentals/home-grown seed producers in real life or medicinals/food and oil producers after the Catastrophe, it might not be a bad idea to wash the seeds before drying/toasting and grinding. Washing, grinding, and cooking can render pretty much any seed, no matter what poppy it came from or how it was harvested, virtually-no-morphine.

People certainly have run into difficulties by failing drug tests due to eating the wrong bagel or roll at the wrong time, despite the absence of physical risk from the minute quantities of morphine conveyed on the seeds' coats. This is a plant where more caution is always better, in real life as in fiction. Plus, the toasting makes them taste nicer. The seeds themselves do not contain any opiates; opiate contamination of seeds is purely what gets stuck to the outer coating during harvest.

There is effectively no risk involved in using large quantities of the oil pressed from the seeds, and none at all if they were washed first to remove any possible outer-coating contamination. Poppy seeds have an extremely high nutritional value (per tablespoon/15 grams, 46 calories and 1.6 grams of protein and 3.6 grams of fat, chiefly omega-3 and omega-6 fatty acids. They are low in vitamins, but contain a number of valuable minerals, being high in iron, copper, zinc (helps increase bone density and overall bone condition), calcium (125 mg per tablespoon, ¼ of the recommended daily adult intake), manganese (antioxidant enzyme co-factor, assists in collagen production), magnesium (improves sleep quality and duration), phosphorus, and selenium, as well as potassium.

Even if your personal beliefs prevent you from using pain control in extreme cases, you will find it worthwhile growing them as a food crop. Poppy seeds are high in oil, over 40%, and their oil is useful as a food ingredient, cooking oil, lamp fuel, fat for a high-quality soft soap, oil paint ingredient, and anti-inflammatory and moisturising element of both medicinal and cosmetic ointments. And if you're Jewish, Purim likely would not feel quite the same without Hamantaschen (a traditional triangular pastry) containing a proper poppy-seed filling. Should your particular post-Catastrophe environment be troubled by encounters with the supernatural, especially malevolent supernatural beings, you will find it useful to know that poppy seeds have a long history as an apotropaic (protective) substance.

Particularly in Poland, poppy seeds were used to break a witch's curse, or scattered around the house or put in coffins in order to distract a witch or spirit (notably the undead), who would be compelled to count every one of the seeds before continuing with any malicious purpose. Vampiric OCD is a common theme in the apotropaic lore of Europe: other seeds used in this manner included millet, mustard, and flax (it is, however, unlikely that the counting-compulsion of the European undead was the origin of a certain vampiric character with the same compulsion in a popular children's television show).

Polish belief also included the use of poppy seeds in aiding the newly deceased's transition to the Otherworld (while protecting against evil spirits who might interfere), and in feasts communing with the dead such as All Saints' Day (November 1), All Souls' Day (November 2), and Christmas Eve. Christmas Eve and the eve of St. Lucia's Day (December 13), are times when witches, at least those of Polish background, are particularly active. Other days which you may find call for the apotropaic use of poppy seeds are Holy Thursday (the Thursday before Easter) for Swedish witches and Walpurgisnacht (April 30) for Scandinavian and German witches.

Poppy seeds may also be used to bring fruitfulness, as was seen in ancient Greece, where they were a significant element of wedding cakes and holy to Demeter; and in Poland, for sprinkling on newlyweds and fruit trees alike (Zemanek et al, op. cit.). If you wish to grow your own delicious seeds in real life or use your poppies chiefly or entirely as a food crop after the Catastrophe, I recommend the varieties "Elka" (a white-seeded sweet heritage cultivar, named after the Slovakian lady who had been growing it in her garden for many years; as mentioned, it does not open vents on its own and therefore does not lose seeds at maturity), "Ziar" (dark-seeded heritage cultivar; like Elka, it was brought to the US by one Slovakian guy who went looking for little old ladies cultivating the special seeds of his childhood); "Pepperpot" (a beautiful bright red with dark blotches at the bases of the petals, commonly used to get that special Eastern/Central European seed taste), "Polish Pulawski" (heritage variety with cream-coloured seeds, a bit darker than most whites); and the fairly common "Hungarian Blue Breadseed".

These are all relatively low-opiate, so toasting and grinding should dispose of any risk of opiate contamination; and are noted for the excellent flavour of their seeds. Poppy seeds come in two main colours, white and blue (sometimes also called "black"); some people also recognise a "brown" seed from Turkey as a separate type. There is some debate among cooks and gourmets as to the relationship between colour and flavour. It is the opinion of some that white seeds in general and possibly brown seeds have a milder and sweeter flavour, while the blue are more "deep" and "nutty" or "almond-like" with a faint bitterness (usually lost in roasting or masked by sweetness in baked goods). Other people claim that there is little or no discernable difference based on colour alone, or that the blue/black seeds are actually slightly sweeter.

Certainly some specific cultivars do have distinctive flavours, and are well worth growing in real life for that purpose if you are legally allowed to. The blue is the most commonly used in Central and Eastern European cooking; the white is generally preferred in Indian cooking. On average, white-seeded poppies appear to have a lower morphine content than blue- or black-seeded cultivars. And on top of all that, poppy seeds are still sometimes used even in modern Western medicine to detect the presence of a fistula between bowel and bladder, for which they are quite effective. Feed the patient whole poppy seeds. If the seeds come out in their urine, there is a passage there, which is probably going to require surgery, because bowel bacteria contaminating the urinary passageways are Bad News...can you say, "Fatal kidney infection"?

Hope that your community has a surgeon and someone who knows how to make ether (not the best anaesthetic in the world – we have many better and safer today – but it can be made in low-tech conditions, albeit gingerly, given its tendency to explode at the slightest provocation. Diana Gabaldon's A Breath of Snow and Ashes describes the production, use, and explosive qualities of ether in extensive and graphic detail, though I wouldn't use it as a manual for making the stuff, and only your author knows if the raw materials will even be available to you after the Catastrophe.

Making and using ether is another of those "hope to your god or gods, Providence, or the universe in general that you never have to use this knowledge, but if you do, things will be bad enough that you will probably be glad you have it" things). Americans, be well aware that US laws on growing P. somniferum do not take account of actual morphine percentages. So if you do grow low/no morphine cultivars (increasingly popular in the commercial poppy seed industry, particularly given the issues re drug testing – and, yes, the wrong poppy-seed roll can cause you to fail a drug test; that "urban myth" has been proven true a number of times), that status probably won't save you if someone decides to prosecute.

2) Harvesting for Medicine

The post-Catastrophe opiate harvest is a whole different box of cats. The common practice was, and in some places still is, repeated scoring of the green pod vertically to a depth of 1 mm (less gets little result; more breaches the seed capsule and allows the latex to leak in, losing latex and contaminating the seed) in the hottest part of the day ca. 2 weeks after the petals have fallen, and collection of the congealed gum (raw opium) the next morning, repeated every 2-4 days for several days. The raw gum must be gently cooked in water for several hours (some boil, but more recent evidence suggests that heat above 85 C /185 F, for any prolonged period of time, degrades the morphine) and the resulting liquid strained well.

The water is then evaporated off, leaving the cooked opium paste, which may be dissolved forthwith into an alcohol (or glycerine) medium, or dried, pressed into flat cakes, and dried thoroughly. This is not a particularly efficient method of extraction, and requires large fields and a lot of low-income people willing to do the work if it is the only method used (it would not surprise me if, when post-Catastrophe civilization has recovered to a certain level, some communities were to use slaves for this purpose...

Or if the slaves in question were to surreptitiously collect some opium of their own, to ease their misery or as part of a plot to drug their overseers and escape). Rain at the time of lancing will wash away the latex and leach a wounded pod more severely than an untouched one. However, there is some evidence that wounding a pod promotes the movement of more alkaloids from the whole plant into the pod (though not more overall synthesis in the plant). Lancing a pod to the correct depth is not known to diminish the quantity of the seed produced, although it may diminish the oil percentage.

Therefore, if and when, and only if and when, the Catastrophe has occurred and processing of poppy pods for home or community medicinal use can be carried out without breaking the law, this may be a method worth considering for maximizing the ease of obtaining the best possible yield from the smaller portion of a year's crop, leaving the larger percentage unscored in the interest of maximum seed oil content. Until then, the totally illegal and demonstrably visible act of scoring poppy pods would be like holding up a big public sign saying, "I am gathering my own awesomely illegal opium", in a way that will completely obviate any potential, "I didn't know they were opium poppies" or "I was growing them solely for decoration/culinary purposes" defense.

Darwin says the character who does this before the Catastrophe probably deserves to get busted for stupidity as much as they deserve to get busted for the actual crime of illegal opiate production/use. Even if lancing is not part of your general post-Catastrophe harvest method, it might be an idea to collect and preserve some of the latex (raw opium) against the possibility that it may be necessary to treat a patient (or, in the case of an outbreak of cholera or similar devastating contagious GI infection, a number of patients – but remember where "food poisoning" from salmonella, campylobacter, and a number of other toxin-producing bacteria is concerned, natural clearance ought not be halted unless a patient is at significant risk of life-threatening dehydration) with severe vomiting as well as pain and/or life-threatening diarrhoea.

As mentioned in the previous section: in such an instance, inhalation is probably a safer means of administering the drug than injecting the opium tincture. Dosage is more difficult to quantify with inhalation of opium, and we know less about inhalation usage in medical terms in general, but the risks of overdose, while always a concern with any type or means of administering an opiate, are significantly less, and titration is comparatively easy. Even many real-life heroin abusers, given the choice, apparently prefer to smoke their drug for those reasons and others, and making that option available is considered an element of harm reduction.

If your weather in any given year does not permit lancing and preparation of the raw opium as described above, a portion of the water extraction from the mature pod may, instead of being dissolved into the alcohol medium, be further evaporated until it can be pressed into cakes and dried completely to set aside in the event that it is necessary to use vaporization/inhalation as a means of administration for the severely vomiting patient. That is not otherwise an optimal storage method, as the medication will keep better in alcohol or even glycerine. Beware of mould inside cakes that have not dried through or been kept properly dry! It can be quite toxic.

Current evidence indicates that the highest morphine/pod ratio is reached in the fairly dry and semi-mature state between 5 and 6 weeks after blooming, which – happily for the beleaguered survivor of the Catastrophe who needs the valuable nutrition and multi-purpose oil of the seed as well as the medicinal use of the pod – is also the earliest point at which the largely mature pod may be harvested and deseeded, with mature seeds suited to cooking or a good germination rate for next year's crop. This is particularly important if you live in a wet area, where you want to harvest the moment the seeds begin to rattle to prevent degeneration (and, if the rains come heavily, water-leaching of the medicinal alkaloids from the pod). If necessary, better to harvest a little earlier and finish the drying/ripening process indoors than to harvest too late and get nothing. If you must harvest early, cut the stem long and sear the end as soon as you cut it.

Glycerine is less effective than alcohol in standard tincture-making procedures. This does not apply to poppy production, since the water-extracted concentrate can be dissolved directly into the glycerine. These extractions may have a shorter shelf-life than alcohol extractions (1 year vs indefinite).

Minimizing exposure to air, heat, and light improves keeping qualities. Food-grade glycerine will be marked with an expiration date, but can keep up to 20 years if stored properly; it neither breaks down readily nor forms dangerous degradation products when it does. If well-sealed, it may dessicate slightly, but will restore its normal qualities upon exposure to air.

The pure form of glycerine is sometimes called "glycerol", but they are effectively the same. Glycerine has been marketed as a "safe" sweetener to people with diabetes, but there is little or no evidence that it is safer than ordinary sucrose, especially for the insulin-dependent. Of course, your insulin-dependent patient doesn't have the greatest post-Catastrophe prognosis...but Eva Saxl, herself insulin-dependent, refined her own in war-torn WWII Japan, saved many lives, and lived to tell the world about it herself.

This prolongs the actual "life" of the cut pod and gives the seed a better chance to mature, in much the same way as cutting the stem of the flower long and searing the end will make it last a bit longer in an indoors fresh flower arrangement. The breeding seeds are resown at some point in late August to early October, depending on your specific climate and how long the flowers took to bloom, after the remainder of the straw is ploughed back in and another healthy dose of aged horse/cow manure plus bone meal is incorporated into the soil.

At this stage of development, the vast majority of opiates are found in the pod and the top 4" (10 cm) of stem. The use of the lower stem and leaves is relevant only for very large-scale production, as in the real-life pharmaceutical industry. The seeds should have reached their final colour, though this is more difficult to determine with white seeds, and be suitable, after a bit more drying, for either food storage/processing or germination.

D) Extraction

There is a great deal of argument in both the scientific and the anecdotal literature as to the most efficient method of extraction from the dry pod. No one is sure whether high-percentage alcohol (ethanol only...remember, this will be consumed by humans, to whom methanol is destructive and easily fatal. Free idea for Ignorant Survivor Tragedy: someone tries to make a poppy extract with methanol instead of ethanol, with the predictable results – or, less tragically, keeps a decoy methanol-extract bottle about for raider/warlord's goon control), water, or something like standard spirits (ca. 40% alcohol/60% mostly water) is more effective. Acidification and warming of the extracting medium has been demonstrated in real studies (as opposed to Internet lore) to make a certain positive difference.

For a final product that is alcoholic enough to be stored for a long time, but concentrated enough that there is minimal or no risk of untowards interactions between the alcohol and the opiate alkaloids in even two to three standard doses, my best guess as to what the Catastrophe survivor might do would be a process that could look something like this: The desired weight of deseeded pods (don't include the seeds; they've got nothing but fatty acids to contribute, especially if they were hand-harvested...most of our poppy seed tea tragedies today came from seeds that were mechanically harvested and ended up with loads of morphine on their outer coats, to the shock and eventual death of the poor folk who drank down large amounts of tea made with an insane amount of seeds), according to best estimate by the average measured contents of the varietal(s), if known, or on an average of 10% of 8% of deseeded dry pod weight (10% morphine per opium – 8% opium overall), are ground as finely as possible and heated to no less than 115 F (ca. 46 C) and no more than 185 F (85 C) in 3x water plus 1x lemon juice or similar acidic liquid such as vinegar, for a period of three to five hours.

There is some anecdotal support for cold-water extraction, but warm-water extraction appears, under actual testing (as contrasted to, "I did it at home and it was pretty strong") to be more efficient. Often the solid material will be strained out and a second water dissolution performed on it before proceeding to the next step. Commercial production often puts dry poppy capsules/stalks/leaves through 4 to 6 extractions to get out every last bit, which is probably worthwhile for people who count their fields in hectares and their yield in kilograms, but is likely to be excessive for the post-Catastrophe survivor unless supplying a whole community, who can then be enlisted to aid in the larger-scale and lengthier process for the sake of the group. The solid material is strained and put in drinking spirits of min. 40% alcohol to cover for a final extraction, while the remaining water is slowly evaporated, being careful not to let the temperature go above 85 C/185 F, until the contents of the pan(s) resemble molasses or thick maple syrup.

E) Extract Preparations

For an alcohol tincture, the alcohol mix is strained again, and used to dissolve the evaporated contents of the pan. If a higher concentration is required after testing, another multiple water extraction/evaporation can be done, and the materials then dissolved into the existing alcohol compound. Retest as before. For those who cannot tolerate even as much as 10 ml (2 teaspoons, 1/3 of a shot) of 30% alcohol, either for personal/religious reasons or physical intolerance (I have known one man who was so sensitive that he even had a bad allergic reaction to the trace quantity of alcohol in "alcohol-free" beer, and therefore could not safely have taken so much as a quarter-teaspoonful of this mixture – and yes, that hypersensitivity did make his life difficult in many ways), water may be used for all extractions and glycerine may be substituted as a medium of dissolution and preservative.

Glycerine is also a laxative (causes osmotic drawing of water into the large intestine, softening the stool), and for prolonged chronic pain use, may help to counter the constipating effects of poppy, although such an extract would be considerably less useful for the purpose of diarrhoea control. A glycerine extract absolutely must not be given to a cholera patient, as the main mechanism of danger in cholera is the loss of fluid through the intestines! In the unhappy event that you are forced to give someone an emergency injection, an alcohol extract, unsafe as it is, is safer than a glycerine extract (except for a patient with the, thankfully extremely rare, hypersensitivity of Mr. Allergic-to-Alcohol above).

Glycerine is bacteriostatic (retards or halts the growth of bacteria, but does not kill them); alcohol is bacteriocidal (kills bacteria). Hence your chances of giving the patient a nasty infection under these circumstances are much lower with the alcohol-based product, and as IM injection of alcohol does not lead to intoxication, it should be acceptable even to those who are religiously and/or personally opposed to the use of the slightest amount of potentially-intoxicating alcohol. In the absence of glycerine, the concentrated water extract may be made into a syrup with large amounts of sugar or honey (hope someone in your area is either growing sugar beets or keeping beehives!), which will not preserve it as long as alcohol or glycerine, but will at least make it possible to make up and test a smaller batch from dried pods every 2 months or so, especially if you have a cold or at least cool place to keep the product.

If you or someone close to you - for whatever reason, physical or religious - cannot use even small doses of medicinal-medium alcohol, I strongly suggest stockpiling glycerine in large amounts. It is a purified product which cannot readily be recreated in a post-Catastrophe environment (though a shorter-lived and impure version may be produced as a byproduct of soap-making, I would be dubious about eating soap-making-produced glycerine myself), but can generally be utilized in most situations for which alcohol is more commonly used as a solvent and preservative, such as the production of herbal tinctures.

Estimating an average of 10 grams (0.35 oz) deseeded pod to 1 dose final concentrate/tincture; assuming that the final volume of your first batch, ca. 30% alcohol by the time everything is mixed together, is 3000 ml. (3.17 quarts), and that the pods used were a lower-opiate cultivar (ca. 200 mg morphine/100 g pod material), then 1500 g (1 lb = 454 grams – going by weight rather than volume measurement here, as I have no idea how the bulk would measure out, and it probably depends on how finely it is crushed or ground anyway) deseeded pod hypothetically, if you could get 100% extraction (which you can't with post-Catastrophe technology), could give a dosage of approximately 10 ml/2 teaspoons "laudanum" = 10 mg morphine. That is, 1/10 the strength of modern opium tincture, 2.5x the strength of modern paregoric.

Or: 2 tablespoons/30 ml = 1 maximum oral pain dose for the opiate-naïve in very serious pain; ¼ teaspoon/1.25 ml equals the amount of codeine in 1 over-the-counter combination codeine/ibuprofen tablet as sold in Ireland/UK; 1 ¼ teaspoon/6.25 ml roughly equals a post-surgical dose of codeine (ca. 60 mg codeine = 6 mg oral morphine). If the pod is a stronger variety, do the maths for yourself. But remember: there will always be a lot of variance. Any given ornamental may be a stronger or weaker producer where you live and when you grew that batch than it was where the original evaluation for the cultivar, if known, was done, in the year that it was done; and pharmaceutical cultivars probably vary even more widely.

Without current testing capabilities, very rough estimations are the best you can get when selecting materials and initiating your process. And never forget: dosage strength per individual batch may vary wildly, not only by strain (remember: a "pharmaceutical" variety is expected to be at least 4 times stronger by weight than the example above, and may be much more powerful than that; other ornamental varieties may be over 3 times stronger than the example here), but by environmental variations, and should not be depended upon based on any theoretical estimate. Such guesswork is only the beginning from which to start testing.

To test strength, you might begin with .75 ml (1/8 teaspoon); check again with a different tester or the next day with the same tester with 1.25 ml/ (1/4 teaspoon); then 2.5 ml (1/2 teaspoon); then 5 ml (1 teaspoon), up to 10 ml (2 teaspoons). This should make it possible to evaluate the specific strength of the batch produced, at least to a degree that allows effective dosage while minimizing the risk of accidental overdose. No given test will apply to any other batch, whether produced by different strains/strain combinations, or by poppies grown in a different year or under different circumstances.

As mentioned above, if the batch is weaker than desired, which could lead to more alcohol intake than is wanted in combination with an opiate (more than 30 ml spirits, which is approximately one standard shot, is probably too much; and definitely too much if a patient needs several 30 ml doses/day), a further water extraction/evaporated concentration can be made and dissolved into it, whereupon the testing process must be redone from the beginning. No testing you can do post-Catastrophe will make your use of this drug even as safe as that provided by pharmaceutical opiates/opioids when properly prescribed and administered by a doctor, and there have been plenty of tragedies associated with those. Your results will still be guesswork; they will just be less dangerous guesswork than if you didn't carefully test each batch.

You are only doing this because there is no remaining alternative in the post-Catastrophe world; not because you were actually ever reckless enough to want to process your own. If you have long-term chronic pain/palliative care patients who have developed a high tolerance and/or have immensely increasing pain-control needs, I would strongly recommend either using glycerine if you have it and avoiding alcohol altogether for that patient, or making separate batches into which more than one batch's worth of water-extracted concentrate are dissolved, or both. Because if your palliative patient requires, say, 200 mg. morphine/day, that's 200 ml. or nearly 7 ounces (30 ml roughly = 1 oz) of 30% spirits...and risks moving from "palliative pain control" to "inadvertent euthanasia" in the context of the patient's weakened condition and poppy dose. The Catastrophe may kill off all or almost all current palliative care patients...but it will not prevent future cases of cancer, COPD, the results of non-fatal but seriously physically destructive injuries, and so forth.

In fact, if people are thrown back on primarily in-house combustion for heating and cooking, even when tobacco has become a rare and special treat if available at all (and if all tobacco production has not been prioritized to insect control on crops), the rates of COPD and possibly lung cancer are likely to go up, as suggested by medical archaeology and the current rates of combustion-household-heating-related lung disease in places such as rural China today. Many native peoples worldwide (including Viking and pre-Viking Age Nordic Scandinavians, Saami, and several groups of Native Americans), living in small groups in harsh environments where there is little margin, developed their own culturally-appropriate methods of dealing with people whom we might consider palliative care patients or just very old and becoming enfeebled. Or rather, encouraging and allowing such people to deal with the situation themselves for the good of their families and tribes.

But that is not our culture, and, hopefully, you will be able to keep it from becoming so after the Catastrophe. As for the chronic pain patient in a survival situation – and I would expect to see more osteoarthritis and far worse rheumatoid arthritis, for instance - appropriate analgesia can help that person to continue contributing to the community: as a worker to a greater degree than might otherwise have been the case, as a teacher, and in carrying out the necessary tasks traditionally assigned to the elderly in order to free up more physically able folk for more physically demanding duties.

Because of the extremely bitter taste, which many find absolutely intolerable, opium extracts back in the day were often flavoured by various other substances, including sugar, honey, various spices, and camphor (probably added chiefly to mask the flavour and possibly for its stimulant effect; see above statements re the combination of stimulants with opioids for improved pain control). However, no matter what you find on the Internet about "camphorated opium tincture", and no matter how historically charming it may sound, don't try making it at home. The risks are far too great. Even in the low quantities used in modern paregoric (4 gr camphor to 1 litre, or 0.4%, in a medication dealt out in quantities of 0.1-0.2 ml/kg), the oral use of camphor has aroused concerns and criticism. Save those camphor crystals or essential oil to put a tiny amount in steam when someone in your family has severely congested lungs. Don't mix camphor with your opiates or otherwise take it orally.

If, after the Catastrophe, you are in a position to need to try extracting opiates from poppies, and you or your patients find the result too disgusting to stomach... add sugar, honey, whatever spices or strong-flavoured herbs you have around; but just do not mess with camphor. You're already going to be taking one big risk in dealing with an opiate that has to be strength-verified by subjective evaluation; don't add another. If you need a stimulant adjunct, use a separate cup of strong coffee...which, thankfully, can be grown indoors without special electric lighting, as coffee plants prefer filtered sunlight to direct, and can be remarkably cold-tolerant. The short varieties Canephora (a Robusta) and Dwarf Catura (an Arabica), in particular, make excellent houseplants. With a bit of forethought and starting your indoor coffee plants early, if your author was kind enough to give you four or five years of growing them before the Catastrophe...You may suffer from plague, war, raiders, or for all I know Alien Space Bats (said I, nodding to S.M. Stirling's Emberverse books once more), but at least you won't be doing it in the throes of caffeine withdrawal.

IV. Back to the Real World: Poppy Species, Strains, and Sources (for those who can legally grow ornamental P. somniferum or want to grow the totally-legal-everywhere non-opiate poppy species)

a) Major Poppy Species

P. somniferum (including var. paeoniflorium) is the only signficant source of opiates. There is some question as to whether the wild P. setigerum may also contain opiate alkaloids, but recently the evidence seems at least to be going against setigerum as the wild forebear of somniferum. If P. setigerum does contain opiate alkaloids, it is at a significantly lower level than P. somniferum.

P. rhoeas - the "corn poppy" which is used in several English-speaking countries as the symbol of remembrance of fallen soldiers - does not contain opiates, but is a functional low-level sedative and analgesic. It has never been reported to be addictive. It grows freely in fields and on disturbed ground of temperate climates. It is also the poppy commonly associated with the goddess Demeter, although the mythological account of it bringing her peace after Persephone's abduction is more suggestive of P. somniferum. Growing and utilizing this plant is legal in all known countries.

Eschscholzia californica, the California poppy, is also a proven low-level sedative, analgesic, and sleep aid, but likewise lacks either morphine or codeine. To my knowledge, there have been no accounts of addiction related to the use of this plant. E. californica is also completely legal to grow, use, and possess in all countries I know of. It requires sandy and usually poor soil, as a result of which it thrives wild in California, and is indeed the state flower. Despite the "illegal to pick the state flower" myth, it is, apparently, actually legal in California to pick wild ones, though illegal to steal them from someone else's land. Nothing except soil and climate issues can stop you from covering your own entire property in this beautiful golden-orange flower - which also comes in cultivated varieties of many colours including cream, bright red, and purple, a delight to the poppy fan who must deal with poor sandy soil and frequent drought - and harvesting it at will. Fortunately, being able to pronounce its Linnean name is not required.

Both P. rhoeas and E. californica will be valuable additions to either your post-Catastrophe or a real-life herbal pharmacopeia. They can be used on their own or as adjuncts to other analgesics/sedatives, including opiates, without risk. And, best of all, no matter where you live, you can start growing, harvesting, and using them now.

Meconopsis (several varieties) is another distant poppy relative without major opiate alkaloids. It can be found in several colours, but the most noted and prized by gardeners are the blue varieties, which are indeed very, very blue. Their recent arrival on the garden scene has been the cause of much interest and excitement. These sapphire jewels are native to the Himalayas, thrive in cold and damp weather only, and are pretty much the only poppies that actually like growing in the shade. They do well in Scotland, Ireland, and cold damp parts of North America. Their medical characteristics have not been investigated by Western scientists.

Traditionally they are considered useful as "cooling", anti-inflammatory and febrifugic plants; but there are no evidence-based studies on this of which I am aware. They are not opiate-alkaloid producers. Be warned: googling "Persian Blue poppy" (a real and quite attractive cultivar of P. somniferum, though rather more purple than blue) may lead one to some pictures of meconopsis and several sites which even claim to be selling "Persian Blue" poppies associated with meconopsis pictures.

Though beautiful in and of themselves, and splendid to add colour to a shady part of a decorative garden, Meconopsis varieties won't give you edible seeds or proven medication of any sort. There are, as yet, no known species of P. somniferum that display a true blue colour, nor has anyone ever been able to cultivate one. I bet if anyone ever does, they'll make an awful lot of money from it; but I suspect the problem is the same as the difficulty of breeding blue roses: the colour just isn't in the species' genetics. Several cultivars can have a blue-ish tinge to their purple-to-lavender in the right light and growing conditions, and include "blue" in the name – Persian Blue, Hungarian Blue Buddha, Hungarian Blue Breadseed. However, "blue" in the name of a cultivar of P. somniferum is usually referring to its seed colour, not its petal colour.

P. nudicaule – a poppy of limited medicinal value but considerable beauty. The leaves can be cooked or eaten as a prevention/treatment for scurvy. This should not be your first choice, nor done in great quantity; the toxicity to humans is relatively low, but present. Also known as the Iceland poppy or Arctic poppy, and, as the name suggests, thrives in cool to cold climates. The flowers can produce red and beige dyes, the pods yellow and brown dyes.

P. orientale – another attractive garden flower. Its potential toxicity to humans is low, but present. Petals may be used in cautious doses to promote sweating.

P. orientale var bracteatum (Iranian poppy, Great Scarlet poppy) - lacks morphine, but is high in thebaine – a potential source of opioid drugs, but only in a proper pharmaceutical laboratory. Otherwise high thebaine levels are a potential source of getting really, awesomely sick and quite possibly dying, as sadly proven by the occasional case in Tasmania where someone has stolen pods for recreational drug abuse out of the wrong field (high-thebaine/low morphine varieties, grown for pharmaceutical production of opioids).

Both P. nudicaule and P. orientale come in an amazing range of colours, and are perennial, a boon to the gardener who gets tired of having to resow their poppies every year. They are legal to grow in all known countries, as are the meconopsis varieties.

P. glaucum (Turkish poppy, tulip poppy). Bright red with black centre. Closely resembles P. somniferum, but the petals grow upwards in a shape similar to a tulip. A truly striking poppy from Anatolia, noted for its extreme hardiness in a wide range of conditions; but only recently attaining popularity in Western gardens. Medicinal uses have not been studied; may or may not contain extremely low levels of morphine, codeine, and thebaine (sources differ). Legal everywhere. An excellent alternative for the American gardener, but save the pack in case it becomes necessary to prove that it is not an opium poppy.

Dendromecon rigida (bush poppy, California tree poppy). A member of the Papaveracae family, but contains no opiate alkaloids. Bright gold flowers, somewhat resembles an E. californica growing as a shrub. No known medicinal or edible uses, but striking nonetheless, particularly if you are focusing on (or limited to) garden plants that can tolerate prolonged drought conditions.

b) Some choice varieties of P. somniferum.

These are a few varieties which, in my opinion, look awesome in the garden, even if the world sails right along without Catastrophe through the entirety of your lifetime... Let me repeat yet again: if you grow them in the US, you grow them at your own risk, and not mine, because while practically every cook in the country would join a revolution if it became illegal to possess P. somniferum seeds, the live plants technically are illegal. And the last place you want to be when and if the Catastrophe comes is locked up in gaol. It would be awfully ironic to die in prison during the Catastrophe as a result of having tried to prepare to survive after it!

Lauren's Grape – A beautiful deep purple, for my money one of the most attractive poppies out there. Sometimes called "Lauren Springer's Grape". Sold by many garden centres; wildly popular as an ornamental. The "bagel story" of this cultivar's origin is proof that it is possible, with a good bit of luck, to develop a true-breeding flower that will take its place in garden catalogues across the world, and sell out very quickly in quite a lot of them, too.

I hope Ms. Springer is receiving the high royalties she deserves on each packet, or however these things are done with new cultivars.

Hungarian Blue Buddha... Grows as a large bush. Many flowers/plant. Sold only by Organical Botanicals, to the best of my knowledge.

Izmir Bush Poppy – there are actually at least two versions of this still extant, the white and the purple. The white resembles the Tasmanian/wild-type (white petals, lavender centre blotches); the purple is lavender with purple centres. The purple, according to the Kykeon Plants site, is about the hardiest poppy ever, especially in damp cool fungus-promoting climates such as Britain; they recommend the white for its flowering beauty and decorative large thick pods.The third variety from Izmir, on which no one has commented, might have been the "Hungarian Blue Buddha".

Allegedly there were three types originally cultivated and sold by Izmir, and Blue Buddha does grow as a large multi-flowered bush; although since Organical Botanicals usually makes a big deal about the strains they got from Izmir originally and doesn't mention that origin for this one, maybe not. Blue Buddha has a deep-purple-to-brilliant-magenta centre edged with lavender. Any fan of bush poppies, with their many flowers and longer overall blooming period, might wish to try all three of these for the sake of attractive aesthetic contrast, in any case. The two named Izmir Bush Poppies are sold by Organical Botanicals and Kykeon Plants.

Izmir Afghan Special ("Galania"). Brought back from Afghanistan by the people at Izmir Poppy Farm some years ago. Alleged to be the headline-making "Chinese GMO" fast-flowering super-opium strain. I cannot determine how much of this might be media hype, or indeed counterculture hype based on media hype. I do know that this Izmir strain is a rich pink and white, and a beauty in the garden. If it is the legendary "Chinese" strain, then one would have the option (in ornamental-poppy-legal areas) to do a late spring/early summer sowing, so as to still have some poppy flowers later in the year when most of them are reduced to the more ascetic look of pods and foliage.

Although, if it were the same strain (unproven and probably unprovable; the original Izmir site, as I recall, only mentioned that they had been brought back from Afghanistan and bred to thrive in southern Canada; and they were available well before 2015, when the first rumours about "new Chinese GMO super-poppies" came out), and if the story about "Chinese-origin GMO" were true (hard to tell for sure, I suspect), and if you are strongly opposed to GMO even for ornamental plants, you might want to just give this one a miss and go for a different pink-and-white such as, say, Queen's or a pink-and-white variant of Giganteum, both of which are commonly sold by many garden centres. There is no shortage of options for this colour combination. Sold by Organical Botanicals and Kykeon Plants.

Afghan White, Persian White, Chinese White, Shyama...pure white flowers. Any of these provide an excellent contrast to the darker-coloured cultivars, particularly the near-black Midnight and Starry Night, the rich red Cherry Glow, and the strong purple Lauren's Grape. I am given to understand that these strains are also white-seeded and thus particularly suited to poppyseed use in Indian cuisine. Nicky's Nursery describes Shyama, an Indian-origin cultivar, as an "improved variety of Papaver somniferum", but I have been unable to determine what they mean by "improved". Shyama sold by Nicky's Nursery; the others are available from various garden centres.

Polish Pulawski...extremely frilly, but single-petalled type (as contrasted to the paeoniflorium varieties); pure white flowers, with seeds of a dark cream colour. If one prefers the classic single-petalled poppy type, this cultivar provides an interesting and highly attractive contrast to the more common smooth-petalled varieties, while still maintaining the lines of a proper poppy flower. Considered an heritage variety, but often grown for its seeds, with the distinct advantage of being notably low in alkaloids. Sold by Organical Botanicals.

Izmir Tasmanian. This particular version was cultivated by Izmir Poppy Farm for a number of years, and – if obtained from one of the reliable suppliers that have taken care to preserve the original Izmir varieties (Organical Botanicals and Kykeon Plants are the only ones I can vouch for) – should be no cause for concern regarding thebaine toxicity if accidentally ingested (opiate-alkaloid toxicity overall would be a concern).

An excellent poppy if one is growing an historical medicinal herb garden and wants display poppies that look like the basal P. somniferum - a few of mine, in some past years, have lived in the fenced Early Major Medicinal, a.k.a. "Do not touch or eat these plants" display area of my mediaeval herb garden, together with henbane, monkshood, black hellebore, deadly nightshade, hemlock, foxglove, and mandrake. Very large pods, also great for crafts. Sold by Organical Botanicals and Kykeon Plants.

Giganteum. Available in several colour combinations. Noted for its huge flowers, which may reach a diameter of 6", and massive pods; by far the favourite source of dried pods for flower arrangements. Variants of this cultivar are sold by just about every garden centre that sells poppy seeds, as it is immensely popular.

Cherry Glow. An intense, brilliant red poppy with darker centre blotches. I always think of the death of Gorgythion in the Iliad when I see this one in bloom. Available at many garden centres, and absolutely the first choice if your ideal image of a poppy is a red flower.

Hen-and-Chicks. Another very popular and very commonly available strain with several colour options. The main flower (the "Hen") is surrounded by a ring of mini-pods (the "Chicks"), adding considerable interest to the poppy patch long after the petals have fallen. This cultivar is much-loved as a source of dry pods for crafting due to its unique appearance. Usually smooth-petalled, but the Izmir variety (Organical Botanicals) has rather pretty fringed petals.

Drama Queen: when you see the picture, you'll understand the name. Possibly the most eye-catching cultivar available today. Highly popular and available at the majority of garden centres.

Midnight and Starry Night: two of the prettiest "black" (or rather, intensely dark, dark purple) poppies available. Excellent for colour-contrast, or growing a Goth garden, together with the pure white varieties described above. For those who like paeoniflorium varieties and want a "black", Black Dragon or Izmir Indian Black would be good choices. Midnight, Starry Night, and Black Dragon (and several other "black" paeoniflorium varieties) are sold by many garden centres; Izmir Indian Black is sold by Organical Botanicals.

I am not personally fond of the appearance of any of the paeoniflorium varieties of P. somnifera, although the "Izmir Indian Black" grew well for me one year. To me, they just do not look like proper poppies; they look like what you'd get if you crossed a chrysanthemum with the late great Andre the Giant. No harm there to Andre, whom we all miss, but he was rather better known for his strength and good humour than for his beauty. However, many gardeners love them, and they are available in a vast range of colours, with petals both plain and frilled, from the vast majority of garden centres in the UK and a great many in the US.

As mentioned earlier and repeatedly: I very strongly recommend against growing any form of P. somniferum in the US as long as there is a functional US and the laws against even ornamental cultivation are upheld. Don't do it. There are plenty of other beautiful poppy species, and it's not worth risking a narcotics conviction just to have a pretty garden plant, especially with the "opioid crisis" and the State, as a result of tightened regulations on pain medication prescriptions and pain clinics with the corresponding rise in illegal opiate/opioid drugs, looking more and more closely for people who might be trying to produce their own major pain-control medications. So, yes, I'm thumping the same drum yet once more, because I really, really do not wish to be responsible for someone's arrest on the grounds of growing the wrong ornamental flower. Nor do I wish for anyone to get the idea that, because I am advising on the most realistic ways for fictional characters to use these plants medicinally in a post-Catastrophe situation, I think or advocate in any manner that anyone should be home-producing opiates now.

c) Seed Sources

Organical Botanicals: Try not to be put off by their crap website. Every time you click on something on their website, you have to scroll down from their screen-covering largely blank brown initial page to see whatever it was you were looking for; the first couple of times I followed a link to them, I thought the site was actually dead. Also, their blog/tutorial "page" was clearly done by the owner's three year-old. Once you get past that, these people have a large number of the strains that the late lamented Izmir Poppy Farm cultivated. They are very pricey compared to anyone else who sells poppy seeds, but have some strains that are difficult or impossible to find elsewhere.

Mainly a poppy specialist, but have a few interesting varieties of pumpkins and maize, as well as some exotics including the Fabled Black Bat Plant, scariest-looking tropical/houseplant the gods ever made and much beloved by Goths with dark green thumbs. If I ever write an horticultural horror story, I know which plant will be playing the starring role; and the Black Bat flower would also make a pretty good visual stand-in for an alien or demon meant to appear frightening. US, but ship to Europe, Canada, UK.

Kykeon Plants: Several of the Izmir strains, and a wide range of other poppies besides. Not to mention just about every herb, in every form, you can think of (with the exceptions of coffee and cannabis...but if you wanted to grow an entire garden of many varieties of native European deadly nightshade plants from this site, you could. I am not sure why you would want to, but if you ever took a notion to do such a thing, this is where you'd go for it). I have literally never seen such a selection in my life. You could stock almost an entire herbal pharmacopeia from these people. UK; ship everywhere except Taiwan, Brazil, and Mexico.

There are a number of e-Bay, Amazon, etc. sources claiming to sell various Izmir Farm poppy seeds, particularly the Afghan Special and the Izmir Tasmanian. Organical Botanicals, to whom the still-extant Izmir site sent me, and Kykeon Plants are the only sources that I personally trust to have kept the strains pure and to be accurate in their advertising. I have a particular affection for Izmir strains because they were imported from various places, but bred in and for southern Canada. They produce some of the strongest, healthiest, and prettiest poppies I have ever seen in my wet temperate Northern European zone, in my garden or anyone else's. If you want to grow poppies in Great Britain or Ireland, or anywhere else with a similar climate where it is legal to do so, I highly recommend any of the Izmir strains.

Seedman: A site highly recommended for both the adventurous real-life gardener and the fictional character making preparations in case of the future Catastrophe. Not just a wide range of poppies, but pretty much anything else you might need or desire, and probably a few things you didn't even know you wanted until you looked at the site. They have several forms of coffee (if you live at sea level, the Robusta may be the only one that works well, but better Robusta than no coffee at all), tea plants (and you wouldn't believe where they thrive), and a very wide range of tobacco seeds plus a guide to growing and processing them (they grow pretty well in places you wouldn't expect, too...and for the non-smoker anticipating the Catastrophe, I have four words: "trade goods" and "pest control").

If growing tobacco in real life for the purpose of smoking/chewing/sniffing, check your local laws regarding home production. Some states and countries legally restrict or forbid the home production of recreational tobacco. Most, if not all, of those states and countries do permit growing Nicotiana species for ornamental purposes. Note: if growing tobacco for any purpose, including the purely ornamental varieties, do not do so anywhere near your tomatoes or potatoes, which are vulnerable to tobacco mosaic virus.

Seedman's biggest fault: the search engine on their website approaches total uselessness. I am not sure whether this is an accidental failure or a subtle marketing technique, since while you're looking for whatever you were trying to find, you're likely to end up adding several more things you never planned to get to your basket. US; ship to Canada, the UK, Germany, Italy, Spain, Norway, and Sweden.

Do not confuse this site with "Seedsman", which is a cannabis seed site. Granted that, these days, cannabis legality is becoming less and less of an issue; and the fictional character will absolutely want and need this valuable medicinal/fibre/food plant to hand after the Catastrophe. However, even possession of the seeds is still illegal in some US states, while others have fully legalized C. sativa for all purposes. Some countries allow for certain amounts of growing for personal use; some do not allow growing at all. Some (Ireland and Great Britain, for instance, at the time of writing), like the US with P. somniferum, allow the "souvenir" selling and possession of cannabis seeds, but germination makes one an immediate criminal. Stay out of trouble: know and obey your local laws!

Fedco: only site that I've found which has both Elka and Ziar, the amazing heritage white- and blue-seeded breadseed poppies. Said by some Central/Eastern Europeans to be the best-flavoured poppy seeds in the world. US, ship only to US. If you live where you can legally grow these poppies, you have to get a friend in the US to receive and mail them on to you. Sometimes the real world is too ironic for fiction. Fortunately, there are many other places which carry one or the other of the two.

World Seed Supply: another site with a very good range of, not only poppies, but many other valuable and seldom-seen herbs and plants, including coffee and some tobacco varieties (though Seedman has a much better selection of the latter). US. Ship internationally, but do not do tracking and will not take responsibility for loss or seizures on international orders, though they warn the buyer in detail.

Nicky's Nursery: a wide range of poppies of all sorts as well as many other herbs and plants. Reliable and excellent germinators; I have stocked a lot of my personal herb garden and flower plots from here, and never been disappointed. UK. Ship pretty much anywhere.

One of the largest problems with current understanding of the benefits of cannabis is that, due to the legal and social circumstances involved, a very high percentage of reports are anecdotal: that is, based on individual personal experience. The problem with anecdotal reports is (1) no way to establish controls, figure in possible confounding issues, etc., and (2) a tendency for self-selection in reporting to present very skewed results. In addition to this, it is human nature to be more affected by, and emotionally if not intellectually, put more weight on an individual's story than on statistics regarding large numbers of faceless strangers.

For instance, one may consider the anecdotal reports of childhood autism "caused by" the MMR vaccine. If there were anything to this beyond psychological factors in regards to assigning "blame" (we'll never know, since the subject is now Officially Toxic in all reputable medical circles)...a rate of 1:100,000, for the 500 million-plus MMR vaccinations given over the last 30 years, would be 5000 cases, the parents of whom would be vastly likelier to speak out than all the parents of children who, as a result of being vaccinated, did not die or suffer severe lifelong damage from the three diseases covered (measles fatality rate according to the Irish HSE's National Immunization Board – 1-2:1000, plus ca. 4:1000 brain damage and other complications; mumps – 50:1000 viral encephalitis, 1:1000 meningitis, plus 1:20,000 deafness).

The results of this skew, if presented without numerical comparisons/confounding issue problems, might be something like a reduced uptake of vaccines, and a corresponding increase in (preventable!) childhood death and brain damage. With cannabis, the skew tends to be in the opposite direction. Those who have benefited are inclined to speak out (and actively support at least widespread medical legalization), but those who have experienced no effects or suffered negative effects are largely unlikely to. The legal and social issues have, until very recently in some places, also made it impossible even to estimate the number of users accurately. In short, while anecdotal reports may point in possible directions regarding the benefits and/or dangers of a treatment, they cannot be relied upon in judging either efficacy or safety.

Part II: Cannabis Sativa

Introduction

This article is written largely for the benefit of the author writing in a scenario following the downfall of modern society who wishes to present the use of herbal medication in such circumstances in a realistic manner. Unlike Part I, which deals with a herbal-origin drug that is incredibly illegal to produce oneself or even to possess/use without a prescription, as well as being dangerous in even the best-controlled legal circumstances (opium), and unlikely to change that status in the foreseeable future, the herb I discuss here is legal in many countries and even US states, and will probably have become legal in more even between the time of writing (November 2018) and the time of publication.

It also has a better safety profile than any over-the-counter medications. I shall therefore confine myself to saying: know the laws about cannabis where you are, as they exist at your current moment, and obey them until they change. As in the previous section, unless specifically stated otherwise, the "you" to whom I write is generally the character in the post-Catastrophe novel. However, if cannabis is legal in real life where you, the reader, are, the guidelines and advice I present may also be relevant to you in real life.

Some people these days use "hemp" for the minimal-THC/low CBD varieties grown for industrial fibre and seed, reserving "cannabis" for the medicinal plant, whether because the latter sounds more dignified or because it sounds more intimidating/alienating, I do not know. If the latter were to be the case, it would not be the first time that this plant's public name has been carefully selected to make it sound more like a dangerous drug than a common staple. Since both words describe the same plant, Cannabis sativa, and since the Catastrophe survivor is not likely to be in a position to make much of a distinction, I use them interchangeably, differentiating the very low-potency fibre/seed strains by the term "industrial hemp". In terms of toxicity, cannabis can hardly be counted as an "extreme herb" of the sort discussed in Parts I and III; quite the contrary. I am including it in this series for four reasons.

First, because it will be such a crucial survivor's staple, for medicine, fibre, and food, after the Catastrophe. I find it extraordinarily implausible that anyone of any intelligence who wants to survive and thrive in the altered world would not do their best to take advantage of it. Even those who reject this plant as a medicine due to personal or religious beliefs about the use of medical plants with psychoactive side-effects will desperately want to grow it for clothing, rope, bedding, and food (the non-psychoactive seeds), and perhaps the non-psychoactive medicinal constituent CBD.

Secondly, hemp may be classed as an "extreme herb" in that it is still illegal to varying degrees in large parts of the world, although this is changing so rapidly that – especially if you live in the US – it may have been illegal in some or all circumstances in your home area while I wrote the piece, but completely legalized by the time of publication. Thirdly, despite non-existent direct toxicity: now that it has become possible to actually study hemp's medical effects and uses, it is slowly emerging that there are some patients to whom it should be given only with caution.

There is increasing evidence regarding possible risks of negative interaction with certain pre-existing conditions, and absolute safety in certain vulnerable populations (children, pregnant women, people with pre-existing cardiovascular conditions) remains, although of course it may be indicated where the relative safety/efficacy, compared to the pharmaceutical options, is superior. Intractable seizure disorders in children are the most commonly accepted instance re efficacy, and it is not unlikely that comparative safety in that population will prove to also be superior to current pharmaceutical options.

Fourthly, there have been a number of extreme anecdotal and anecdotally-based claims made regarding the medical efficacy of cannabis in some life-threatening disease situations, particularly cancer. If these prove true in clinical studies, cannabis will absolutely be the most valuable medicinal herb possible after the Catastrophe (and maybe in real life). But, while evidence-based medicine may well, in the course of time, prove some of these life-saving uses to be truly effective, we do not have that evidence yet.

We only have a wide range of laboratory studies and anecdotal evidence suggesting a potential highly worthy of serious evaluation in a number of regards. Advice gained by random Internet searching does not suffice to make recommendations which might lead anyone with a potentially fatal condition to go for an unproven substance as a complete replacement for treatments the efficacy of which, though tragically imperfect and often traumatic to the patient, can at least be estimated to a relative degree. There is, of course, no reason whatsoever why cannabis should not be used as an adjunct to proven cancer treatments, and every reason what it should. It can certainly improve quality of life, and there is a strong possibility that it may have curative capabilities, with little risk and limited concern about side effects in the vast majority of patients. It just should not, at this time, be used instead of current treatment modalities. There are two things you may notice about this section of Extreme Herbalism (and Appendices III and IV) in contrast to the others.

Parts I and III deal with herbs that have either been extensively studied for a very long time, present a limited range of effects with (usually) known mechanisms of action, or both. When dealing with plants that have not undergone extensive scientific and clinical studies yet, I will cite a great many more sources, some of which appear to be mutually contradictory; and spend a lot of time saying, "maybe", "possibly", "potentially", and "more research needs to be done". At the moment, given the long enforced hiatus in medical research on cannabis, this is the song sung by the vast majority of real-life health-care practitioners regarding the vast majority of possible uses for medical hemp. Hope that the Catastrophe holds off until we have learned more!

Cannabinoids: A Quick Overview

THC – psychoactive, anti-nauseant, analgesic, appetite stimulant, nervous stimulant in pure form, contributes to sedative effects when combined with other constituents.

CBD – anti-epileptic, anti-convulsant, smooth muscle relaxant, anti-inflammatory, anti-bacterial, analgesic, appetite stimulation. Also counteracts psychoactive effects of THC. Now in third-stage trials as the medication Epidiolex.

CBN (cannabinol) – breakdown product of THC; potential uses include sedation, analgesia, appetite stimulation, anti-bacterial, anti-inflammatory, anti-convulsive, anti-fungal.

CBG (cannabigerol) – a precursor to THC and CBD.-2 adrenergic receptor agonist (stimulator): vasoconstriction, reduces bowel motility, suppresses adrenaline release, sedation, improves concentration; induces glucagon, inhibits insulin secretion. Similar drugs include clonidine. Also anti-protozoal, anti-bacterial, and an appetite stimulant.
CBDV (cannabidivarin) - demonstrated anti-epileptic and anti-convulsant effects; in clinical trials at this time.

CBC (cannibichromene) – antagonist (blocker) to TRPA-1 receptors, which contribute strongly to various forms of pain sensation. Potentially useful in treating and mitigating pain from irritation and destructive inflammation.

I. Recent History, Effective Components, Cautions, and Medicinal Uses

a) A Bit of the History

Cannabis was an important drug in the US pharmacoepia until the 1930s, when it was made illegal against the strong advice of the American Medical Association. Harry Anslinger's largely one-man campaign against cannabis was at least in part motivated by racism, and he used racism as his primary tool in getting the new laws passed, possibly including his most infamous alleged statement: "Reefer makes darkies think they're as good as white men" (reported as having been said during a Narcotics Bureau conference, along with other remarks of a similar nature.

Though in fairness - a concept apparently alien to Anslinger regardless of the facts regarding this particular quote - there were no recording devices going at the time and he did not put the comment in writing, so, often repeated as it is, it cannot be proven that he really said it). One of his main, and most effective, techniques in getting the change in laws past the US public was certainly adopting the Mexican slang term "marijuana" for the herb.

The average American had no idea that this terrifying new headline-bait drug abused by the fictional hordes of unpleasantly stereotyped Mexican immigrants was the same thing as the over-the-counter cannabis tincture that Mom doled out in spoonfuls to Grandpa for his rheumatism and to his teenaged granddaughters at That Time Of Month. Cannabis became illegal for general sale in the UK in 1928; illegal to grow in the UK in 1964; but continued to be available by prescription there until 1971. Prior to the 1930s in the US, and for decades longer in the UK, cannabis had been used as a low-to-mid level analgesic and in the treatment of migraines (for which Sir William Osler considered it the best remedy then available, an opinion shared by many migraine sufferers even today), as well as for many other purposes.

It was first introduced to the English-speaking world by Sir William Brooke O'Shaughnessy, an Irish physician who became familiar with the drug while working in India. His history will be of particular relevance following the Catastrophe, as he was able to successfully treat tetanus with high oral doses of the Indian strain (likely to have been high in CBD). While Dr. O'Shaughnessy was unable to save the life of a patient with rabies using this drug, he was able to at least provide palliative care with it, making it possible for the patient to swallow liquids and relieving pain and anxiety to some extent. Although hemp had been used to treat seizures in India for centuries, Dr. O'Shaughnessy was the first Western physician to realize its value and use it for this purpose.

What are terpenes and terpenoids?

Terpenes are aromatic hydrocarbons which plants produce as defences against pests and attractants for pollinators. Terpenoids are modified terpenes (usually with the addition of oxygen functional groups), produced from terpenes when a plant is dried.

Terpenes and terpenoids are major components of essential oils, and contribute to the variance in effect of different cannabis strains with similar cannabinoid profiles. A few of the major ones include:

Beta-caryophyllene – anti-inflammatory, antioxidant, analgesic
Camphene – may reduce elevated triglycerides and plasma cholesterol
Humulene – anti-bacterial, anti-inflammatory, possibly anti-tumour
Limonene – anti-depressant, anti-fungal, anti-bacterial
Linalool – also found in lavender and thyme. Sedative, anti-depressant, anti-inflammatory, immune booster.
Myrcene – potent analgesic, anti-inflammatory, sedative, antibiotic, anti-mutagenic. Inhibits the formation of gastric and duodenal ulcers.
Pinene – stimulant, anti-inflammatory, bronchodilator, expectorant, counteracts memory loss.
Pulegone – sedative, fever-reducing, stimulates brain function by breaking down acetylcholine.
Terpineol – relaxant, anti-oxidant, anti-malarial, acetylcholine inhibitor.

b) Cannabinoids, Terpenes, and Terpenoids

The two cannabinoids which have been most thoroughly studied at this time are THC (tetrahydrocannabinol) and CBD (cannabidiol). Cannabinoids are terpenophenolic compounds (contain both a terpene group and a phenol group) which are specifically, though not exclusively, found in C. sativa.

THC is the source of the psychoactive and anti-nauseant effects of cannabis, some of its analgesic qualities; and preliminary studies indicate its potential efficacy as an anti-cancer drug.

The FDA has approved synthetic THC (dronabinol and nabilone) for treating nausea and stimulating appetite. CBD was largely unrecognised until relatively recently, when its potency as a smooth-muscle relaxant and treatment for intractable epilepsy became known.

The FDA recently approved an oral CBD solution for use in certain forms of epilepsy. CBD is also showing efficacy as an anti-inflammatory. CBN (cannabinol), a breakdown product of THC when exposed to light and oxygen or left to degrade, is now also being examined for potential uses including sedation; anti-bacterial, anti-inflammatory, and anticonvulsive effects; analgesia; and appetite stimulation.

The study of CBN is still, even comparatively to the study of THC and CBD, in its infancy; but it is worth maintaining awareness of it, especially after the Catastrophe when you have grown more hemp for fibre than you can possibly use medicinally in a year. Note that even in some places where the whole herb and THC-containing extracts are still illegal, products containing CBD without THC are perfectly legal. In Ireland at the time of writing, for example, although cannabis is barely and very grudgingly beginning to be accepted for certain medicinal uses, one can purchase extracted CBD over the counter at many health-food stores and pharmacies.

In other places, the status of CBD-only products may be a gray area. CBD products are Federally legal in the US, but states vary: in Texas at the time of writing, industrial-hemp derived oil is legal, but CBD oil with even trace levels of THC (0.5%) is only legal with a Compassionate Use prescription, which is only available for intractable epilepsy. Again, know your local laws! Contradictory results in preliminary studies regarding the safety and efficacy of cannabis in various conditions may also be due at least in part to the wide range of active constituent levels between different strains. A high THC/low CBD strain might be suspected, due to the stimulant effects of THC, to carry a higher risk in regards to cardiovascular conditions and perhaps a lower efficacy in regards to controlling epilepsy; but THC has also specifically been identified as the primary effector in the anti-nauseant and appetite-stimulating effects which have already proved their value in modern medicine.

For both ethical and practical reasons (mostly because the studies done are retrospective population studies), it has not been possible for researchers to identify individual strains and concentrations of constituents in their subjects' histories. It is rare, if it ever occurs, for the medical user to have limited themself primarily to a single strain for the course of their treatment; expecting the recreational or spiritual user to have done so would be like expecting a wine-drinker to have limited themself to a single grape and vineyard for an ongoing period. The issue is further confounded by the high level of cultural emotional involvement both for and against this drug, which might raise suspicion of some studies' interpretations in either direction. Secondary descriptions of studies in the general media are even more problematical in this regard, on both sides.

Finally, it has not until very recently started to become common practice even for those few medicinal researchers in a position to provide their volunteers with selected and consistent cannabis to actually cite the strain utilized. As discussed at the end of this section, THC, CBD, and CBN are far from the only constituents of cannabis with known or potential physiological effects; terpenes and terpenoids, aromatic compounds in which cannabis is exceptionally rich, may affect the user in a variety of ways, directly and via synergy with the main medicinal components.

This range of content presents a considerable potential obstacle to any full whole-herb study which does not include at least a small selection of strains being evaluated separately (and, in a more general sense, is another reason why many physicians prefer isolated pharmaceutical products to whole herbs overall: plants are extremely chemically complex).

It has frequently been suggested that THC and CBD often modulate each other's effects by their opposing actions, but may in some regards also have a synergistic medicinal and/or psychoactive effect. The term "entourage effect" is often used as shorthand for "co-modulating or synergistic effects between phytocannabinoids, terpenes/terpenoids, and possible other plant constituents".

No studies have been performed examining this effect specifically. In an interview with Scientific American, Ethan Russo (pharmacological researcher, medical director of biochemical research company Phytecs, and psychopharmacologist) observes that 10 mg of THC causes temporary psychosis-like symptoms in ca. 40% of patients, whereas 48 mg of THC administered in a preparation with a 1:1 THC:CBD ratio (MS palliative drug Sativex (Russo was the study physician for three Phase III clinical trials of this drug) caused this result in only 4 out of 250.

Russo has been one of the most significant promoters of the "entourage effect" in regards to both cannabinoids and other constituents. But the same interview quotes neurobiologist and cannabis researcher Margaret Haney stating that such studies as have been done on THC isolate vs the whole plant show no significant difference between the two.

Cannabinoids: A Quick Overview

THC – psychoactive, anti-nauseant, analgesic, appetite stimulant, nervous stimulant in pure form, contributes to sedative effects when combined with other constituents.

CBD – anti-epileptic, anti-convulsant, smooth muscle relaxant, anti-inflammatory, anti-bacterial, analgesic, appetite stimulation. Also counteracts psychoactive effects of THC. Now in third-stage trials as the medication Epidiolex.

CBN (cannabinol) – breakdown product of THC; potential uses include sedation, analgesia, appetite stimulation, anti-bacterial, anti-inflammatory, anti-convulsive, anti-fungal.

CBG (cannabigerol) – a precursor to THC and CBD. ⋄-2 adrenergic receptor agonist (stimulator): vasoconstriction, reduces bowel motility, suppresses adrenaline release, sedation, improves concentration; induces glucagon, inhibits insulin secretion. Similar drugs include clonidine. Also anti-protozoal, anti-bacterial, and an appetite stimulant.

CBDV (cannabidivarin) - demonstrated anti-epileptic and anti-convulsant effects; in clinical trials at this time.

CBC (cannibichromene) – antagonist (blocker) to TRPA-1 receptors, which contribute strongly to various forms of pain sensation. Potentially useful in treating and mitigating pain from irritation and destructive inflammation.

However, a comparison test done on the high CBD/very low THC Israeli medical strain Avidekel (identified by name, but described as "Clone 202" throughout the majority of the study) and a pure CBD extract showed a greater anti-inflammatory effect from the whole plant than from the pure extract, suggesting that even a slight presence of one constituent may influence the overall effects of the dominant one. Other phytocannabinoids (cannabinoids from plants, as contrasted, say, to the endocannabinoids such as anandamide which the human body produces naturally, synthetic cannabinoids, or any that might be extracted from animal sources in the future) have also been identified, but little testing has been done on them. One study (see section 1, part 4, under "Anti-bacterial, anti-fungal, anti-parasitic") included nine various plant compounds derived from cannabinol (CBN), cannabichromene (CBC), and cannabigerol (CBG).

The potential medical functions of these and other phytocannabinoids – in isolation or in combination with terpenes, terpenoids, and other constituents of the whole plant – largely remain to be determined. CBDV (cannabidivarin) is undergoing clinical trials by GW Pharmaceuticals in regards to its anti-epileptic/anti-convulsant activities. The ability of CBG alone to stimulate appetite, valuable in situations such as cancer and late-stage HIV infection, has also been demonstrated, as has the absence of psychoactivity/neuromotor impairment from CBG. Something to keep in mind if you are choosing seeds as part of your pre-Catastrophe preparations, or using hemp medicinally in real life: different strains, even if their THC:CBD ratio is identical, may differ in a wide range of other constituents.

Terpenes and terpenoids (derived from terpenes) are not only responsible for an aromatic plant's odour, but may have physiological effects as well. Cannabis contains over 100 terpenes. In practice, this means that, although the primary medical components of two strains may be the same, they may have different effects on any given individual. Lacking sophisticated laboratory equipment, some terpenoids may still readily be identified by the use of the Human Chemical Analyzer Mark I, a.k.a. "senses of smell and taste". Menthol and camphor are both terpenoids; the terpene D-limonene contributes most strongly to the scent of oranges; linalool is a major factor in the aroma of lavender, basil, some thymes, and, indeed, cannabis; pinene is characteristic of pine (and other conifers') resin.

Vitamin A is a diterpene. Some terpenes and terpenoids are isolated for medicinal use, and it is strongly suspected that part of the difference between isolated THC and/or CBD, and whole herb usage, is due to the absence vs. presence of these compounds, and possible synergies between terpenes/oids and the major cannabinoids. Allergies and sensitivities to specific terpenes and terpenoids are known, so – although one must always use great caution when investigating allergies, especially after the Catastrophe when you can't just buy a new Epi-Pen – it is possible that the person who got a headache from cannabis of one strain (which does not constitute "being allergic") would receive only positive benefit from a different strain.

Probably the best approach for your own use, if legal where you live, is to try out small quantities of a number of different strains for effect, paying particular attention to see if there is any relationship between types of scent (grassy, citrus, flowery, pine, etc.) and how you respond to a given strain. The issue of toxicity in dosage is seldom if ever a concern with this plant, as its therapeutic index (the range between "minimal effective dose" and "LD50, = kills 50% of test subjects in the species to which it has been administered"") is so great that it has literally been impossible to measure.

Short of a massive allergic reaction, it is impossible to poison a patient by administering excessive amounts of cannabis. It is, however, quite possible to cause them significant psychological distress with excess dosages, particularly with lipid-medium oral administration. In such cases, it is recommended to put the patient in a quiet environment and reassure them as often as necessary that the effects of the medication will not harm them and will pass off in a few hours. High levels of CBD can cause very significant, though not life-threatening, sedation and even impair voluntary muscle control; high levels of THC have been known to cause severe anxiety, temporary paranoia, and signs of sympathetic hyperactivity (elevated heart rate, sweating, etc.). CBD mitigates the latter effects of THC, making it preferable to use a strain with a reasonably balanced THC:CBD ratio in any circumstances where higher dosing may be required (see section below, "The Plant").

3. Potential Side Effects and Cautions

a) Cardiovascular Side Effects

Despite its virtual non-toxicity in acute doses, cannabis should not be thought of as the perfectly-safe-in-all-circumstances cure-all touted by many advocates. While direct toxicity is not a concern with cannabis in humans (or cats, positively notorious for their love of this herb), there are some cautions which should be kept in mind when administering this medication. Inhaled cannabis usually causes a spike in blood pressure and a rise in heart rate and stroke volume; the latter are also seen with oral ingestion. Some evidence is now emerging that this additional stress on the cardiovascular system may be a factor of concern in patients who have cardiovascular problems, particularly ischaemic stroke risk or a previous stroke history.

It has also been suggested that regular usage may increase overall stroke risk, especially in younger patients - although there is also emerging evidence that cannabis may help in neurological recovery after the stroke has already occurred, as well as following traumatic brain injury and in neurodegenerative conditions. The blood pressure spike and other common temporary effects such as tachycardia (fast heartbeat) are also of concern regarding patients who suffer from uncontrolled hypertension and have a known or suspected propensity towards cardiac arrhythmias.

Until more is known, cardiovascular issues should be considered as relative contraindications to the use of whole higher THC-strain cannabis or THC/synthetic THC alone, particularly by means of inhalation ("relative contraindication" = be aware of risks and do not administer unless potential benefits significantly outweigh potential dangers; "absolute contraindication" = do not administer under any circumstances). This side effect is a worrying one, but comparable in kind to the substantial risks of caffeine usage in people with cardiovascular problems (whether it is comparable in degree remains to be evaluated).

CBD alone has been shown to either have no effect on blood pressure or heart rate, or to actually reduce resting blood pressure and stroke volume (while increasing heart rate slightly to compensate for decreased stroke volume). Therefore, if whole cannabis is otherwise indicated for a patient with potential cardiovascular vulnerabilities, an evenly balanced or high-CBD/low-THC strain is likely, from what we currently know, to be the safest choice.

b) Cannabis in Pregnancy

The full effects of cannabis in pregnancy are unknown and difficult to test even in a retrospective study, as confounding factors such as the use of tobacco and caffeine are common in mothers who utilized cannabis during their pregnancies. However, the recent discovery that the endocannabinoid anandamide is a significant regulator of embryo implantation raises a possible cause for concern. While lower levels of anandamide stimulate implantation, higher levels inhibit it.

Both mouse models and venous blood tests on women suffering ectopic pregnancies have revealed a consistently high level of endocannabinoids, suggesting that elevated cannabinoid receptor signalling may interfere with embryo transport; there is also evidence to suggest that the same mechanisms by which cannabinoids inhibit the migration and proliferation of some cancer cells may be significantly harmful to a developing embryo. Chronic THC use further appears to impair uptake of folic acid (vitamin B9), which would increase the risk of folate-deficiency birth defects; if this medication is required for the expectant mother, she should considerably increase her folic acid intake. After the Catastrophe, when the vitamin pills have run out, this means a lot of leafy green vegetables, beans, whole-grain breads/cereals, and citrus if available.

While the significance of these potential dangers has not been proven yet, as with all drugs that have not been clearly proven to be safe for use in pregnancy, cannabis should probably be avoided during pregnancy and conception attempts if possible until and unless it is proven pregnancy-safe. We also lack substantial information about the effects of cannabis in the later portions of pregnancy. As with other relative contraindications, the issue of whether a pregnant woman should take cannabis for any purpose is also a matter of judging what approach is likely to cause the least harm to the patient (and her developing baby).

It is generally accepted that even the use of the more dangerous drugs commonly used for epilepsy treatment, although they are known to carry a risk of harm to the fetus, are less potentially harmful than allowing the mother's epilepsy to go uncontrolled during the course of her pregnancy. Since drugs such as valproate, phenytoin, and phenobarbitol are unlikely to be available for very long after the Catastrophe, cannabis and valerian will be among the only options available for preventing and controlling epileptic seizures, and the real-life use of harsher drugs as a preferable option in pregnancy should serve as at least a temporary guide to risk evaluation regarding cannabis for pregnant women after the Catastrophe (in real life, we have options which probably aren't safer, but at least are better understood).

THC has also been detected in breast milk for periods ranging from six days to six weeks after use. Although the data on potential consequences is still very limited, animal studies and one small human study suggest that there may be some dose-dependent retardation of motor development in the infant ingesting THC through breast milk, although no adverse consequences in regards to mental development were reported in the small studies dealing with a human population. More evaluation regarding the actual risk level still needs to be done in order to accurately weigh the benefits and hazards of THC in breastfeeding (vs. formula bottlefeeding) and what the optimum choice or choices are for the care of any given infant – but as with the use of any insufficiently tested drug in pregnant or breast-feeding patients, it is generally considered wiser practice overall not to introduce cannabis to a developing foetus or infant if avoidable.

c) Immune System Effects and Viruses

The anti-inflammatory effects of cannabinoids are the proverbial double-edged sword. While suppressing the inflammatory response can be highly beneficial in various circumstances, that also means suppressing a good part of the immune system functions. The suppression of virus-related or –stimulated chronic inflammatory conditions, which possibly includes a number of auto-immune diseases, is a good thing: at that point, the inflammation has become a pathology in itself, not a part of the viral clearance process.

The suppression of acute virus-related inflammation is a very bad thing, since it impairs the body's ability to destroy and clear the virus. Cannabis inhibition of calcium activity in neurons permits a greater level of viral replication and disease progression: the death of the rabies patient that Dr. W.B. O'Shaughnessy treated palliatively with cannabis was quite likely hastened by the drug (although its palliative effects, in a disease that was 100% horribly fatal at the time and very close to it now if adequate vaccination does not occur in time or the Milwaukee Protocol fails, probably still made it a worthwhile choice in terms of quality-of-life vs quantity-of-life).

Cannabis- or cannabinoid-increased, sometimes greatly increased, viral load, shedding, and replication have been demonstrated variously in herpes simplex virus (HSV) 2, Kaposi's sarcoma herpes virus (KSHV), and HIV-1; worse disease progression and outcomes have been shown in HSV-2, KHSV, influenza, and hepatitis C. It has been also been suggested that the suppression of immune responses in the brain by endogenous (native to the body) activation of the CB2 cannabinoid receptor may allow easier blood-brain transmission of HIV and contribute to HIV encephalitis. But curiously, cannabis also inhibited HSV-1 and inhibited reactivation from latency in Epstein-Barr virus (mononucleosis) and KSHV, possibly due to suppressing inflammatory stimulation.

Overall, cannabis is relatively contraindicated in acute viral infections. In HIV at this time, it is relatively contraindicated until a palliative-care stage (where the comfort and nourishment of the patient take precedence) is reached. Since modern anti-retrovirals have gone some way towards reducing HIV to a chronic disease rather than a death sentence, the large majority of HIV patients in real life should probably avoid cannabis until and unless evidence to the contrary is gained. After the Catastrophe, when pharmaceutical medications run out...you may soon, sadly, be back to the tragic decade between the mid-'80s and '90s.

People who are currently taking any drug with immunosuppressant effects, including corticosteroids (prednisone, prednisolone, hydrocortisone, and beclomethasone are the most common) should only use cannabis – for any purpose – after discussing it with their GP. Cannabis is contraindicated to varying degrees in people with immunodeficiencies. However, if you need immunosuppressants after the Catastrophe when pharmaceuticals have run out, cannabis may be your best option for that purpose. This does not apply to people taking corticosteroids to treat adrenal insufficiency – cannabis does not replace cortisol/cortisone in body functions – but the need to consult your GP as long as you are using those drugs certainly does (when you have run out of your replacement corticosteroids, then you may have a very serious problem).

D) Adolescent and Adult Psychiatric Conditions and Cognition

Concerns have been repeatedly raised about the potential hazards of cannabis in children and adolescents. Neurological development in humans continues until roughly the age of twenty-five, so there is at least a possibility that frequent use in younger patients, unless it is necessary to deal with a life-threatening condition such as intractable epilepsy, or a situation of chronic pain, could present a hazard. Specific genetic polymorphisms which appear to be associated with the development or exacerbation of schizophrenia in young people, particularly those who frequently use cannabis, have been identified. It is more difficult to be certain of causality in regards to the cannabis-schizophrenia association.

A Norwegian study from 2012 showed that brain function was improved in older patients with schizophrenia who were also frequent cannabis users (the authors of the study attempted to interpret this as "the cannabis-users weren't really schizophrenic originally, this was an effect caused by cannabis use", but there were no indications favouring that interpretation above "improves function in adult schizophrenics" in the actual data produced. Norway did not legalize medicinal cannabis until 2016, and the debate on allowing it was raging in 2012; it would be interesting to see if the same data received the same interpretation there now).

One investigation in 2009 determined that the number of cannabis users who would have to cease use altogether in order to prevent one case of cannabis-associated schizophrenia, in the most vulnerable group evaluated (male heavy users in the 20-24 year age range), is approximately 2,800...whereas in the least vulnerable group (female heavy users in the 35-39 year age range), 10,870 would have to cease use in order to prevent one case. For heavy cannabis use and psychosis, the most vulnerable groups' numbers needed to prevent a single case is 1,360 in male heavy users aged 20-24, and 2,480 in female heavy users aged 16-19. The figures are four to five times higher in regards to light users.

In contrast, the number of people who would need to be screened to prevent one case of lung cancer is 320 individuals, which is considered an ineffective ratio. High doses of cannabis or isolated/synthetic THC can produce temporary symptoms similar to some of the symptoms of schizophrenia, but the same can be said of many pharmaceutical drugs. For instance, carbamazepine, most common brand name "Tegretol" – used as an anticonvulsant and for treating trigeminal neuralgia, one well-defined and one strong potential indication for the use of cannabis as well – can in some people cause auditory and visual hallucinations; derealization; depersonalization; behaviour changes and loss of control; and anhedonia...in short, an excellent match for many schizophrenic symptoms.

Carbamazepine is also occasionally used for treatment of or as a treatment adjunct for patients suffering from schizoaffective disorders (schizophrenic symptoms plus a mood disorder), schizophrenia, and mood disorders. It therefore remains uncertain to what degree there is a real association between cannabis use and young people developing schizophrenia; and if there is a real association, whether it is the result of cannabis acting as a triggering or contributory factor to the psychiatric disorder, or an attempt to self-medicate in the early stages. The use of tobacco by the same patients is also considered to be a significant confounding factor. No similar studies have been done, to my knowledge, on the use and abuse of alcohol or other recreational drugs in this regard, which might assist in clarifying the question.

Having said that, I would consider that the unproven nature of the safety profile of cannabis for the under-twenty-to-twenty-five population in this regard is cause enough to consider age a reason for caution regarding the ongoing use of cannabis in a younger patient, especially where there is a family history of schizophrenia and/or related disorders, except when not using it actually presents a greater hazard to such a patient's life and well-being. Again, I point to the current epilepsy drugs of choice, the potential dangers of which can be significant and side effects quite unpleasant, but which are far preferable to not controlling the seizures. It is also improbable that the occasional short-duration and lower-dosage use of hemp in even a genetically vulnerable young patient is likely to present a significant risk. There is also the issue of THC-related effects vs CBD-related effects. The psychotomimetic qualities associated with the use of some hemp strains in some people, and hence the potential risk of speeding the progression of schizophrenia in genetically vulnerable teenagers, seem to be primarily or exclusively associated with THC.

CBD administration has been shown to block the psychotomimetic effects of THC, and initial studies are indicating that CBD alone may have significant potential as an anti-psychotic medication in general. In general, significant mental disorders of any sort should be considered a relative contraindication to the use of cannabis until more study has been done on the matter, and particularly on the varying effects of the different cannabinoids. If cannabis is required for a potentially vulnerable patient, a high CBD/low THC strain is likely to be the safer choice. There are mixed conclusions on the relationship between cannabis and mood disorders, particularly depression and bipolar disorders.

Some indications suggest that cannabis has antidepressant effects; others suggest that it may exacerbate depression. Results in studies on bipolar disorder and cannabis are similar; some studies report exacerbation and worse outcomes, while others have observed a mood-stabilizing effect. The matter is, once again, made more difficult by the question of, "Is the cannabis contributing to the patient's mood disorder, or is the patient self-medicating a mood disorder via the use of cannabis...or possibly both?" A multiplicity of potential confounding factors make this a very problematical question to answer.

Again, however, I may compare the use of carbamazepine in treating mood disorders with its occasional mood disorder-generating side effects. It is quite possible that a drug which is beneficial to some patients in such regards may have the contrary effect in some others, especially when the drug, like whole hemp, is essentially a cocktail of several constituents, some of which may have opposing effects. There is, at any rate, some good reason to consider cannabis as a potential avenue of enquiry for anti-depressant effects. In recognition of the relationship between cannabinoid-receptor activation and appetite stimulation, a selective CB1 blocker, rimonabant, was developed as an anti-obesity drug. It proved to be an effective appetite suppressant – but was never approved by the FDA due to serious safety concerns about depression and other psychological disorders associated with the drug, and had to be withdrawn two years after its approval in Europe. Approximately 10% of people taking it developed depressive or other mood disorders; 1% developed suicidal ideation.

This does not prove that agonists (THC) stimulating CB1 activity beyond the physiological norm are effective anti-depressants, but does open possibilities of research regarding a possible role of endocannabinoid levels and cannabinoid supplementation in the causes, diagnosis, and treatment of depression. The issue of lasting effects of cannabis on executive cognitive function remain questionable due to contradictory study results. No one particularly questions the presence of varying degrees of acute (while the patient is still directly under the influence) impairment from cannabis. Studies focusing on recreational users indicate the possibility of both short-term and ongoing deficits. However, in one instance, medical marijuana patients, after three months of treatments, improved task function and showed brain activation more comparable to that of healthy controls than to their pre-treatment state.

The authors of the latter study suggest that the difference may be age-related, as recreational users are often below the threshold of adult brain development, whereas the majority of medical cannabis patients at this time are mature adults. Baseline health may also play a role: in the medical patient, cannabis could counteract illness/pain-based impairment of function to restore the patient to normal.

E) Enzyme Inhibition/induction and Drug Interactions

THC and CBD both have a limited ability to inhibit the CYP450 enzymes, though less powerfully than grapefruit juice and other citrus fruit (specifically inhibit CYP450 3A4). They may, thus, slightly raise the concentration of drugs which are metabolized by enzymes in this family. It is particularly important for patients on warfarin to be monitored carefully if also being treated with cannabis or cannabinoids; in one case study (patient receiving CBD oil for intractable post-stroke epilepsy), the CBD use reduced the optimal dose of warfarin by ca. 30%. Smoked, but not oral, cannabis induces CYP182, speeding the metabolism of drugs such as theophylline. Monitoring is advised when using cannabis together with drugs metabolized by these enzymes (warfarin, simvastatin, prednisone, buspirone, and others).

F) Gynaecomastia, Sperm Count, and Fertility

It is startling how many legitimate medical sources list cannabis use without qualifications as a cause of gynaecomastia (breast development in men). So far: there was one study in 1972 which indicated a relationship, and another in 1977 which indicated no relationship. Some degree of gynaecomastia normally occurs in ca. 35 percent of men, with higher prevalence ranges in adolescents (may be up to 60%) and men in the 50-69 age group. The main reasoning for the medical claim that cannabis causes gynecomastia is that a study done in 1974 suggests that heavy chronic use may lower plasma testosterone – although later studies indicated no relationship, and one study, done in Denmark and published in 2015 (Gundersen et al), indicated that cannabis use could slightly raise testosterone levels.

The most recent investigation (large population-based sample representative of the US, Thistle et al, pub. 2017), concluded, "Our results were similar to those of Gundersen et. al., however, recency of marijuana use was better correlated with testosterone level than was frequency of use". In short, while your doctor (or medical school tutor) was probably not deliberately lying to you about the presence of a largely unexamined possibility that cannabis might cause gynaecomastia, they were certainly either the victims of unexamined misinformation in their own medical education (excusable in the pre-Internet era, especially before "evidence-based" became the standard for medicine; not so excusable now), or acting irresponsibly in stating a highly unproven possibility as a certainty and making confident recommendations based on it.

While much lesser in degree (few have died of gynecomastia by itself), this is the equivalent in kind of, for instance, telling a patient straight-out (at this time, with what we have been able to prove) that cannabis or any of its isolated constituents will cure cancer. "It appears plausible" is not a substitute for "evidence-based", and there have been many medical tragedies when "plausible in theory" was enacted to the significant harm of the patient population. Which is also why one should remain cautious about the more exciting possibilities of cannabis or any of its constituents as a curative until the more extensive research that the preliminary studies indicate appropriate has been done.

From the evidence that we now have regarding direct cannabis/gynaecomastia and the theorized mechanism of cannabis influence on androgen production, we can say with reasonable certainty that the trope "cannabis causes moobs" is folklore plus straw-grasping speculation, not good science or ethical medicine. A young man has a better chance of developing gynaecomastia from drinking a daily beer (assuming it was flavoured with hops, which do contain a high level of phytoestrogens) than from using cannabis...and an adolescent male has a far better chance of showing a little temporary gyno (60%, remember! – normally mild and self-resolving) as a result of his powerful flood of endogenous androgens naturally converting, as they do, to oestrogens.

This is why androgenic steroid abusers also have concerns about developing this condition; a close look at the chests of many professional bodybuilders reveals the swelling of that telltale "button" or "bulb" beneath the nipple (known to some by the charming term "bitch tits"). One could, of course, argue that if cannabis raises testosterone levels temporarily, it could theoretically be associated with gyno in that manner – but the degree of increase noted by Gundersen et al and Thistle et al was described as statistically significant (consistently enough to indicate that a finding is probably real), but slight; and, according to Thistle's study, temporary.

Just as a minute possibility exists that cannabis-related increases in testosterone could cause gyno in the same way that male adolescent hormonal production and androgenic steroid use or abuse are sometimes known to, this could be a possible mechanism of lowered sperm count among male cannabis users, assuming that further studies confirm current evidence in that regard. A direct effect of cannabis constituents on sperm production seems more likely, but neither possibility can be ruled out until more research has been done. There are reasonably solid indications for regular cannabis use lowering male sperm count. For instance, Gundersen's large 2015 study which found raised testosterone also found a 28-29% decline in sperm count among male regular users.

This is consistent with earlier studies' findings. Several recent studies also indicate a substantial possibility that sperm motility and shape are affected negatively by regular cannabis use. Does this affect male fertility? A normal male sperm count ranges from 15 million to 200 million sperm cells in a given sample. If the user's original count were at the low end, his fertility could be significantly affected. If in the lower-middle to high ranges of normal – probably not.

Certainly if a man already had a low sperm count, low motility, and/or an unduly high percentage of deformed sperm (an healthy percentage of normal-shaped sperm is 4-14%. Below 4% normal morphology, conception may become more difficult), adding a further factor could make his issue or issues more severe. The rare man with Klinefelter syndrome (XXY) who retains any fertility, for instance, would be well-advised to avoid anything that would have a negative impact on his sperm quantity, motility, or quality.

However, a large study done in North America indicated that neither male nor female use of cannabis had any perceptible impact on fertility rates overall - an interesting result considering that it has been suggested that hemp might have the potential to disrupt implantation and embryonic development, discussed above (3b). Whole cannabis is never going to make it as a male birth-control pill (or a morning-after pill, for that matter), and looking for a sperm-suppressive constituent would probably be considered a very long shot by the pharmaceutical industry (as in: they haven't even tried checking it out yet to my knowledge, and they'll try almost anything). No significant investigations of the effect of hemp usage, whole or isolated-constituent, on pubescence and/or puberty outcomes have yet been done. This has been identified as a major research gap.

g) Allergies

As with all herbs, the potential for severe and, indeed, possibly fatal allergic reactions cannot be ignored regarding cannabis. It is true that the phrase, "I'm allergic to cannabis" is often used in real life to mean anything from, "I don't want to try any/don't want the smell of your smoke in my clothes, but I don't want to sound like a wet blanket or criticize you in your own home", to "it gives me mild headaches" or "I tried it once and didn't much like it". However, some people really are allergic to cannabis. Some people are allergic or sensitive to specific terpenes and terpenoids, the character and percentage of which differ by strain and may be altered significantly by growing conditions. A few people are extremely allergic to all forms of C. sativa (including the "indica" and "ruderalis" variants).

Ephinephrine dosing in anaphylaxis

Ephinephrine (adrenaline) normally comes in ampoules diluted at 1:1000, which is 1 mg/ml. It is injected intramuscularly; the deltoid and the large thigh muscle are favoured sites.

Children <5 = 0.15 ml (150 mcg)
6-12 = 0.3 ml (300 mcg)
12-18 = 0.5 ml (500 mcg)
18+ = 0.5-0.6 ml (500-600 mcg)

This can be repeated every 5-10 minutes up to three doses if necessary. Maximum effect is seen in 10 minutes; if necessary, perform CPR while medication is taking effect and be sure to keep assessing the airway.

An adult Epipen contains 0.3 mg of adrenaline. An Epipen Jr contains 0.15 mg. In real life, only two doses should be given without medical supervision; and even if the patient appears to recover, they should go to the hospital for evaluation after using an Epipen, as more medication and supportive care may be required.

After the Catastrophe, you may just have to give multiple Epipen doses to reach the higher dosing levels if required.

As with any drug or other substance, unless there is a strong reason otherwise (e.g., differentiating between a genuine allergy to a specific antibiotic and a sensitivity to/dislike for the less pleasant side effects in circumstances when that antibiotic truly would be the best choice if not risking an allergic reaction), such statements should be taken at face value.

A simple statement that one would prefer not to use any particular medicament (or recreational drug, for that matter), for any reason or no reason, so long as the benefits and risks of using vs. not using are understood, is always perfectly acceptable. One cannot ethically administer any form of treatment to a competent adult who understands the risks involved if they choose not to accept it.

The same is true for recreational usage, only more so because recreational usage, by definition, is not potentially life-saving, so there should be no possible consequences of any sort for refusing a recreational substance. Having said that, know something important about allergy in regards to any drug! Allergy is a type I hypersensitivity reaction with very clearly defined symptoms resulting from specific cellular reactions.

It is characterized by itching, skin reddening and/or welts ("hives"), copious discharge from nose and eyes, soft tissue swelling which may compromise the upper air passages, and constriction within the airways of the lung, the latter two of which may very well prove fatal if not treated promptly with an IM dose of ephinephrine (adrenaline). The symptoms of allergy do not include headaches or diarrhoea, and seldom include nausea. It is not uncommon for patients to claim a penicillin allergy when what they really wanted to say, if armed with the appropriate knowledge, would have been, "It gives me headaches and/or stomach and bowel distress" (a common reaction to many antibiotics).

This misidentification is potentially hazardous if the best antibiotic for the specific infection is in the penicillin family. After the Catastrophe, it may also be crucial to be able to distinguish between genuine food allergies (potentially fatal!), food intolerances (should be avoided, but unlikely to be fatal, and preferable to starvation), and food extreme-dislikes (if the taste of something really makes you or one of your survival group gag, study different methods of processing and preparation to minimize that effect...or prepare to eat fried slugs. Unless you're allergic to shellfish, in which case, totally don't eat fried slugs or other molluscs – anaphylaxis will kill you faster than starvation). When growing your own field of hemp after the Catastrophe, you should also monitor allergy reactions in your general community during the blooming period.

As with ragweed or any other form of windblown pollen, cannabis pollen can and does cause the full range of allergic reactions, from sniffles to anaphylaxis... and cannabis produces a lot of pollen, in great clouds that can travel a long way. If hemp pollen allergy becomes a significant problem in your survivor group or community, you may have to confine yourselves to wool and flax (or cotton if it grows where you are), and figure out something else you can produce to trade for medicinal cannabis for those who aren't allergic, or keep the medicinal plants in a greenhouse and grow flax for fibre and seed.

It should also be noted that allergic cross-reactivity has been observed between cannabis and a number of other plants, including various weed pollens, and some fruits such as peaches and tomatoes. All parts of the plant, including seeds, and irrespective of cannabinoid levels, have the potential to evoke serious allergic reactions in people who are sensitive to it; cases have been noted of reaction to the dust of industrial hemp, which has also been implicated in the development of byssinosis ("brown lung disease"; caused by inhaling the dust of cotton, flax, or hemp fibres).

h) Asthma and Other Lung Conditions

The potential effects of hemp on asthma are mixed. On the positive side, its anti-inflammatory and smooth muscle-relaxant capabilities offer possible benefits in regards to easing the inflammation and spasming of an asthma attack. On the negative side, any form of inhalation, especially smoking, is irritating to the lungs and can trigger or exacerbate an asthma attack; even a mild allergy to any of the cannabis constituents can severely potentiate this risk.

The concerns about lung irritation and damage also apply for other pulmonary conditions for which hemp might be used, including COPD (chronic obstructive pulmonary disease, which often results from the ongoing irritation and inflammation caused by tobacco smoking) and lung cancer (many forms of which are also strongly associated with tobacco-caused irritation, inflammation, and genotoxicity).

In short: where a pulmonary condition, especially one stemming from smoke-related damage to the lungs, exists, the inhalation route is contraindicated unless there is no other means of administration possible and not using hemp would endanger the patient's life or significantly decrease their quality of life. Obviously this covers smoking, with or without a tobacco admixture; but vapourizing and dabbing (the inhalation of extremely high-powered concentrates such as hash oil and rosin) are also potential lung irritants and should be avoided if at all possible.

The pulmonary patient who requires cannabis may be treated with oral lipid extracts (most commonly in the form of cannabis-infused butter used for preparing baked goods), tincture taken orally or as a spray in the mouth, a topical infused oil, a suppository or pessary, or an essential oil/concentrate mixture. Unless you are in an emergency situation after the Catastrophe and have not had time to prepare or a chance to access any of the alternate routes of delivery, there should be no need for the pulmonary patient to inhale this medication.

H) Addiction and Use-vs.-Abuse

Cannabis is not physically addictive in the sense that serious physical withdrawal symptoms are rare in humans if present at all (although the simultaneous use/cessation of other substances is not infrequently a confounding factor); various aspects of tolerance may develop to different degrees. The regular user, for whatever purpose, is also likely to develop a more practiced set of mental, psychological, and physical compensations for effects that may be startling to the naïve user.

It has been observed that the level of tolerance to different effects of hemp is variable even for a single user, dependent on the variable expression of CB receptors in different parts of the brain; that tolerance is heaviest in regards to the less-desirable side effects; and that this may be a significant benefit allowing up-titration of the medication while minimizing unwanted side effects. Hemp is psychologically habituating: sudden cessation after a period of regular heavy use may cause disappointment, usually non-clinically-significant depression, disordered sleeping patterns, and crankiness, if not to the same degree as withdrawal from the genuine addiction of nicotine...or the demi-addiction of many anti-depressants (patients taking drugs such as escitalopram are strictly warned not to discontinue abruptly due to untowards physical, as well as psychological effects; tolerance requiring increased dosage does not occur, but tolerance to the initial effects has usually developed by the time the therapeutic effect is established, usually four to six weeks after initiation).

The term "cannabis addiction" is often inaccurately used even by health-care professionals (and often by health-care professionals working in addiction-treatment clinics, who, it must be said, have a certain interest in classifying cannabis as "addictive") to mean "regular heavy usage with significant psychological habituation".

Tetanus (Clostridium tetani) is a bacterium commonly found in dirt, saliva, and manure. It can enter through any breach in the skin, but is most commonly associated with penetrating wounds: "stepped on a rusty nail" is the classic case history.

This bacterium produces toxins which cause the characteristic intense spasms of skeletal muscle which often tear muscles and fracture bones, and the distinctive facial grimace (from whence the name "lockjaw").

In real life, tetanus is prevented by vaccination and regular booster shots, and treated with tetanus immunoglobulin, magnesium sulfate, and oral, IV, or continuous IV diazepam (a benzodiazepine).

The whole object of treatment is to control the extreme muscular spasming; a trachaeotomy and mechanical ventilation may be required.

The less prejudicial term "cannabis use disorder" is defined in DSM-V by roughly the same criteria normally applying to the misuse of a psychoactive substance, including aspects such as persistent use of more than is desired; social and lifestyle consequences related to cannabis use or preoccupation with obtaining and using it; physical harm as a result of cannabis use; inability to cease using cannabis; development of tolerance; the presence of withdrawal symptoms (however subtle) when the drug is discontinued. "Use vs abuse" is a difficult distinction to make.

The lines between recreational use/abuse, entheogenic use/abuse, and medical use/abuse are fine and exceedingly wobbly. Regarding hemp: for over fifty years in the US, the recreational user whose dosage and frequency were comparable to the "light social drinker", the person using cannabis solely for entheogenic purposes, and the medical user were all classed as "cannabis abusers" by the bulk of the general population and the majority of health-care practitioners alike.

Currently, some responses to the "opioid epidemic" involve reclassifying some patients using opioids under the careful direction of a physician and/or licensed pain clinic as "opioid abusers". One seldom hears the term, "caffeine abuser", but it applies to nearly every university student who is not a practicing Mormon trying to achieve an all-nighter (and people have died from caffeine overdoses). The redefinition of "smoker" (of tobacco) as a moral perjorative seems to have precluded the term "tobacco abuser".

It is generally accurate to say that a substance is being abused if it is being used for pleasure to a degree which significantly endangers mental, physical, and/or social health, or if it is being used in an inappropriate context (e.g., the use of anabolic steroids to win a competition unfairly might be construed as abuse).

Any substance which activates the brain's reward system has the potential for abuse, including food. Toby Moore's novel Death by Chocolate presents a humourous dystopia in which certain foods and going over your recommended BMI are illegal – a response to local legislation taxing such items as sugary sodas in response to the "obesity crisis". So cannabis certainly can be abused; but there is no reason to think that the risk is particularly high, and (excluding the cases where side effects or primary uses contraindicate hemp usage) the level required to abuse the drug is higher than that of many other common reward-stimulating substances which are less frequently recognised as drugs of abuse, such as caffeine.

4) Medicinal uses

a) Tetanus

Perhaps the most spectacular demonstrated medical use of cannabis to date has been Dr. W.B. O'Shaughnessy's success in curing a tetanus patient with this drug in the pre-vaccination, pre-immunoglobulin era. Knowing about this will certainly be a lifesaver after the Catastrophe, when everyone's tetanus boosters have run out and no immunoglobulins are available. After the Catastrophe, your chief options for treating tetanus will be maximal doses of cannabis of a high-CBD strain, plus valerian, the mechanism of action of which is similar to that of a benzodiazepine. You will need to maintain nourishment and hydration through a nasogastric tube (best feeding option available after the Catastrophe, and also allows the administration of oral medication directly into the stomach.

A tetanus patient is expending vast amounts of energy in the spasming, and hence requires 3500-4000 calories a day, including at least 150 gr. protein!). Opiates may be given for pain, and may be required at dosages up to WHO pain pyramid level 3 (morphine). If so, and if also using valerian, monitor the patient with extra caution, as the intrinsic opiate risk of respiratory depression can be potentiated by adding what is, for all effects and purposes, a benzodiazepine.

Cannabis does not affect the vital signs even in conjunction with WHO level 4 drugs (IV fentanyl), and has been determined safe to use with opioids. This total-care regimen may need to be maintained for as long as three to four weeks; total recovery time may take several months. Human-to-human transmission is rare, most usually via faecal spores, or if the patient bites someone and the bitee is extremely unlucky (very, very rarely, tetanus spores can be found in the mouths of humans and other animals), but the sporulated bacteria are common worldwide.

The stump of the umbilical cord is particularly vulnerable to tetanus invasion, and the greatest care with hygiene should be taken at all times until it has dried up and fallen off naturally. If you are a Masai following (or returning to) ancient traditional ways, do not use cow manure to stop the bleeding of the umbilical stump. No matter how much spiritual might and future prosperity this could bring the child, the risk of killing them with tetanus before they ever get a chance at those benefits makes the practice definitely not a good idea.

B) Cholera

As well as O'Shaughnessy's previously mentioned use of cannabis as a palliative measure to comfort the patient dying of rabies, he also experimented with it in the treatment of cholera. While cannabis does assist in diarrhoea control to some degree (especially regarding bowel cramping and spasming), in the case of a severe secretory diarrhoea such as cholera, it proved of more value as an analgesic and calmative than as a cure.

It is worth remembering, however, that in the event of a cholera epidemic after the Catastrophe – assuming that you still have the means of opiate production – cannabis can safely be used at all levels with opiates, which are effective in treating cholera, although the most crucial lifesaving treatment is and shall likely remain the maintenance of hydration and electrolyte homeostasis (detailed discussion in Part I). You are strongly advised to keep an especially close watch on the fluid output/replacement of a cholera patient who is receiving analgesic cannabis, as discussed below re the use of cannabis to lower stomach acid, which can increase diarrhoea volume in cholera.

C) Multiple Sclerosis

Cannabis is proving valuable in relieving some of the symptoms of multiple sclerosis. This was the first indication for which a cannabis product (Sativex, an oral-spray tincture with a 1:1 THC:CBD ratio) was legally approved in Ireland. Despite that approval, it is not used here as the process of medication review determined that the specific drug was excessively expensive for the amount of relief afforded. In fact, the pharmaceutical version was grotesquely over-priced compared to the cost of production, though a number of patients who had previously found relief from severe MS spasticity by the use of illicit cannabis strongly questioned the decision that the price was not worth the benefits.

The price/benefit decision was not made by MS patients. A mouse study from 2011 demonstrated that, at least in mice, CBD specifically reduces the clinical signs of experimental autoimmune encephalomyelitis (the experimental mouse analogue of MS), diminishing axonal damage, inflammation, and spinal cord microglial activation and T-cell recruitment, all of which play a significant role in the pathology of MS. This suggests the possibility that hemp could prove not only to reduce the symptoms of MS, but might have potential in terms of actually treating the disease.

As well as its demonstrated efficacy against MS spasticity, a recent meta-analysis of cannabis, cannabinoids, and the synthetic THC equivalents in multiple sclerosis patients disclosed that it was also effective in aiding bladder control, as well as being safer and better tolerated than the anticholinergic drugs normally considered the primary choice for MS incontinence. The ability to reduce spasticity was shown to be similar to that of the current front-line treatment, corticosteroids, with less difficulties regarding negative side effects.

The authors comment unequivocally that, "(the cannabinoids) can be considered safe drugs, with no serious complications regarding withdrawal syndromes or drug dependence effects." Surprisingly, it has been determined that the use of Sativex spray does not generally impair the ability to drive in MS patients, and appears to actually improve the driving of some patients with moderate to severe MS spasticity. In the EU, the drug comes with a label warning against driving or operating heavy machinery, etc., if one suffers somnolence, dizziness, or other possible safety-impairing side effects.

But that is not the case for the large majority. It has been variously theorized that the driving improvement is related to improved cognition; the reduction of spasticity; and/or reduction of the polypharmacy which many MS patients require to control their symptoms.There is some concern that the use of Sativex might increase the plasma levels of THC above the legal-driving maximum permitted in many countries and therefore have the potential to cause legal trouble for the patient.

Whether these policies will change as testing for cannabis levels becomes more common and more detailed information is gathered on the topic is unknown. Sativex dosing is certainly considerably lower than the usual quantities administered in even mild recreational dosing: one dose = 2.5 mg each of THC and CBD, whereas the average joint is likely to contain around 30 mg. THC, often with negligible CBD content.

D) Inflammatory Bowel Disease

Cannabis is showing very well as a treatment which improves the quality of life in patients suffering from inflammatory bowel disease (Crohn's, ulcerative colitis) and irritable bowel syndrome (mechanism still unknown). Endocannabinoids play a significant role in protecting the internal intestinal layer from inflammatory destruction. It is, in fact, suspected that an endocannabinoid deficiency may actually play a role in inflammatory bowel conditions, which, if so, would lead to cannabinoids as the obvious pharmaceutical replacement. Cannabis is currently considered an option for symptomatic control of IBD, and suitable for large-scale controlled trials with a view to establishing safety, dosage, and efficacy, particularly when the serious long-term risks of established treatment methods (corticosteroids, biological medications, and immunomodulators) are taken into account.

E) Lowering Stomach Acid

There is some indication that regular cannabis use (more than 2 days/week) may lower the level of stomach acid. Whether this is a good thing or not depends on the individual patient and circumstances. Low stomach acid renders one more vulnerable to infective GI conditions and more prone to copious diarrhoea resulting from those conditions (the study in question actually used cholera as one of the challenging agents), which will be a real and present danger after the Catastrophe. But the patient who was on anti-acid treatment such as proton-pump inhibitors prior to the Catastrophe may be well-advised to use cannabis regularly as a replacement, remembering that a bleeding ulcer is also a potentially severe and perhaps fatal danger, in real life right now, and much more so after the Catastrophe. As Lois McMasters Bujold observed in

The Warrior's Apprentice (Baen, 1986) a hole in one's body with blood pouring out is equally dangerous whether it's on the outside or the inside. And if you can't operate...In real life, the standard treatment for Helicobacter pylori, the primary cause of stomach ulcers in humans, is "triple therapy": a proton-pump inhibitor, clarithromycin or metranidazole, and either amoxicillin or (for the penicillin-sensitive) clarithromycin plus metranidazole.

The antibiotics are chosen specifically to cover both Gram-positive and Gram-negative bacteria, although H. pylori itself is Gram-negative. After the Catastrophe, you may be dependent on cannabis plus whatever bacteriocidal herbs (such as Verbena officinalis, the ethanol extract of which indicated a significant broad-spectrum potential covering both Gram-positive and Gram-negative bacteria) and/or homemade penicillin you can find. The apparent efficacy of cannabis against S. aureus and MRSA (both Gram-positives) may be of some assistance as well. Stomach acid does not cause ulcers, as used to be believed before the discovery of H. pylori's role, but it most certainly does exacerbate them.

F) Cancer Management

Cannabis is playing an increasingly important role in both the management of treatable cancer and of palliative care cancer patients, and may offer the hope of significant possibilities in regards to future treatment options. One of the main motivating factors in the re-recognition of this plant's medicinal uses and its return to legal status has been its demonstrated efficacy in managing cachexia and iatrogenic nausea in both cancer and HIV patients – which in turn became obvious when it became clear that patients who are wasting away and dying in great discomfort and pain tend to be rather less than concerned about legal issues in regards to substances which offer them effective relief.

Laboratory studies thus far have shown various cannabinoids to have a wide range of effects which may be of value in treating cancer, including pro-apoptotic, anti-mitotic, and anti-angiogenic effects (causing cancer cells to die, discouraging their division, and preventing the growth of new blood vessels necessary for a tumour to grow beyond a certain size). In vitro (artificial environment) and rodent studies have shown diminished tumour size in lung carcinoma, glioma, thyroid epithelioma, leukaemia, lymphoma, and skin carcinoma; apoptosis (programmed cell death) of cancerous cells in glioma, leukaemia, lymphoma, and skin carcinoma and (in vitro only) prostate carcinoma and neuroblastoma.

Cell-growth inhibition was seen in vivo (mouse) and in vitro for lung carcinoma, and (in vitro only) uterine carcinoma. Cell-cycle arrest appeared in vivo (mouse) and in vitro for thyroid epithelioma, and (in vitro only) breast carcinoma. Cannabinoid receptor involvement was demonstrated in glioma, thyroid epithelioma, leukaemia, lymphoma, skin carcinoma, and breast carcinoma. Despite the demonstrated high likelihood that cannabinoids have very significant benefits in treating cancer, there has not been adequate clinical investigation of efficacious cannabis usage for this purpose in humans yet, although the increased medical awareness of the potential medicinal values of hemp and the growing rate of legalization are moving towards making the appropriate investigations possible.

Biotech firm Cannabis Science has already selected basal cell carcinoma (a very common form of skin cancer) as the object of clinical trials on the combined grounds of multiple anecdotal reports of cannabis extracts having been used successfully to treat tumours, the widespread prevalence of basal cell carcinoma, and at least one case study by a physician on the effective treatment of a basal cell carcinoma by means of a topical cannabis extract. Cannabinoids, terpenes, and curcumin (from turmeric) have also shown potential activity in slowing the progress of glioblastoma, a particularly nasty and aggressive form of brain cancer.

While cannabinoids are still a long way from being proven curative or preventative for any form of cancer in real life, let alone having appropriate dosage and treatment regimens investigated...after the Catastrophe, in the absence of proven treatment modalities which require the full capabilities of current technology, the use of cannabis in cancer patients will at worst aid in maintaining quality of life and carrying out palliative care, and might offer some hope of increased survival time or even recovery.

g) De-generative Neurological Diseases, Ischaemic and Traumatic Brain Damage, and Autism.

Cannabis appears to be markedly neuroprotective in terms of treating degenerative neurological diseases such as Alzheimer's, Parkinson's, Huntington's chorea, and amyotrophic lateral sclerosis ("Lou Gehrig's disease"). As mentioned above, it is also showing considerable promise in treating the neurological damage caused by ischaemic strokes, and may be useful in treating neonatal ischaemia (another condition where, if cannabis or one of its constituents proves out, the benefit of administering the drug to an infant might well outweigh the risk).

KN38-7271, an agonist which activates the dual CB1/CB2 endocannabinoid receptor (as whole cannabis does), when administered within 4.5 hours of a severe traumatic brain injury, showed significantly improved survival rates at one month from the injury, and a decrease in the occurrence of critical intracranial and cerebral perfusion pressure. No adverse effects were reported.

Whether the varied constituents of whole cannabis would detract from or enhance the neuroprotective effects of activating the dual endocannabinoid receptor in regards to traumatic brain injury remains to be seen. A small preliminary study indicated potential benefit of CBD in autism management. Using a 20:1 CBD/THC ratio oral solution and titrating up to a maximum of 10 mg/kg CBD per dose, significant improvement was seen in a number of the patients in regards to behavioural outbreaks (61% of patients), anxiety (39%), communications problems (47%), and disruptive behaviours (29%). It was determined that the results of this study solidly justify further and more extensive research into the potential usage of CBD or CBD/low-dose THC for managing autism.

H) Pain Control

In terms of pain control, depending on dosage and means of administration, cannabis is considered to achieve levels 1 and 2 of the WHO pain pyramid (described in detail in Extreme Herbalism, Part I). In other words, it can provide analgesia ranging from the equivalent of a dose of aspirin, ibuprofen, or acetaminophen to the equivalent of a weak opiate such as codeine or a strong non-steroidal anti-inflammatory drug such as diclofenac.

Unless you actually administer enough to sedate your patient into unconsciousness, it will never be a substitute for WHO 3 drugs (morphine and other strong opiate/opioids), except perhaps in severe neuropathic pain, for which it seems to be particularly effective. However, in areas where medicinal use is legal, cannabis has proven to be a valuable replacement for codeine and an adjunct allowing marked reduction in the need for other opiate/opioid drugs, particularly in chronic pain patients, who are especially vulnerable to developing tolerance and addiction as the price of receiving enough analgesia to allow them a reasonable quality of life and degree of function.

The insulin plant, Costus igneus, is also showing considerable promise in the treatment of type II diabetes. But it probably won't replace insulin either, though one small study reported that insulin-dependent patients treated with fresh leaf or leaf-powder (1 fresh leaf or 1 tsp powder, on an empty stomach in the morning), were able to reduce their dosage by 50% within sixty days of beginning treatment (reference in text).

This reduction could be a life-preserver over the time between the Catastrophe and when animal-pancreas insulin production gets rolling. Costus igneus is native to South America and hardy only along the southern US borders and California coastline. If you think you might need it, and don't live where the winters don't freeze, stock up on the dried material and start thinking about possible trade routes.

It has been demonstrated that cannabis does not depress vital signs even in combination with IV fentanyl (WHO level 4), and that it is safe to use in conjunction with opioids, as well as possibly offering therapeutic assistance in treating opioid addiction. It has been shown that CBD alone significantly enhances the analgesic effect of morphine in mice, and most probably in humans, via its antagonism of the sigma-1 receptor (which may also be implicated in neurodegenerative and some psychiatric conditions).

There is some evidence that cannabis is particularly effective against neuropathic pain (typical of diabetes and possibly the main contributor to fibromyalgia pain, among other causes). Cannabis as an adjuvant to spinal cord stimulation achieved good pain control in treating even severe cases of chronic refractory pain from failed back surgery syndrome.

1) Diabetes

The surprisingly high likelihood of benefits provided by cannabis in weight and blood-sugar modulation may seem counter-intuitive, given that everyone who hasn't been living under a rock in the Antarctic for the last fifty years has heard of "the munchies". However, to the rather considerable startlement of the researchers who have been looking at this issue, regular cannabis users consistently had a lower degree of obesity, as well as smaller waist size (one of the most reliable easily-measured indicators of both body fat level and cardiovascular risk) and lower fasting glucose levels than non-users. The likeliest mechanism for these results is the role of human endocannabinoid receptors in metabolic control.

Obesity is unlikely to be a major problem for most people after the Catastrophe... getting enough food to survive will probably be far more of an issue, and the glycaemic control of survivors with type II diabetes is likely to improve overall as a result of circumstance-enforced lifestyle changes (diet and exercise). But for the patient with more advanced orally controlled type II diabetes who can no longer get their daily doses of metformin, sulfonylureas, GLP-1 agonists, DPP-4 inhibitors, and SGLT-2 inhibitors – none of which you can make at home, and I don't recommend encouraging Gila monsters to bite you just because their venom contains the original GLP-1 agonist! – cannabis may offer significant survival benefits. In the more advanced patient with diabetes of any sort, cannabis has also shown marked promise in treating the neuropathic pain sometimes associated with this condition.

The cause of "the munchies", incidentally, seems to be a brief but marked drop in blood sugar shortly after absorbing cannabis. The patient with diabetes who still has the use of drugs associated with hypoglycaemia (insulin, sulfonylureas such as gliclazide/"Diamicron") is advised to be aware of this fact and to have at least a sugared drink ready if they start experiencing hypoglycaemic symptoms. There is also a small risk that the subjective experience of cannabis may mask these symptoms; so remain careful and aware, and, if possible, try not to utilize cannabis by yourself if you are taking drugs that can cause hypoglycaemia.

Unfortunately, cannabis is no substitute for insulin. Cannabis in diabetes is appearing to be very similar to cannabis in pain control: useful for mild-to-moderate needs, but won't do the job when a major drug is needed. Nor will the insulin plant, despite quite impressive preliminary results (see sidebar). Trials in mice have indicated the possibility that CBD may slow the type I diabetes autoimmune attack on the beta cells of the pancreas and reduce destructive inflammation in the early stages, prolonging the time until insulin is required.

J) Anti-Inflammatory and Anti-Auto-Immune Diseases

The anti-inflammatory efficacy of both whole hemp and individual cannabinoids (THC, CBD, and probably CBN – separately or as interactive combinations) has recently come to considerable prominence, and is one of the best-studied medical uses for this herb and its constituents. Activation of the CB2 cannabinoid receptor, which is now being proposed as a significant therapeutic target for pharmaceutical drug development, causes strong anti-inflammatory effects, reduces pain, and protects the liver (the CB1 receptor is, among other things, responsible for the psychoactive effects of cannabis).

Ascites (fluid collection in the abdominal cavity) is easy to determine, by checking for "shifting dullness". With the patient lying flat, place the middle finger of one hand on the middle of their belly and tap sharply with the middle finger of the other. You should hear a resonant thump.

Continue tapping every inch or so down to the flank. Eventually the resonant sound may become dull. Mark the point (or get the patient to put their own finger on it) and turn them to lie on the opposite side. Wait two minutes. Tap at the same place and the areas immediately around it.

If the thump is now resonant on the flank, the fluid has shifted and ascites is present. This may indicate congestive heart failure, liver failure, severe hypervolaemia, or a number of other conditions; what it confirms depends on what other signs and symptoms had you looking for it in the first place.

The cannabinoid sesquiterpene beta-caryophyllene, which comprises 12-25% of cannabis essential oil (and is also found in the essential oils of many other plants, including cinnamon, black pepper and oregano – though you still can't get high from smoking oregano), binds selectively to the CB2 receptor. CBD has been shown to have a powerful anti-arthritic effect in mouse collagen-induced arthritis (simulating rheumatoid arthritis in humans).

CB1 and CB2 control immunomodulation in a number of ways, affecting cytokine production, T-cell activation, and macrophage migration, among other significant elements of the immune-inflammatory response. This function is suspected to explain why cannabis and cannabinoids are beginning to prove or strongly indicate efficacy in the treatment of multiple sclerosis, inflammatory bowel conditions, inflammatory liver conditions, and those types of cancer with significant inflammatory components.

Another proposed mechanism is THC-induced histone modification (a means of activating or suppressing certain genes) of T-helper cells. As mentioned above (section I, part 3, "Immune System Effects and Viruses"), this strong and multi-functional anti-inflammatory effect also means that cannabis is contraindicated in the presence of acute viruses, although potentially extremely useful in the damaging chronic (pathological) conditions caused by the failure of acute inflammation to resolve properly, regardless of aetiology (viral, bacterial, traumatic).

In regards to treating auto-immune diseases, CB2 stimulators including cannabis and specific cannabinoids have the potential both to address the inflammatory damage and pain directly, and to decrease the overall immune system response in order to prevent further problems. In other words, by operating through multiple pathways, cannabis appears to act as both an NSAID and as an immunoregulator which may possibly prove out to be comparable or superior to corticosteroids (a common treatment for some autoimmune conditions) in terms of efficacy, safety, or both, and which may also prove protective against types of cancer which are mediated by inflammation.

The degree of potency required for this purpose has not been quantified, not least due to the fundamental problem of evaluating complex whole herbs. There would be many advantages to replacing the chronic administration of corticosteroids, which may cause iatrogenic Cushing syndrome (central obesity, muscle wasting, impaired glycaemic control, skin thinning, characteristic "moon facies" and "buffalo hump", depression, and steroid psychosis), with a less harmful drug. However, until probable dosage levels and large double-blind trials comparing the efficacy and side effect profiles of whole cannabis and individual cannabinoids to the major pharmaceutical corticosteroids have been done, such a replacement cannot yet be commonly introduced into clinical practice.

As mentioned earlier in this article: after the Catastrophe, cannabis might be the only readily available substitute for immunosuppressive use of corticosteroids (though not a treatment for adrenal insufficiency, a critical indication for these drugs). Until the latter stages of sepsis, cannabis/cannabinoids may be useful in controlling the exaggerated inflammatory response and limiting damage. However, late sepsis shows a marked down-regulation of the immune system, possibly as self-modulation in response to the immune hyperactivity of the early stage, and this leaves the patient more vulnerable to remaining pathogens. Therefore, whether cannabis or other CB2 receptor agonists are beneficial in treating sepsis or not may depend on the severity of the condition and the stage at which it is administered. After the Catastrophe, best practice might be to administer cannabis early and often when an inflammatory over-reaction is suspected, but cease when it becomes severe.

In real life, given our other proven options, this needs to wait until more research has been done. One case report also suggests that, as the increased release of vasopressin (anti-diuretic hormone) in sepsis is modified by the endocannabinoid system, the hemp user may be at an increased risk of severe hypervolaemic hyponatraemia (dangerously low salt due to water retention). This may be difficult to judge without the standard electrolyte lab tests. Marked puffiness, particularly about the ankles, and especially if a finger pressed firmly just behind the inner ankle bone leaves a visible dent (pitting oedema), abdominal fluid swelling (ascites), and difficulty breathing (dyspnoea) due to increased lung fluids would indicate this condition, but may not be seen in very acute conditions such as sepsis. Cannabis seed oil is rich in omega-3 and omega-6 polyunsaturated fatty acids (PUFAs), with a 3:1 ratio of omega-6 to omega-3 (a ratio shown to inhibit inflammation in rheumatoid arthritis – the normal Western diet maintains a ratio of 15-16.7:1).

> Note well: you don't have to be in a tropical zone to contract malaria! It was a serious health problem in Northern Europe until quite recently; one of the worst epidemics ever was in the Soviet Union in the 1920s (13 million cases/year at peak), with transmission particularly high in Siberia, and 10,000 deaths recorded in Archangel (near the Arctic Circle.
>
> In fact, I once studied with a man who contracted malaria in a Siberian prison camp during WWII. Malaria was largely wiped out in Northern Europe and North America by human activity. And when the levels of human land use, pesticides, and land drainage change again after the Catastrophe, it will probably come back.
>
> Stock up on purified quinine and artemether; trade for cinchona bark ("Jesuit bark" – the original herbal source of quinine); grow Artemesia annua ("sweet wormwood" – a traditional Chinese malaria remedy which is the source of the first-line drug artemether; and don't forget your mosquito netting and avoidance of stagnant water!

Omega-3 is noted for its anti-inflammatory properties; although omega-6 (arachidonic acid and its predecessor lineolic acid) is a substrate for the primary inflammatory pathways, it does not appear to increase inflammation and may reduce it; a Finnish study correlated higher levels of the omega-6 lineolic acid with a lower serum inflammatory marker (C-reactive protein), and it is noted that the omega-6 PUFAs also act as substrates for some anti-inflammatory compounds. A low ratio of omega-6 to omega-3 (defined as lower than 4:1) also prevents the overproduction of pro-inflammatory cytokines (cell signalling agents); the 3:1 ratio is considered optimal for metabolic conversion of these two PUFAs.

Oral hemp seed oil (6 weeks treatment) has been shown to decrease eczema (atopic dermatitis), a condition often associated with hypersensitivity immune reactions in general, notably in the "atopic triad" of eczema, asthma, and hay fever. Hemp seed oil, therefore, may be a useful oral anti-inflammatory adjunct, as it works by different pathways than the other plant constituents. Cannabis roots were also used traditionally in a range of anti-inflammatory therapies. They do not contain any THC.

While a swift Internet search will reveal many claims that they contain CBD, the exhaustive analysis done by Ryz, Remillard, and Russo (cited below) indicates that this is not the case. Darcy Stoddard at Tierra del Sol Farm (Hemp-EaZe) also sent roots for chemical analysis to personally establish the truth of the matter, and commented, "Happily we have learned that no THC was detected. Surprisingly no cannabinoids were either."

So, there you have it: no THC, no CBD, and no other cannabinoids. What the roots do notably contain is friedelin (anti-inflammatory, analgesic, anti-pyretic, and hepatoprotective; served well as oestrogen-replacement therapy in ovariectomized rats) as well as a range of terpenes, terpenoids, alkaloids, and phytosterols with known anti-inflammatory activities. Like the seed oil, the roots might thus be gainfully combined with cannabinoids in order to treat inflammation and aid in analgesia via multiple directions.

K) Anti-bacterial, Anti-fungal, Anti-parasitic

Five of the cannabinoids present in hemp (THC, CBD, CBG, CBN, and CBC) were described in one study as showing "potent activity" against a variety of MRSA strains. A more exhaustive analysis of some of the less-researched cannabinoids showed that: Cannabinol (CBN) derivatives had good activity against Candida albicans ("yeast infections" or "thrush") and Staphylococcus, and moderate activity against Mycobacterium intracellulare (a cause of atypical pneumonia). Not tested against other mycobacteria (tuberculosis, leprosy, M. avium). Cannabichromene (CBC) derivative activities were weakly anti-candidal, mildly anti-malarial, and moderately anti-leishmanial. Leishmaniasis is a common protozoal disease transmitted by sandflies.

It can variously cause skin ulcers which may take up to a year to heal (cutaneous type); ulcers and disfiguring erosion of the nose and mouth (mucocutaneous); and damage to the liver, spleen, and bone marrow which is normally fatal without treatment or if not treated quickly enough (visceral type; also called kala-azar, black fever). Even a brief visit to endemic areas can risk any of these: cutaneous leishmaniasis has not infrequently been seen in soldiers returning from the Middle East, and there was a tragic case in Ireland some years ago of a young patient dying of visceral leishmaniasis contracted during a weekend visit to Turkey. Cannabigerol (CBG) derivative activites were moderately to strongly anti-leishmanial, with mild anti-malarial and anti-MRSA activity.

All of these constituents are present to some degree in whole hemp, though, as always, varying in level and percentage according to strain and growth circumstances. These findings indicate that various cannabinoids could be valuable targets of pharmaceutical research in regards to anti-fungal, anti-parasitic, and anti-bacterial usage. They also suggest that the post-Catastrophe character might not do badly to keep a flask of cannabis alcoholic tincture for wound disinfection, or cannabis medications for general use when dwelling or travelling anywhere that sandflies and mosquitoes live. In regards to MRSA, Russo notes the strong anti-MRSA effects of both CBD and CBG as well as the terpene pinene (source of that "piny" smell in many strains), and suggests, "Given that CBG can be produced in selected cannabis chemotypes, with no residual THC as a possible drug abuse liability risk, a whole plant extract of a CBG-chemotype also expressing pinene would seem to offer an excellent, safe new antiseptic agent."

As recent history, particularly in Russia, has taught us, malaria will also be a concern even in Northern regions. The neuroprotective qualities of CBD in general discussed above, and an initial mouse-model study in specific, indicate that CBD may have significant neuroprotective capabilities in regards to cerebral malaria, improving survival and full recovery. Cerebral complications are the direct cause of approximately 50% of deaths in malaria, and often have severe long-term consequences for survivors as well. CBD offers a potential treatment for reducing the harm done by malaria in real life, especially considering the increasing level of resistance to anti-malarials shown by Plasmodium spp; and will be even more crucial after the Catastrophe. Regrettably, cannabis seems to have no demonstrable activity against Gram-negative bacteria.

L) Anti-Nauseant

The efficacy of THC as an anti-nauseant and appetite stimulator for chemotherapy and HIV patients was the first characteristic of hemp to be re-recognised in the Western medical system, leading to the production of the synthetic THC drugs nabilone and dronabinol (Marinol). Both prior to legalized medical use and after legalization in many countries, these medications have often been prescribed for chemotherapy patients when standard anti-nauseants have failed. It should be noted that many patients find that they prefer whole cannabis for any of several reasons, including the difficulty of taking pills while vomiting; faster action and/or greater ease of titration with inhaled hemp; and the different effects of other cannabinoids and terpenes.

The pure THC-analogues appear likelier to cause a stimulant "speedy" or "paranoid" reaction, which is probably mitigated by the presence of CBD and certain terpene profiles. The director of the Drug Policy Analysis Program (UCLA's School of public affairs said of Marinol that, "It wasn't any fun and made the user feel bad...so it could be approved without any fear that it would penetrate the recreational market, and then used as a club with which to beat back the advocates of whole cannabis as a medicine." Sativex, a whole-cannabis tincture with a 1:1 THC/CBD ratio, used as an oral spray, has regularly received positive reviews from the patient population, particularly for its primary indication in treating symptoms of multiple sclerosis.

This is possibly not least because the even balance is often reported to mitigate the psychoactivity level of the medication, making it less likely to disrupt activities of daily living than either the synthetic THC-analogues or high THC/low CBD strains (the low dosage probably helps there too); the speed of absorption through mucous membranes is slower than smoking, but much faster than digestive absorption; the ease of titration is fairly comparable to smoking; and it can be administered even when there is severe nausea and vomiting. CBD also contributes to the anti-nauseant effect of whole cannabis, probably by means of its action on the somatodendritic 5-HT1A autoreceptors in the dorsal raphe nucleus of the brain, which diminishes the release of 5-HT (serotonin)

m) PTSD Treatment

Post-traumatic stress disorder (PTSD) is essentially a trauma-induced rewiring of neurological pathways causing extreme negative emotional reactions in response to trigger factors which most people would find innocuous. Symptoms include panic attacks, nightmares and sleep disturbance, general anxiety, "flashbacks", a hypervigilant/hyperaroused state in which the sufferer is unable to relax and has a startle response to even ordinary stimuli, and often an inability to perform daily activities or tolerate ordinary occurrences which evoke the original event (e.g., someone with PTSD from a severe automobile accident might be unable to drive the route on which the accident took place, or unable to drive, or even ride in a vehicle, altogether; even before PTSD was recognised as a condition, one of the classic descriptions was the veteran who drops flat and reaches for the weapon he used to carry when he hears a car backfiring on the next street). Some degree of PTSD may occur in 25% of people who suffer severe trauma.

The combat/immediately post-combat prevalence in veterans varies according to many factors (the nature of the war and their individual part in it, the medical and social support received during and following the traumatic period), but seems to run between 2-20%; lifetime prevalence in veterans is estimated as 6-31%. After the Catastrophe, you may expect PTSD to become a veritable epidemic. It is unlikely that many will make it through the Catastrophe and its aftermath without significant trauma of some sort (and most of those who are able to avoid severe psychological trauma will already be or have been in professions that have forced them to develop coping mechanisms if possible: some veterans and combat military; some police officers; some medical personnel, especially those in fields where emotional stress is more severe and often more likely to occur unexpectedly, such as ER work; etc.).

A total prevalence two years after the Catastrophe might well run even as high as 1 in 3 of the general surviving population. This, in turn, will increase the level of danger survivors risk from themselves and others in a number of ways, ranging from conscious or unconscious self-harm and suicide to general bad judgment and physical aggression-reaction. If the supernatural is a part of your post-Catastrophe world, PTSD may also open characters to supernatural contact or invasion, particularly by predators of any sort your author is pleased to imagine and you're not so pleased to deal with (though it could also be a trigger or means for developing supernatural capabilities, in a shamanic-initiation-by-death-dismemberment-rebirth sort of way – for either protagonists and their associates, or antagonists who might or might not have gone a little mad or hooked up with nasty beings in the process). The psychological mainstays of PTSD therapy are trauma-focused cognitive behavioural therapy (CBT: in which the therapist guides the patient in identifying and coping with the triggers which also reinforce the underlying neurological pathways, and managing their various symptoms), and EMDR (Eye Movement Desensitization and Reprocessing) therapy.

Although the mechanism of the latter is not fully understood, and the whole concept sounds frankly wooly on the face of it, there have been a number of clinical trials done which proved EMDR to be strikingly effective. A 2014 review cited twenty-four randomized control trials out of twenty-five as showing benefit, and seven of ten which indicated that EMDR was more rapidly-acting and/or effective than trauma-focused CBT. EMDR is accepted by the medical world in general as an efficacious form of therapy for PTSD, on the grounds of, "we don't know how or why it works, but it definitely works". Currently, the primary pharmaceutical treatment for PTSD is antidepressants.

The efficacy profile for these is not good: 9 patients must be treated for every 1 who receives benefit from them, and the remission rates are low (20-30%). Where it is legal for medicinal use for PTSD, cannabis is receiving increasing attention as a drug which may have the potential to be more efficacious and safer than antidepressants. Antipsychotics, though not generally recommended for this purpose, are nonetheless sometimes used as a second-line treatment when antidepressants have not worked. The evidence for these, while indicating the possibility of reasonable efficacy, is still limited, and the side-effects of antipsychotics can range from the annoying (hypersalivation, sometimes requiring an additional anticholinergic drug to dry the mouth) to the disabling (drug-induced Parkinsonism) and the long-term health-threatening (induction of metabolic syndrome leading to type II diabetes) to, in rare cases, the short-term potentially fatal (agranulocytosis, GI paralysis).

In theory, cannabis is well-suited to the treatment of PTSD in many regards. The endocannabinoid system interacts with many systems implicated in the pathology of PTSD: hippocampus (a brain area strongly associated with memory) and amygdala (a brain area strongly associated with fear/anxiety responses); cortical regulation of memory processes; and the hypothalamic-pituitary-adrenocortical or HPA axis (hormonal and cortical steroidal control of stress adaptation and general metabolism, among other things). Appetite, addiction, memory, anxiety, and pain responses are also affected by the endocannabinoid system.

Particularly important for PTSD treatment is the role of the endocannabinoid system in the extinction of aversive memories: a deficiency in CB1 receptors or receptor activation diminishes the ability to recover from fear-conditioning, whereas activation of CB1 (the main target of THC) is required for negative memory extinction, and appears to have a selective activity in controlling amygdala function regarding the extinction of fear/trauma memories.

Both the hippocampus and the amygdala have, or should have, particularly high levels of CB1 receptors; activation of these decreases excitation, and is likely to directly diminish the hypervigilance/hyperarousal typical of PTSD. Dysregulation of the HPA axis, leading to increased adrenal cortical hormone release, is increasingly being identified as a common factor in the development of PTSD and other anxiety-related (as well as depressive) disorders. In terms of clinical trials, much information is still lacking. Shisko et al review the various studies that have been done, all of which had significant flaws in method and/or execution.

For instance: one study found significant benefits, but their patient-selection method was predisposed towards a positive outcome; another which found significant benefits (and was the only one to actually use cannabis in a controlled fashion – up to 5 mg THC in infused olive oil, 2x/day) was very small and further confounded by the use of pharmaceutical drugs, including in some instances benzodiazepines (contraindicated in PTSD), and the lack of verification that other drugs were not also being used.

One found worse outcomes for patients diagnosed previously with cannabis use disorder, but the study participants were not currently using cannabis, and the nature of the study (observational) meant that no causality could be established; another that identified exacerbation rather than benefit did not verify the use or non-use of other drugs, and the clinical significance was dubious. None of the studies reviewed by Shisko et al – the results of which were often contradictory – were carried out in such a manner as to present solid evidence in either direction. The first clinical pilot study on cannabis for PTSD in veterans (headed by Dr. S. Sisley, Scottsdale Research Institute) only approached completion of patient enrolment in August of 2018. As a pilot study, the numbers are fairly low (estimated 76 candidates in total, two different sites), but should suffice to demonstrate the scope of potential for cannabis regarding this purpose. Sisley's trial is arranged in such a way as to correct for previous cannabis trials difficulties regarding varying THC/CBD levels, by dividing the patients into four groups: high THC/low CBD; high CBD/low THC; high THC/high CBD; and placebo.

The synthetic THC nabilone was the object of a clinical trial in regards to nightmare control and sleep improvement in patients (general population) diagnosed with PTSD. 72% received either complete cessation of nightmares or a significant reduction in intensity; some patients also observed improved overall sleep time and quality, and diminishment of night sweats and daytime flashbacks. Terpenes such as myrcene (also found in mangoes and, at a high level, in hops) and linalool (lavender, particularly the essential oil), which have significant anti-anxiety properties on their own, may contribute to the efficacy of whole cannabis in controlling the symptoms of PTSD, while THC appears thus far to be the primary actor in regards to neuroemotional reprogramming of trauma-induced brain pathways.

Current strains high in myrcene include: Blue Dream, White Widow, various Kush hybrids; strains described as "primarily indica" characteristically contain more than "primarily sativa". Linalool is notably found in White Widow, Amnesia Haze, Super Lemon Haze, Granddaddy Purple, and Lavender, among others; it is characteristically higher in sativa-dominant strains. While still awaiting the outcome of Dr. Sisley's pilot study, not least in regards to any findings regarding the most effective THC/CBD balance for the purpose, it seems likely that the many US states which have approved hemp for PTSD treatment are justified in having done so.

As well as probably being the main drug suited to the purpose, and certainly the most readily available after the Catastrophe, it is entirely possible that, upon further testing, cannabis may prove to be superior to current pharmaceutical options for PTSD in regards to safety, efficacy, and side effect profile. Not certain yet, but the bulk of the evidence is pointing in that direction.

n) Other Potential Human Uses

One recent study indicates that regular use of THC appears to be a protective factor against lower urinary tract infections in young men. Regarding fibromyalgia, in a very small (26 patients) study in Israel, all patients reported significant improvements in all parameters from the use of cannabis, and 50% discontinued taking any other medications for fibromyalgia. 30% reported very mild adverse effects; none reported moderate or severe adverse effects.

o) Veterinary Uses

The use of cannabis in veterinary medicine is only now being explored. No recommended dosages have yet been set for cats, dogs, or horses. As of the time in writing, it was illegal for veterinarians in any state to prescribe cannabis to an animal, but in cannabis-legal states, it is permitted to give cannabis to your own animals. In dogs and horses, a high CBD/low THC ratio of the base material is almost certainly preferable, not least to avoid distressing an animal who may be frightened by the unfamiliar psychoactive effects. Cats seem to like their THC, although the benefits of CBD should not be ignored in these creatures. Even given the relative uncertainty of cannabis metabolism in dogs, cannabis is, as with humans, a valuable or potentially valuable adjunct in cats, dogs, and horses alike for supplementing the analgesic effect of the (far more dangerous) opiates and allowing a reduction in opiate dose while maintaining good pain control.

i) Cats

Cats are famously known, not only to tolerate cannabis well, but often to enjoy it. Cats have been caught actively invading purses or backpacks in search of a hidden stash of dried hemp flowers, then self-administering it in the same manner that they use catnip (roll, writhe, purr, nibble a bit, wave paws in the air, imitate catskin rugs, and generally act like stereotyped happy hippie cats. “So mellow...prrrr...so mellow, man...”).

I have personally seen cats shove their faces against the mouth of a cannabis smoker to beg for their own dose. This is not, however, a good way to dose a cat, as the smoke from any burning plant material is not good for their lungs. A weight-appropriate small amount of infused butter or oil may be given to the cat to eat directly, mixed into its food, smeared on paws to be licked off, or administered as a topical smeared on the inside of the cat’s ears, where the skin is thin and absorption takes place readily.

There is little concern about cannabis toxicity in cats, though it is wise to start low and go slow, especially with higher THC-containing compounds, until you are certain that your cat responds like the majority; some cats, after all, even dislike catnip. Because of the anti-inflammatory effects of CBD, CBN, and THCa, cannabis may well prove to be a particularly safe and effective substitute for toxic or low-therapeutic-range pharmaceutical NSAIDs in cats (there are NSAIDs compounded specifically for cats, available through veterinary prescription).

Do not use NSAIDs made for humans, which include aspirin, ibuprofen, and diclofenac, on cats. Do not ever use acetaminophen (paracetamol) for cats: one standard over-the-counter tablet is more than sufficient to kill a cat. Do not give a cat any compound in any form, cannabinated or otherwise, which also contains pure essential oils. Cats are extremely sensitive to essential oils, even when highly diluted, but can tolerate low doses (ca. 1-3 drops topical, diluted in a carrier oil, or diffused in moderate amounts into a room's air as long as the cat can escape the room at will) of the vast majority of essentials.

II) Dogs

Little research has been done in real life regarding either the safety profile or the efficacy of cannabis in dogs. The issue is further confounded by the number of accidental canine ingestions where the cannabis was part of a chocolate-based product, leaving the issue of whether the cannabis played any role in the toxicity uncertain. Because of differences in liver function, it is generally accepted that lipid-medium ingested cannabis has the potential to be more problematic for canines than for humans or felines. In severe cases of over-ingestion by dogs, IV hydration and cardiac monitoring may be required. Gary Richter, author of Ultimate Pet Health Guide, observes that dogs have higher levels of endocannabinoid receptors in their brainstems than humans, so are extremely sensitive to THC.

While, as with humans, no definite LD50 can be established for dogs, this sensitivity indicates that when calculating dog doses, one cannot simply scale human doses down (assuming the dog is less than human-weight to begin with). In short, considerable caution is required in administering THC to dogs.

There do not seem to be significant issues with CBD. For animal conditions in general, Richter recommends the CBD/THC balances as follows:

- Seizure disorders, chronic pain, inflammatory conditions, neuroprotective (regarding head injuries and other forms of brain damage), cancer, anxiety, sleep disorders: high CBD/low THC (defined as 4:1 to 20:1).
- Inflammatory bowel disease, pain, inflammation, cancer, possibly spinal cord injuries: approximately a 1:1 ratio.
- Severe pain, advanced arthritis, cancer: higher THC/lower CBD.

He advises administering 2-3 times daily, starting at ca. 0.1 to 0.25 milligram/kg (2.2 lbs) of bodyweight per day total (1/2 to 1/3 the total at each dose) and very gradually titrating up. Richter notes that up to 5 mg/kg has proven beneficial in difficult seizure cases, but warns that it is important to be very cautious with THC. Evidence suggesting that high CBD/very low THC whole cannabis or isolated CBD may be helpful in many canine conditions, particularly seizure disorders, inflammatory conditions, some cancers, arthritic problems, is increasingly accumulating, although vets will probably not be able to prescribe it until considerably more clinical studies have been done. THCa is also strongly anti-inflammatory and non-psychoative, suggesting that it might be fruitful to investigate the effects of raw or undecarboxylated whole cannabis in dogs.

III. Horses

Anecdotally, horses are observed to respond well to either whole cannabis extracts (lipid medium) or extracted CBD, used to treat neurological problems, neuropathies (including very severe ones such as trigeminal neuralgia), and inflammatory disorders. The optimum dosage seems to be approximately 1/2 of human medical dosage by weight: that is, a 1500 lb horse would receive ca. 5 times the amount that a 150 lb human would require. It is probably wise to assume that a hungry horse (or other hooved livestock) can wreak immense devastation on a hempfield simply for the fresh greenery.

It has been demonstrated that THCa is not converted into a psychoactive form in the rat digestive system, and that it shows no psychomimetic effects in several other species, including mice, rhesus monkeys, and dogs, so it is fairly likely that it would not affect a horse. However, you are relying on that field for fibre, food, and medicine, so make sure your fences are strong, because horses, cattle, and sheep will absolutely eat your growing cannabis! If you have goats...good luck to you. As a goat-owning friend once said, "You can have a goat or a garden, but you cannot have a goat and a garden". Goats can not only jump, but climb with quite unreasonable skill and agility for hooved creatures; and personal experience suggests that they also teleport when humans aren't watching.

Another point to keep in mind in regards to livestock getting into the hemp field: horses and other single-stomached mammals do not decarboxylate THCa to any significant degree by digestion. There is a significant possibility that this is not the case for ruminants, given the prolonged processing period in a warm environment and the microbial fermentation process. While chowing down on enough cannabis to make it act alarmingly and pass out might not hurt a cow (unless the owner loses their temper as well as their crop), it would probably cause significant distress to the animal. Also, mammals can and do concentrate and excrete THC in milk, as a result of which even feed made from whole fibre hemp has been a matter of some concern to the European Food Safety Authority.

Breeding for Autoflowering and for CBD

The autoflowering trait is a simple Mendelian recessive. Thus, if an autoflower is crossed with an autoflower, the results will always be autoflowering. If crossed with a photoperiod, the results are:

aa x PP
aP aP aP aP
(F1 – all photoperiod-dependent)

In the second generation,

aP x aP
aa aP aP PP
(F2 – 1 autoflower, 3 photoperiod-dependent, 2 of which carry the recessive for auto.)

High THC/low CBD and high CBD/low THC are codominant traits, expressed equally. A high-THC plant crossed with a high-CBD plant yields:

TT x CC
TC TC TC TC
(all progeny moderate levels of 1:1 THC:CBD ratio)

A strain with a moderate 1:1 ratio, bred to itself, produces:

TC x TC
TT TC TC CC
(1 high THC; two moderate 1:1 ratio, 1 high CBD)

THC and CBD are produced by the plant in exactly the same manner until the last step of conversion, where THC-synthase, CBD-synthase, or both determine the final ratio of these two substances. The prevalence of one enzyme or the other is largely genetic – and is co-dominant, as mentioned above - but may also be influenced by growing conditions. This is why we see ratios as high as 20:1 in either direction, but 1:1 strains tend to run at ca. 10%:10% or less, give or take some individual variance.

5) Cannabis and the Supernatural

As with poppy products, no clinical studies have been published detailing the effects of cannabis on various types of supernatural beings. One may, however, safely assume that methods of oral administration to vampires as known from a wide range of fictional sources are similar to those of any other orally-ingested drug: that is, at second hand by means of consuming the blood of a living person who has recently taken the drug themselves.

The efficacy of inhaled cannabis in vampires will depend on their lung-circulation status, which in turn is likeliest to depend on how recently they have fed, plus or minus the issue of whether lung absorption of anything, including oxygen, is possible for your particular vampires. Similarly, topical administration of cannabis to vampires should be expected to depend on their general circulation status.

Cannabis administration to zombies of any description other than the toxin-and-ritual-induced Haitian type is probably a complete waste of both time and cannabis. If zombies are at all susceptible to drugs, you will probably want something considerably stronger and faster-acting to sedate one... say, a large animal tranquilizer dart. But the majority of reports indicate that they are not thus susceptible.

It is reasonable to expect that the response of shapeshifters to cannabis will fall somewhere in the range of what might be expected in a normal human (though due to increased metabolic rate, higher and more frequent dosing may be required for full efficacy) to what might be expected of their animal shape in the natural world.

Judging by the multitudinous reports of cats with a passion for cannabis, I would expect that shapeshifters with a feline side would tend to be particularly fond of this drug as a recreational substance, with little or no risk entailed by using it in either shape. Cannabis might also prove to be an effective calmative/analgesic to the distressed or injured feline shapeshifter in their animal form. (It has not been determined if shapeshifters with a primary feline form are able to get high on catnip in either or both of their shapes, although since large cats are affected by catnip in exactly the same manner as small cats, it seems plausible. If you manage to verify for certain what the answer to this question is, Enquiring Minds Want To Know.)

In regards to werewolves: the above cautions regarding cannabis in dogs apply, because a canid is a canid (except for Chihuahuas, which I suspect to have been planted on Earth by space aliens. No, just kidding. Mostly). Werewolves are often considered to be more toxin-resistant overall (excluding species-specific toxins such as, for some, silver and possibly certain herbs) than either humans or non-supernatural canids. Nonetheless, until there is more information on cannabis safety in non-supernatural canids, caution is advised in dosing werewolves with it, at least when they are furry.

At the very least, they are likely to require much lower doses to achieve the psychoactive effects of THC. If possible, inhalation should be preferred to oral ingestion for werewolves due to shorter effect and safety/ease of titration. If the Dire Wolf in the Grateful Dead song of the same name was able to sit down and play cards with the narrator, it is not unreasonable to assume that a werewolf retaining all or most of their human consciousness in shifted form could take a hit from a pipe or vapourizer. Concerns about lung damage and carcinogenicity from inhaled smoke probably do not apply, assuming your werewolf patient has the super-healing factor often ascribed to lycanthropes and other animal-shifters. Little has been written, in real life or fiction, regarding the effect of cannabis upon ghosts.

I recall only one (otherwise quite forgettable – in fact, I can't remember title or author) urban fantasy novel which suggested that the aroma was a deterrent to spirits. Googling "cannabis supernatural" mainly leads to reviews of the cannabis strain called Supernatural (sativa-dominant hybrid; THC content ca. 22%, which is considered highly potent; no information on CBD content available) and discussions of cannabis use being mentioned in the TV series of the same name. Historically, however, cannabis has been used for a very long time throughout most of the world to facilitate living human interaction with the spirit realms, a usage still practiced in real life by many modern mystics working in both traditional and recently invented belief systems. One of the (possibly; accurate dating and authorship is considered highly problematical) earliest medical texts to mention cannabis, the "Divine Farmer's Herb Root Classic", attributed to Emperor Shen Nung (ca. 2838-2698 B.C.E.), indicates that overuse of this plant can cause one to see spirits.

The Caucasian Gushi "shaman's grave" found in the Yanghai Tombs (Gobi Desert, ca. 700 B.C.E.) contained 789 grams (slightly over a pound and a half) of high-THC, well-prepared hemp flowers, and the accoutrements of the younger woman in the Oseberg burial (Norway, early 9th century) included a small bag containing cannabis seeds, as well as four cannabis seeds inside one of the burial-pillows. While the latter has been the cause of much speculation about Viking Age entheogenic use. It is probable that the Vikings, both by direct experience and through interaction with the Islamic world, were aware of this plant not only as an analgesic and anti-inflammatory (common medical uses in Northern Europe at the time), but as a psychoactive.

The question of whether or not the Oseberg woman used cannabis as an entheogen remains unanswered. However, the bag of seeds she wore and the inclusion of seeds in the pillow-stuffing does suggest at least the possibility of some form of amuletic usage for cannabis seeds. Unlike the henbane seeds found in the "Fyrkat witch's" burial (Viking Age Denmark), which were very probably meant to be used directly for their psychoactive and medicinal properties (though these cannot be separated from the purely spiritual uses of a plant in the traditional mind), cannabis seeds are only relevant medically in regards to their mildly anti-inflammatory oil and nutritional value.

But Scandinavian folklore does include the scattering of flaxseeds as an apotropaic and distractor of malignant supernatural beings; were the seeds of hemp, the other major fibre plant, believed to have a similar effect? The question may be of value to both the author of post-Catastrophe fiction and the author of fiction set in Viking Age Scandinavia. It is, of course, also possible that the Oseberg woman's seeds were simply put in the grave with her to assure her of a supply of hemp fibre in the Otherworld, although the small personal bag is more suggestive of magico-religious use.

Although nature spirits and other forms of elementals are seldom mentioned in the context of their interactions with cannabis, it might be worth noting that it was the custom in Norway through the 19th century (recorded in the valley of Gausdal) for men, when passing a field of hemp plants, to doff their hats as a sign of respect, since "The plant was known to house a vette, a nature spirit best treated with respect". A seafaring country such as Norway could hardly have survived without this crucial fibre for ropes – in fact, through the nineteenth century, it was legally required for all farmers to plant at least a patch of hemp – so the high degree of respect shown to the plant and the being whom it embodies should hardly be surprising.

6) Means of administration and preparation

Cannabis (aerial parts excluding seed) may be administered through inhalation (smoking or vapourization), absorption through oral membranes (usually in the form of an alcoholic tincture used as a spray, as per the above-mentioned pharmaceutical drug Sativex), topically as an infused oil or salve (cream or ointment), or orally as either an alcoholic or a lipid extract. Neither THC nor CBD is water-soluble. Cannabis tea is only effective if whole milk or cream is added at the same time as the plant material is put in to steep, and this is an extraordinarily ineffective means of extraction, as only the fat content of the milk makes it possible to achieve any extraction at all.

a) Decarboxylation

Before utilizing cannabis in a tincture or lipid extract, it must be decarboxylated. This is achieved by drying it and/or subjecting it to a certain level of heat. Cannabis can be dried in the same manner as any other herb: slowly by putting in a dark dry environment, or more quickly by heating at very low temperatures. CBD first begins to evaporate off at 150 F/66 C, and boils at 185 C/365 F. THC decarboxylates at 50 C/122 F, and boils at 200 C/392 F. Water boils at 100 C/212 F. Generally the temperature issues are not a problem in baked goods made with cannabis-infused oil or butter, as the dough or batter heats more slowly and affords a certain amount of insulation.

There is some question as to whether drying/curing plus combustion or heat-preparation suffices to decarboxylate all of the a-THC and a-CBD (the inactive forms which must be transformed in order to bind to human cannabis receptors); and more question as to whether a long steeping time at a sub-boiling temperature in the case of butter or oil will do the job effectively. The simplest common estimation of heat/time appears to be ca. 100-105 C (212-221 F) for ca. 60 minutes,which converts the vast majority of cannabinoids to active form while preserving the maximum percentage and number of terpenes and terpenoids. A more specific chart regarding the means and nature of material, and the focus on THC or CBD:

Temperature =/- 5 F or 3C	300 F/149 C	HOT OIL	212 F/100 C (WATER BOILS AT SEA LEVEL)
Means of Heating	OVEN	---	BOILING WATER (BATH OR DOUBLE BOILER MAX)

High THC (plant)	10-18 MIN	---	90-120 MIN
High CBD (plant)	15-25 MIN	---	2-4 MIN
High THC (kif or hash)	5-10 MIN	--	90-120 MIN
High CBD (kif or hash)	10-15 MIN	--	--
Infused cannabis oil	--	UNTIL BUBBLES DIMMINISH OR CEASE TO FORM	---

B) INHALATION

There is some question as to whether smoking cannabis involves an increased risk of lung cancer. A recent population-based study indicated that this was not detectably the case. Smoking cannabis does, as does inhaling any other form of burning plant material, irritate lung tissues and may increase the risk of COPD or aggravate existing pulmonary conditions. Vapourizing – heating the material to slightly below the point of combustion and inhaling the compounds released – is safer, and preferred by many medical personnel, especially for patients whose lung function is already compromised. This is normally done by means of plug-in or battery-powered devices designed for the specific function; some even have temperature controls that allow the user to alter the proportions of THC and CBD inhaled (CBD vapourizes between 66-185 C/160-365 F; THC does not boil until 200 C/392 F).

After the Catastrophe, if vapourization is preferred, it will probably be necessary to use either a manual vaporizer (a small pipe terminating in a glass bulb where the plant material is placed; the bulb is then heated from below with a candle) or something more resembling an opium pipe or the two-foil method used by smokers of heroin, where the material is placed on one piece of heavy foil and heated from below, its vapours then being quickly sucked up through a tube rolled from the second piece of foil.

c) Alcoholic Extracts: Tincture, Wine, and Beer

Cannabis tincture may be made with either alcohol or glycerine (see Part I for a full discussion of the storage and use of glycerine in the post-Catastrophe world. Short version: if you or any of your prospective patients can't or won't use small amounts of medicinal alcohol, stockpile glycerine: it can last up to 20 years if kept in a dark cool place, and does not become dangerous even when it does degrade). Alcohol is a more efficient means of extraction; glycerine requires frequent agitating and may never be as strong as an alcoholic tincture made with the same amount and potency of plant material. The dry plant material is crushed and covered with alcohol or glycerine. The higher the percentage of alcohol, the more efficient the extraction will be, although perfectly acceptable results have been reported not only from the use of standard spirits (40%/80 proof), but from wine and even strong beer, particularly if the cannabis is introduced at the same time as the hops or other flavourings and not strained out until it is time to move the beer into its final bottles or keg.

One ounce (30 grams) of high-quality dried cannabis flowers, in a standard 5 gallon/40 litre batch of homebrewed beer, is said to produce approximately the same effect per bottle as smoking a single joint, and to give a rather pleasant dry herbal flavour to the beer. Given the close relationship of hemp to hops, and the number of terpenes some strains share with hops, perhaps this is not surprising. The Canadian company Province Brands is shortly to release a non-alcoholic, gluten-free beer brewed from the stems and roots of cannabis plants, containing ca. 6.5 mg THC or, according to the brewer, a potency by which one cannabis beer = roughly the effect level of one standard alcoholic beer. How they managed to evolve a recipe that didn't taste like lawn clippings remains their own secret, but one gathers it wasn't easy.

The plant material is left in the tincture for up to a month (maceration) in a dark place before straining and rebottling. It may be beneficial to shake it once or twice a day with alcohol, and is virtually necessary with glycerine. Any aerial part of the plant may be used (no cannabinoids in the roots), but varying parts give varying potencies. The flowers are the most potent and richest in the small resin glands where a majority of THC is stored, followed by the small leaves growing from the aggregations of flower buds; then the larger "fan leaves"; and finally the stems. Many home producers prefer to reserve the flowers of this plant for inhalation, while making tinctures or lipid extracts from the leaves and perhaps the stems.

This decision will probably be a matter of the quantities of plant available to you, your expected medicinal uses, and your other uses. It is highly likely that the stems will be of far, far more benefit as a source of fibre for ropes and clothing than they could ever be as a low-potency source of medicine. If the potency of your finished tincture is insufficient to your expected usage, maceration may be repeated with more dry plant material.

D) Lipid-medium Extracts: Oil and Butter

An infused oil for oral or topical use may be produced by maceration in the same manner as a tincture, or it may be prepared by means of gently heating the plant material in the oil for 3-12 hours, paying close attention to the temperature guides given above. Any food-grade oil is suited for this purpose. While hempseed oil contains neither THC nor CBD, it does have anti-inflammatory action of its own when taken orally. Hempseed oil should never be heated above 150 C/300 F, and cannot be used for frying. It is better taken as a supplement or used as a basis for salad dressings. Cannabis-infused butter is often used in producing medicinal edibles.

A common ratio is ½ oz (14 grams) of hemp flowers to one pound (454 grams) of butter; though it is more common to make butter with the large fan leaves, while reserving the flowers for inhalation. Butter-making is done in the same manner in which oil production by heating is carried out. Some producers recommend the use of a double-boiler to keep the butter from getting too hot, or else mix it with water to ensure that the temperature never rises above 100 C/212 F. After straining, the bowl with the butter/water mixture is set aside. The butter will solidify on top when cool and can then easily be scooped off and used for baking in the same manner as ordinary butter.

Some people recommend using ghee, or clarified butter, especially in situations where you do not have a refrigerator: clarified butter keeps a good deal longer at room temperature than whole butter does. To clarify your own butter, melt it gently in a pan. You will observe it separating into a clear layer and a layer of solid whitish particles. Gently pour the clear layer off; that is your clarified butter. The particles can be spread on bread (though it may be salty if you didn't start with desalted butter), or incorporated into cheese; they are quite edible. Either dried or fresh cannabis can be used in the warmth-method infused oil or the butter, since the heat used is sufficient to decarboxylate the herb; however, fully decarboxylating first is said to produce a more efficient result.

Many people have also reported that dried herb is preferable if the intention is to eat or cook with the product, as fresh cannabis, especially if the leaves are the main part used for the purpose (common in oil and butter infusion), also contributes quite a bit of chlorophyll. This notoriously results in a "green" taste (those lawn-clippings again). The mild heating used for this method does not melt or evaporate THC/CBD into the oil; it merely speeds the normal process of dissolving these substances. Butter, of course, has to be liquid to achieve an infusion effect.

E) High-Potency Concentrates: Hash Oil, Rosin

After the Catastrophe, you will retain the option of making a "hash oil" or "honey oil" extract. The safest way to do this, and the way that is most likely to be available to you, is to make an extremely powerful and concentrated tincture in high-percentage (60% +, and higher is better) ethanol, then evaporate it slowly and carefully (remember, ethanol and its vapours are very flammable) to further concentrate the medicinal constituents. The result is reported to be a somewhat "tarry" substance of extremely high potency, which can be vapourized or dissolved in alcohol or a lipid.

If you have the capability to distill essential oils – and if you had the good luck to get or learn how to make a home essential oil still before the Catastrophe or if your survival group is producing its own spirits, you should - it is said that one of the most effective anti-nauseants known to humanity is one batch (ca. 1 oz dried flowers) of cannabis extract dissolved in 10 ml (roughly two teaspoons) peppermint essential oil. A single drop on the tongue is all that is likely to be required, or that drop can be dissolved into a teaspoon of food-grade oil and applied topically, with the essential oil causing quick absorption.

Undiluted peppermint oil can cause unpleasant burning sensations and even raise a welt on sensitive skin, so dilution is very much recommended. Another, though far more hazardous, means of making such an extract requires that you either have stockpiled or found somewhere a quantity of high-purity lighter fluid (the Newport brand is perhaps the best-known), and also prepared yourself beforehand with the small simple device known as the Honeybee (available at many shops which specialize in cannabis-related products) and some coffee filters. Dry plant material is powdered into the Honeybee until it is full; the perforated bottom, in which a circle of coffee filter or equivalent sits to keep crumbs out of the product, is positioned over a glass or ceramic bowl, and the lighter fluid is sprayed into the top as if refilling a lighter, dripping down through the plant material and extracting the medicinal components on the way.

Be warned: butane vapour is extremely flammable, and highly unhealthy to breathe. Do not even think about trying this except in a well-ventilated area where there is no risk of stray sparks! The most minute spark caused by static electricity or the hobnails of your boot scuffing on a stone could completely obviate all the effort you have put into surviving the Catastrophe and living this long...and, in fact, obviate your remains as well. Your author may want to put this on the list of, "How characters can kill themselves by stupidity or carelessness even if they survived the actual Catastrophe" plot options. Assuming that you did actually manage the highly dangerous part of the process without blowing yourself up, which may or may not be something that can be assumed, leave the bowl with the extract in a safe place with good ventilation for twenty-four hours to ensure that all the butane has evaporated. Ideally, it is best to put that bowl inside a bowl of hot water to increase the rate of butane evaporation.

The result has been described as a "honey-coloured" substance with the texture of slightly sticky lacquer. It may be either scraped up with a knife or dissolved by alcohol or oil; the same technique mentioned above for producing an alcohol extract/essential oil blend should be equally effective for a butane extract. Rosin is a recently evolved substitute for the more difficult and potentially dangerous process of making butane hash oil.

The basic idea is that either slightly dried buds or a quantity of hashish are subjected to heat and pressure, causing the expulsion of a small quantity of extremely powerful concentrate. There are now commercial rosin presses available, though they are rather expensive; a more common means of producing one's own involves the use of a hair straightener.

The raw material is wrapped in parchment paper and put inside a hair straightener at the lowest setting (280-330 F/138-166 C), with pressure exerted for 3-7 seconds. A faint sizzle should be audible. The flattened plant material is then removed for reuse in tincture, butter, or oil; the rosin itself is scraped off the parchment paper. After the Catastrophe, if electricity is no longer available to you, it will be more of a challenge to gauge the temperature of a hand-operated press or vise, but the convenience of using the concentrated extract (and the absence of risk in making it, unlike butane hash oil) may make the effort worthwhile.

"Live rosin" is a term used to describe rosin that has been pressed either from buds that have only had two or three days to dry (just enough so that they don't explode in a cloud of steam when subjected to heat and pressure) or from "bubble hash" (ice water separation of fresh-frozen resin from plant material. Both bubble hash and rosin are highly prized where legally available in real life, as these methods of extraction preserve the highest percentage of the valuable but volatile medicinal terpenes (and are said to contribute considerably to the user's enjoyment as well).

Hash oil and rosin may be mixed into lipids or alcohol; added in small quantities (1 minute drop) to smoking herbs of any sort; or inhaled via a vapourizer or dabber. A dabber is a long, heatproof tool with a point or tiny spoon on the end, designed to transfer concentrate to the hot surface on which it will vapourize. The simplest version of the latter would be a large flat-headed nail heated up with a small torch; many more efficient "dabber rigs" are available on the market today, with the nail being enclosed in glass or ceramic to collect the vapour and make it easier to inhale efficiently.

F) Ointments and Creams

For the base, room-temperature-liquid food-grade oil (4-5 parts – more oil makes a softer ointment) and wax (1 part; preferably beeswax, but paraffin will work) are gently melted together. A double boiler is optimal to keep the temperature from ever getting high enough to cook the cannabinoids out of your materials. If you want to avoid straining, you can use a pre-infused hemp oil. Otherwise, you can put the plant material in now, enough that the oil/wax mix covers it by one to two inches. Flowers or any of the hemp's leaves can be used for this purpose.

They can be either fresh or dry, since the heating will decarboxylate the main cannabinoids; but again, pre-decarboxylating may have more efficient results. Fresh material, because of its liquid content, will make a slightly softer ointment. Warm until all the wax has melted into the infused oil or the dry herb has steeped for 2-3 hours at a low heat. To test the texture, dip a spoon or knife-blade into the mix so that the bowl/blade is coated.

Pull it out and allow it to solidify, then rub the result on your skin. If it is too gloppy, add more wax. If it is too hard, add more oil. Continue until either you are satisfied with the texture, or run out of space in the pot. If you used any whole herbs, strain now. You may also stir in any other essential oils you wish to add at this time. Bottle quickly, seal, and label.

A cream is softer than an ointment and absorbs into the skin much more easily, without leaving the greasy texture characteristic of ointments. As well as oil with lipid-soluble ingredients and wax, a cream will include water and water-soluble ingredients. Therefore, as oil and water proverbially do not blend, making a cream requires an emulsifier (a substance which binds to both). Most people in real life order these from a natural cosmetic supply or health food store.

There are a wide range, but the two likeliest to be available to you after the Catastrophe (depending on where you live) are carrageenan and soap (usually a "castile" soap, which is properly made with olive oil as the fat, though any oil can be used). These are added to the oil/wax phase of the process at a ratio of approximately 5-8% of the total. So: 1/2 cup of wax, 3.5 cups of oil, and 6 cups of water (a .5 to 3.5 to 6 ratio) would require .5 - .8 cup of castile soap or carrageenan. A lotion is relatively liquid. The proportions are roughly 1 part oil to 6 parts water or water-based substance.

How to make Castile Soap

» 37.5 oz. vegetable oil (traditionally olive, but any vegetable oil will do)
» 9.4 oz. potassium hydroxide (KOH)
» 20.2 oz. water, preferably distilled
» 8 oz glycerine.

Warm oils on low heat. Mix water with glycerine. Add KOH to the mixture. Do this in a well-ventilated place and wear safety goggles, long sleeves, hat, and gloves; the mixture will heat up.

Always add the KOH to the water and not the other way around! Do not inhale the fumes! Add the mixture to the oils and stir until your soap becomes opaque and thick.

Continue to cook on low heat for several hours, until the mixture becomes translucent. Essential oils or powdered herbs may be added at this point.

This recipe produces 4-4.5 lbs of concentrated soap paste, which can be diluted to 1-2 gallons of liquid soap.

> Potassium hydroxide, a form of lye, is simply obtained by:
>
> 1) Drilling holes in the bottom of a watertight wooden container such as an old barrel.
> 2) Covering the bottom of the barrel with a layer of gravel, then a layer of straw.
> 3) Filling the rest of the barrel with hardwood ashes.
> 4) Pouring rainwater into the barrel and allowing it to drain through into an iron or steel pot (do not use this pot for any other purpose afterwards!).
> 5) Repeat until the solution is strong enough to float an egg in (roughly a nickel- to quarter-sized, or 5-cent to 50-cent for Euro-based coinage, should be visible above the top of the liquid.
>
> This liquid can be used directly in place of the KOH-powder/water mixture in the recipe above, at a total of 29.6 oz.

Aloe vera gel is often used for both its textural and its skin-care functions; a common proportion for such a lotion would be 1 part oil to 1 part aloe vera gel to 5 parts water, plus ca. 3-4% emulsifier. To produce carrageenan: this substance is dissolved from seaweed via hot water. A proportion of roughly 5 ounces (150 grams) of the base seaweed (Irish Moss, common on shores on both sides of the North Atlantic) is boiled and stirred in 8 quarts (7.57 litres) of water for ten minutes. 2 more quarts (1.9 litres) of cold water are added; the whole is strained when it becomes cool enough (a jelly bag will do nicely) and left to cool until it gels.

The gel can then be dried by simple evaporation and powdered. This is not as fine or pure as the more elaborate means of processing commonly used by real-life producers, but it will serve the purpose. A topical hemp cream would get its cannabinoids via the use of an infused oil or replacing part of the water/water-based ingredients with an alcohol or glycerine tincture. If herbs with water-soluble constituents are to be added to the cream, it is generally best to steep them in the water beforehand as if making an infusion. Aloe vera gel (the gel inside the leaf) may be substituted for part of the water in order to achieve a smoother texture and gain the benefits of this herb for conditions such as eczema, psoriasis, and burns.

g) Suppositories and Pessaries

Suppositories are inserted into the rectum. Pessaries are inserted into the vagina. Both are designed to slowly dissolve, delivering both local and systemic effects. They are used locally for pain, inflammation, and infections (fungal and bacterial); systemically when a patient is badly nauseated and cannot tolerate oral medication, but IV treatment is not optional. A very small study (2 patients) indicated that rectal bioavailability of THC alone was ca. 50% higher and 25-50% more effective than oral lipid bioavailability, probably due to avoiding the first-pass metabolism transit through the liver.

The doses used (2.5-5 mg synthesized THC rectal) were effective at reducing pain and spasticity, and showed no noticeable psychoactivity or cardiovascular sequelae. The best medium for a suppository or pessary is an oil which is solid at room temperature, but melts at body temperature. Coconut oil is particularly favoured, having the optimal melting qualities and, in cases of yeast infection, having its own anti-fungal benefits. Cocoa butter is also good; it melts more slowly, which may be of advantage to the person who can't administer it immediately before having a lie-down. Beeswax by itself does not melt at human body temperature (its melting point is 145-47 F/63-64 C).

However, it may be mixed with a food oil such as olive, flax, hempseed, or any other suitable for human consumption at a rate of 1-2 parts oil to 1 part beeswax in order to produce a solid insertion that will slowly dissolve. Dosage may be roughly calculated as per the guidelines given below. There are no clear guidelines for specific dosing. The hemp (leaves or flowers) may be infused directly into coconut oil or cocoa butter by means of slow heating (121 C/250 F until bubbles stop forming or for ca. 45 minutes); or, if using a beeswax/food oil mixture, one can use a food oil that has already been hemp-infused.

Strain the infused oil/butter or stir the beeswax/oil mix thoroughly together. If desired, a few drops of appropriate essential oils (calculate as 1 drop/dose) may be stirred in at this point. Lemongrass and oregano are recommended, in particular, for yeast infections. A quarter-teaspoon of honey per dose may also be useful if the intention is to treat bacterial infections (not such a good idea where there are yeast infections; yeast thrives on sugars!). Pour into moulds. There are a number of options here. The thing is to size the insertion appropriately so that it will go in comfortably and stay in until it melts; and to avoid sharp edges.

Anything from an ice cube tray that does round cubes to a small hollow romantic aid is excellent for the purpose. Lining the mould with parchment paper or a small amount of lubricant may aid in removing the insertion from the mould. Freeze, or at least chill as best you can. Remove insertions and keep them well-sealed in a cool place until they are needed. Insert into the appropriate orifice just before bedtime, or plan to lie down for an hour or so while melting and absorption take place if you need to apply more than 1x/day.

h) CBD Oil

There is some general confusion as to what "CBD oil" actually is. The term is used for the extract – the CBD equivalent of "hash oil" - for products with the extract dissolved in a carrier oil; and carrier oil infused with industrial minimal-THC cannabis. The issue is further confused by the use of the popular and legal-looking term "CBD" oil for extracts or infusions which actually contain THC as well; some people distinguish between "hemp CBD oil" (industrial cannabis, negligible amounts of THC) and "marijuana CBD oil" (medicinal hemp, varying amounts of THC). There are a number of sites on-line which purport to instruct in "how to make CBD oil". I looked at every one of these I could find.

Not one described how to make an oil in which the THC (or other cannabinoids) could be separated from the CBD. Without exception, they were simply descriptions of how to make full-spectrum cannabis oils by every means from simple infusion to butane extraction. Useful in producing a whole-cannabis product; potentially dangerous if one were to attempt such a method in the belief that one would achieve a non-psychoactive result and, say, attempt to drive after using it (plus, see above cautions regarding the suspected role of THC in cardiovascular risk).

The only way to get a CBD oil by any of these methods would be to start with plant material which contained only trace amounts of THC (industrial or special CBD medicinal strains); and the only way to do it efficiently at home, given the low percentage of CBD in industrial cannabis (< 3.5%), would be to use a specially bred high-CBD/minimal THC medicinal strain such as Avidekel (< 1% THC:15-18% CBD) or Candida CD-1 (0.5% THC:11-15% CBD). Even then, a high concentration would mean that, say, a toxicology test might well find measurable amounts of THC in the bloodstream, although such a product would probably suffice as a CBD oil in all practical terms. Keeping the temperature as low as possible, ideally below 66 C/150 F, is crucial for maximum CBD retention; remember that your CBD starts to evaporate before your THC!

Regrettably for the survivor of the Catastrophe who would like to produce a true CBD oil from the one or two strains they have acquired randomly by whatever means possible after the Catastrophe – this is not a simple process. Hypothetically, a very prolonged steam distillation (maximum 100 C/212 F) might slowly melt and evaporate the majority of the CBD along with the aromatic constituents, leaving the THC in place. But I am not aware of this method ever having been tested; there is no data suggesting how effective it might or might not be; and a random strain might not have enough CBD to make it worthwhile.

Given that the maximum CBD level of industrial (fibre/seed commercial use at this time) hemp seems to be ca. 3-3.5%, and most industrial strains are lower than that, their value in CBD oil production is primarily to the large producer who can readily extract and concentrate the low percentage of CBD from a high volume of plant material, and uses industrial hemp for this purpose because of legal issues and availability in quantity. Having said that, if you have no richer source of CBD available, or need a largely-pure CBD oil and do not possess one of the aforementioned CBD-rich strains (and if the hypothetical long-steaming doesn't get enough CBD out to be worthwhile), the whole-cannabis methods I have mentioned could be used on industrial hemp for this purpose.

I) Cannabis Roots

Traditionally, cannabis roots were juiced (fresh), extracted with hot water (fresh or dried), or pulverized and mixed into wine for an alcoholic solution. The majority of the historical uses were topical (Ryz, Remillard, and Russo, op. cit.). Friedelin, one of the chief anti-inflammatory components of the root, does not mix well with water and has a very high melting point (503.6-509 F), but it is soluble in alcohol. For the full profile of anti-inflammatory and analgesic components, hemp root could reasonably be juiced and used fresh, the juice mixed with alcohol, or an alcoholic tincture made from the fresh or dried root. It is also possible to use the fresh juice to make a cream or lotion, as described above, simply by substituting it for the "water" component of the mixture.

J) Timing and Potency of Different Forms of Administration

Inhaled cannabis, whether smoke or vapor, takes effect quickly and passes off relatively quickly, from 2 to 4 hours depending on strength and quantity. It is, however, not recommended to do anything that might be the equivalent of driving or working with heavy machinery until at least 6 hours after the last inhaled dose.

Cannabis extract in an alcohol medium takes effect very quickly when absorbed through the membranes of the mouth; quickly (less than half an hour) when swallowed as an oral medication. Its potency is generally considered, dose for dose (and always depending on how strong the tincture was in the first place), to be comparable to that of inhaled cannabis. This is certainly the potency for which you are aiming in your preparation.

Topically-applied cannabis in a lipid extract (including ointments, creams, and lotions) also takes effect quickly. Its potency in terms of psychoactive effects is generally lower than that of any form of ingested cannabis medication; but its anti-inflammatory capacities as a topical medication compensate for that, making this a preferable means of administration when a lesser degree of psychoactivity is desired, as well as for treating a patient who is too badly nauseated to tolerate any form of oral dosing. It would be particularly effective for the treatment of chronic pain/inflammatory joint conditions.

Oil-or butter-based oral cannabis takes effect slowly; it may be as long as two hours before the full effects are felt. It also lasts longer, usually 6 to 8 hours in perceived effect, with a recommendation of no less than 12 hours before taking part in any potentially hazardous activities.

The delta-nine THC (natural form) taken in a lipid medium is processed into 11-hydroxyl THC, a significantly more potent form, by the human liver. Some of the nineteenth-century European descriptions of eating extremely large doses of hashish mixed with butter, nuts, and spices (Fitz Hugh-Ludlow; Théophile Gautier and other members of the Parisian "Club des Haschishins", which was just what the name sounds like – a club of hashish eaters, which included such notables as Baudelaire and Victor Hugo) are more comparable to more recent accounts of major psychedelic drugs than to the usually-expected effects of cannabis. However, low doses of lipid-medium cannabis, assuming that one does not have to drive, ride, run a chainsaw, or similar, are more useful for ongoing chronic pain control due to the prolonged duration.

Pessaries and suppositories take effect in a psychoactive sense more swiftly than oral lipid hemp, but more slowly than mucous-applied alcohol-based remedies. The drug passes straight into the bloodstream without being processed through the liver (the lower 2/3 of the rectum drains directly into systemic circulation, whereas the GI tract above that drains into the portal system which leads into the liver). Like topical preparations, the psychoactive effects are generally comparatively low. However, inserted delivery mechanisms will mostly be administered for their local effects on pain, inflammation, and fungal infections.

The above-described method of dissolving a concentrated cannabis extract in peppermint oil is said to take effect very swiftly. This is particularly marked when it is used to control nausea and vomiting, although whether the swift initial relief is due more to the peppermint oil, the cannabis, or a synergy between the two remains undetermined. For new or inexperienced users, the recommendation is usually to start with one of the methods that is quickly absorbed and quickly metabolized, such as vapourizing or sublingual/buccal spray, at a minimal dose (one to two inhalations from a vapourizer, or a single spray). The full effects should be clear within half an hour, at which time the patient can titrate up slowly if required, or wait for the effects to diminish if needed. It is also advised, if possible, to have a fast-acting preparation of CBD (or high CBD/low THC) available for the cannabis-naïve user: as CBD can counteract the psychoactive effects of THC, it is useful as an antidote for excessive psychoactivation.

K) Raw Cannabis

Many claims regarding the potential health benefits of eating or juicing raw cannabis have recently been made, though solid documentation is difficult to find. There do not seem to have been any clinical studies done. However, the most probable benefits of raw cannabis include:

1) Fibre supplementation. Yes, raw hemp leaves certainly do provide dietary fibre, which is important for proper bowel function (especially in a patient who requires opiate pain control).
2) Terpenes. Raw fresh hemp contains the maximum potential terpenes in the plant, as it has not been subjected to the heating and/or drying which causes the more volatile terpenes to evaporate even as it transforms the primary cannabinoids into their active forms.
3) Vitamins and minerals. Like the majority of leafy green vegetables, cannabis contains folate (B9), iron, calcium, vitamin C, and vitamin K.
4) Potential anti-cancer effects. This requires further study, but the initial investigations appear quite promising, at least in regards to prostate cancer.
5) Greatly lowered psychoactive effects while retaining many of the active benefits of the herb. While a small amount of THCa converts to THC very readily, it is generally not to a degree which causes significant effects. This is of no small importance in treating a patient whose duties, lifestyle, or religion do not permit psychoactive drugs, but who may benefit from the THC-a, CBD-a, and terpene content.

THCa, the non-decarboxylated predecessor of psychoactive THC, has shown protection of dopaminergic neurons, as does THC itself. THCa, however, is a stronger agonist (activator) of PPAR□ than decarboxylated THC. Thus, it is more highly neuroprotective for diseases characterized by dopamine dysregulation such as Huntington's and quite possibly Parkinson's and other neurological diseases characterized by inflammation and degeneration. In this regard, THCa also may be better suited as an agent of glucose and lipid metabolism regulation in type II diabetes, actually outperforming rozaglitazone, one of the drugs currently used for this purpose, in terms of both PPARy metabolism and safety profile. [cxxvii]

In rodent studies, THCa has been shown to be a more powerful treatment for nausea and vomiting than THC, as well as lacking the psychoactive side effects which can be inappropriate and/or distressing for some. Making smoothies from or juicing raw cannabis has become something of a health fad in areas where growing is legal. Dr. William Courtney, one of the main advocates for raw cannabis, suggests up to 15 fresh fan leaves and 2 large buds harvested early (when trichomes are clear, as described in the section below on harvesting medicinals). Fresh buds in this state would have to be frozen to maintain a regular supply, as otherwise there is a relatively short window (< 1 month) in each spate of growing; dried herb is said to lose some of the alleged benefits (some terpenes lost to drying process; THCa and CBDa converting into activated THC and CBD). Most people who use raw cannabis mix it with other vegetable or fruit juices, as the flavour of cannabis juice alone is reported to be not particularly nice.

L) Determining dosage and potency

Fortunately for your patients - since you, after the Catastrophe, no longer have access to either real pharmaceuticals or the means of directly measuring the active components of your herbal medications - precision in dosage is seldom if ever required in administering medicinal cannabis. Depending on the patient, their condition, and how tolerable they find the psychoactive side effects, a single dose may range from 1 mg THC/1 mg each of THC and CBD, to 2000 mg or even more. The same rules that apply to herbal medications in general apply to cannabis: because of variances in weather, etc., you cannot depend on any given batch being of the same potency or even the same THC:CBD ratio as the one before it, even if the method of preparation does not change.

A good general guide to your goals regarding convenient potency for practical usage, however, is: If starting with a strain that you roughly know the THC content of, it is easy to calculate within a general range. Since, unlike the rest of the herbs in this book, even a large error on the positive side of dosage is unlikely to be harmful, going by rule-of-thumb is good enough with cannabis. If you don't know the THC level, you can generally best-guess range by testing the batch (the best tester being someone who has had extensive experience with medicinal and/or recreational hemp):

< 10% - low potency for most modern strains, though often seen in 1:1 THC:CBD cultivars.
11-14% - moderate potency
15-20% - high potency
> 20% - very high potency

For convenience, the example I give will be for a modern high-powered strain of 20% THC.

» Trim (the small leaves with all the little resin-heads that are trimmed off the bud when it is prepared for drying or inhalation): ca. 10% THC by dry weight. 1000 mg (0.035 oz) trim = 100 mg THC, or 10 10 mg doses of cannabutter or oil in a batch containing one gram of good trim.
» Buds: 20% THC by dry weight. 1000 mg flowers = 200 mg THC.
» Fan leaves (the big spreading ones): 5% THC by dry weight. 1000 mg fan leaves = 50 mg THC.
» Tincture: 1 litre ethanol (40-70%) = 1000 ml. At 10 grams (ca. 1/3 oz, dry weight) of trim (est. 10%), 1 ml = 1 mg THC. At 100 gr of trim (roughly 3.3 oz), 1 ml = 10 mg THC. Double estimates for buds.
» Rosin – ca. 3-4x percentage of cannabinoid in flower (20% THC, 5% CBD in flowers = 60-80% THC, 15-20% CBD in rosin)
» Hashish – high-quality resin, such as bubble-hash or the best dry-sifted, may be up to 3x percentage of cannabinoids in flower.
» 1 gram rosin from 20%/5% = 600-800 mg THC, 150-200 mg CBD
» 1 gram hash from the same plant = 400-600 mg THC, 100-150 mg CBD
» 1 gram flowers = 200 mg THC, 50 mg CBD
» 1 gram trim = 100 mg THC, 25 mg CBD
» 1 gram fan leaves = 50 mg THC, 12.5 mg CBD

As mentioned before, dosage levels are only beginning to be established, particularly for THC. The common estimated strength of a gentle inhaled recreational dose is ca. 30 mg THC, or ca. 1/7 of a gram of strong dried buds. For lipid-medium oral dosage, 2.5 mg THC is considered a solid starting point, and many commercial edibles use 10 mg as their dose standard; but far higher doses can be tolerated and are often desired by more experienced users.

CBD can be calculated in a similar manner if you roughly know the CBD percentage of your strain. Unfortunately, not being psychoactive, CBD levels are more difficult than THC to gauge by subjective testing. Fibre hemp flowers range between 0.5 and 3.5% CBD, but there are concerns about using these plants for human intake, as they are often grown in areas of high industrial pollution to help the ground recover, and may contain various toxins. The most common recommendations for CBD dosage:

» General health: 2.5-15 mg CBD
» Chronic pain: 2.5-20 mg CBD
» Sleep disorders: 45-60 mg CBD.

In most studies regarding, for instance, epilepsy, oral CBD is given in very high doses. Oral CBD has quite low bioavailability, so higher dosing is needed for efficacy. Cannabidiol doses of up to 300 mg daily have been used safely for up to 6 months. Higher doses of 1200-1500 mg daily have been used safely for up to 4 weeks. Cannabidiol sprays used under the tongue have been used in doses of 2.5 mg for up to 2 weeks.

The Mayo Clinic's recommendations show the wide range of therapeutic dosages available, particularly for CBD:

» Loss of Appetite in Cancer Patients: 2.5mg of THC (orally), with or without 1mg of CBD for six weeks.
» Chronic Pain: 2.5-20mg of CBD [with or without THC] (orally).
» Epilepsy: 200-300mg of CBD (orally) daily.
» Movement Problems Due to Huntington's Disease: 10mg of CBD per kg of body weight daily for six weeks (orally).
» Sleep Disorders: 40mg-160mg of CBD (orally).
» Multiple Sclerosis (MS) symptoms: Cannabis plant extracts containing 2.5-120 milligrams of a THC/CBD combination daily for 2-15 weeks.
» Patients typically use eight sprays within any three hours, with a maximum of 48 sprays in any 24-hour period.
» Schizophrenia: 40-1,280mg oral CBD daily.
» Glaucoma: A single sub-lingual CBD dosage of 20-40mg (>40 mg may increase eye pressure).

An alternate dosage chart for CBD by body weight and pain levels:

BODY WEIGHT	<25 lbs 11 kg	26-45 lbs 12-20 kg	46-85 lbs 21-38 kg>
PAIN LEVEL 0-3 NONE-MILD	4.5 MG	6 MG	9 MG
PAIN LEVEL 4-6 MODERATE	6MG	9 MG	12 MG
7+ SEVERE	9 MG	12 MG	15 MG

BODY WEIGHT	86-150 lbs/39-68 kg	151-240 lbs/68.5-109 kg	241 lbs/109.5 kg>
PAIN LEVEL 0-3 NONE-MILD	12 MG	18 MG	22.5 MG
PAIN LEVEL 4-6 MODERATE	15 MG	22.5 MG	30 MG
7+ SEVERE	18 MG	27 MG	45 MG

Sativex spray (an alcohol-based 1:1 compound for oral spraying) - 1 dose = 2.5 mg CBD/THC; repeat and titrate up as needed. You could kill yourself uptitrating too much and too quickly with paracetamol or other over-the-counter painkillers. You cannot kill yourself with Sativex, even if you drank the whole bottle on a oner (unless it were an industrial litre-sized bottle, I guess...but the cannabis wouldn't be what killed you; that would be the alcohol).

Estimating CBD (or THC) in tincture administered by dropper:

- •1 dropper normally contains 1 ml of liquid. Calculate specific cannabinoid dose per ml for the batch of tincture as described above.
- •1 ml, for practical purposes, equals roughly 20 drops from a standard medicinal dropper.

Bioavailability

THC has a higher bioavailability than CBD via almost every route of administration. As mentioned above, the oral bioavailability of CBD is pretty low, with studies measuring a range between 4 and 20%. A 1986 study reported a bioavailability rate of 6%, while a 2009 study reported it between 4% and 20%. While both findings differ significantly, both are pretty low, with a 20% bioavailability rate being the most optimistic scenario (of a 100 mg oral dose, only 20 mg will be absorbed and effective).

» Sublingual consumption of CBD and THC - reported rates range from 8-40%.
» Smoking – 2-56% THC absorbed.

The only exception to THC absorbing more readily than CBD is transdermal administration, in which the absorption of CBD (and CBN) are 10x higher than THC. Both delta-8 THC (very similar to d-9; also psychotropic; generally included in overall THC percentages) and CBD absorptions were significantly enhanced by a 30-33% ethanol medium.

Guidelines for estimated strength:

These are easy and convenient units to work with, and if you have a rough idea of the cannabinoid contents of your medicinal material, you should be able to calculate how much and what type of plant material is needed per batch to achieve appropriate strength.

- •1 dose of tincture = 1 teaspoon of alcohol-medium or 2 teaspoons of glycerine-medium.
- •1 dose of topical infused oil = 1 to 2 tablespoons
- •1 dose of oral infused oil or butter = 1 teaspoon. After the potency of the lipid batch has been experimentally confirmed, the amount of oil or butter desired in a batch of baked goods can then easily be calculated. If the recipe calls for more oil or butter than the cannabis dosage required, it can of course be topped up with ordinary oil or butter.
- •1 dose of extract-containing essential oil of peppermint, topically or orally = 1 drop

- 1 dose of inhaled cannabis = roughly the equivalent of 1 joint or small pipe-bowl full; basically a large pinch. If you still have a working vapourizer or have been able to MacGyver a functional equivalent, vapourizing is markedly more efficient than smoking, since a significant percentage of the essential constituents are lost in direct combustion. Start with half the smoked dose in the vapourizer. If that doesn't do the job, you can always vapourize more.

The optimum tester is a healthy adult with experience in the effects of at least inhaled and lipid-medium cannabis. Because cannabis tolerance is not developed in the same way that tolerance to drugs such as alcohol and opiates/oids is, there should be little or no concern that such a tester, even if they are a regular user, will underestimate the comparative effect of a preparation upon a cannabis-naïve patient, although lengthy experience and increased comfort with effects that might unnerve the novice may incline them to prefer stronger dosages for their own use.Inhaled and oral-membrane-spray cannabis are the easiest forms to titrate up at need (or if the patient finds the dosage uncomfortable, the swiftest to wear off), followed by peppermint oil and alcohol/glycerine tincture, then topical oil/ointment.

Oral lipid-medium cannabis, because of its very long duration, is extremely problematical regarding titration. It might be advisable, if the oral dose seems insufficient after two hours, to titrate the overall level upwards by means of inhalation or administering tincture, rather than giving the patient more lipid-medium oral cannabis. All tinctures and oils, if their potency is insufficient upon testing, may be strengthened by adding more dry plant material and repeating the process as necessary. Microdosing (1-2.5 mg of each desired cannabinoid) is increasingly gaining in popularity, as many people receive therapeutic benefit (inflammation, nausea, anxiety, and some pain all appear to respond well to microdosing) at a dose below the quantity required for psychoactive effects.

Since it is so easy and safe to titrate upwards, there is no risk in beginning with a microdose and, if symptoms are not showing enough improvement within half an hour, gradually increasing the level bit by bit until the optimal balance is reached. If you have been able to grow both high-CBD and high-THC strains (or, in real life, if you have high-CBD products available), even more fine-tuning in this regard is possible, given both the counter-psychoactive CBD effects and the fact that CBD itself is significantly therapeutic for many of the conditions for which this herb is used.

III. The Plant

Cannabis sativa, a.k.a. hemp, has been a vital source of fibre, food, and frequently medicine for nearly as long as humans have had agriculture and textile arts. It is a dioecious plant, which means that an individual plant will usually be either male or female, though hermaphroditism does occur, usually as a response to lighting-period stress. The gender division of cannabis is crucial in many regards: only females produce seeds or large quantities of high-potency flowers; males are often either largely culled or, for fibre, harvested early; and the quality of fibres produced is different.

In common usage, cannabis is divided into two major sub-groups, called "sativa" and "indica". The latter is more accurately described as "cannabis sativa var. indica". There is also a third variant, C. ruderalis, discussed below. In real life (and hence undoubtedly in realistic fiction), no one cares even slightly that all three are technically the same species. Most people simply speak of "sativa, indica, ruderalis, and hybrids", and inaccurately separate industrial cannabis from C. sativa var. sativa.

Those varieties called "sativa" are generally taller-growing, often with a "leggier" phenotype, considerably better suited to fibre production because of their greater height, and tend to be higher in THC and lower in CBD. "Industrial hemp" is simply a generic term for those strains of C. sativa which show an intense sativa phenotype and minimal THC/low CBD content (bred specifically for central stalk height without regards to cannabinoid content over hundreds of years, and for minimal THC over the last three human generations or so).

The "indica" varieties are commonly shorter and more compact, and tend to have a higher CBD:THC ratio, although many variants also produce a high level of THC. C. indica was the approved source of medicinal cannabis for the British and American pharmacopiae, and would have been the variety used by Dr. W.B. O'Shaughnessy in his spectacular early discoveries. The breeding of hybrids for the purpose of producing plants with the desired characteristics of both...generally a more indica-like phenotype (easier to grow indoors), but with the higher THC levels plus or minus high CBD...is extremely common among both professional and hobby growers.

The third subspecies, Cannabis ruderalis, is a wild variant that is never seen on its own in practical usage. It is a small plant – little to no fibre-production value - with very low levels of the primary active constituents – little to no medicinal value. Its one significant trait, which has led to it being bred into the more valuable varieties to produce the increasingly popular high-potency "dwarf" or "auto-flowering" strains, is that it reaches medicinal harvest-stage maturity within eight to ten or twelve weeks of sprouting regardless of light levels (as described below, non-autoflowering varieties of cannabis are photoperiod-dependent).

This allows both for multiple harvests in the course of one year, and for keeping a medicinal strain with specific properties (the dwarf) separate from a strain grown chiefly for fibre and seeds (a tall medicinal or industrial "sativa" strain). As with the preference for the indica phenotype among many indoors growers, the smaller size of these plants makes them easier to grow in a restricted space and/or provide light for.

1) Site, Soil, and Sowing

a) Sizing and Siting Your Hemp Patch

i) Sizing

Thomas Jefferson noted that one worker could tend three acres of hemp/year. He was, of course, speaking of experienced workers. It would probably be imprudent to assume that you will be able to do as well as Jefferson's farmhands (free or slave) in the first year or two. S.M. Stirling describes, at some length, the difference between "what people with real traditional farming experience can achieve" and "what can be managed by modern, often previously-sedentary, novices" (Island in the Sea of Time and Dies the Fire). His portrayal is, if anything, optimistic. If, and only if, it's legal where you live, you would be very well advised to take at least a small patch of cannabis from sowing through fibre, seed, and medicinal harvests before the Catastrophe happens, so that you don't lose your crop or its products through ignorance when it really matters. Yields from industrial cannabis can range from two to six short tons (4000-12000 lbs, or circa 1800-5500 kilograms) of dry stalks per acre, depending on climate and soil.

You might reasonably expect that cannabis originally bred for medicinal qualities would tend towards the low end, especially the shorter indica or hybrid types, though some of the tall medicinal sativas, when grown outdoors, may rival the industrial sativas. The amount of useful textile fibre is generally in the neighborhood of 12-20% of the dry stalk weight. Hemp yield ranges from 25% to 50% greater than that of flax when grown on the same land. Cannabis seeds grown commercially have been cited, per acre, as producing anything from 800 lbs (ca. 318 kg), to ten times that amount.

This yields a possible minimum of 30 gallons (ca. 113.6 litres) of oil, plus up to 600 lbs (about 272 kilograms) of flour, and a possible maximum of three times that. If the maths don't sound like they add up, remember that oil is lighter than water, and water is the basis of 1 litre = 1 kilogram. The amount of any hemp product produced by professional commercial growers and their modern large-scale machinery will probably be greater than you can manage growing on your own in a post-Catastrophe environment. If you are a pre-Catastrophe prepper, I would definitely advise planning for the low end rather than the high end of those yields. And there is, of course, always a chance that any crop will fail completely in any given year.

Sometimes they all do, which is how people end up sacrificing their kings to the gods or burning sinners (terminology and victims change, human behaviour doesn't) in hopes that the harvest will be better next year. And when you get hungry and frightened enough because the weather went bad, the livestock died, and the grasshoppers ate all your grain or whatever, that sort of thing might start sounding like a good idea to you too. Along with eating what the Icelandic Landnámabók, in such circumstances, discreetly described as "many abominable things...which ought not to be eaten" (ch. 30). And they probably didn't mean slugs, as Iceland was blissfully slug-free until the invasion of Spanish slugs in 2003.

II) Siting and Fertilizing

Cannabis prefers light and warmth. It has often been observed that any situation and fertilizers which suit tomatoes will also suit cannabis. Tomatoes are not related to hemp; they are close kin to deadly nightshade, tobacco, and potatoes. Nonetheless, the habits and needs are very similar. Cannabis is also suspected of being vulnerable to tobacco mosaic virus, so do not plant it near tobacco, tomatoes, or deadly nightshade if you can avoid doing so. Aside from that, cannabis is said to serve well as a companion plant, since the powerfully aromatic terpenoids ward off many pests that affect other plants.

Your hemp field should be sited, if possible, in full sun. A rich, but well-drained soil, with a relatively neutral to mildly acid pH (no higher than 7, no lower than 6) is ideal. Standing water encourages fungus among the roots; excessive humidity encourages fungus in the flowers; both are very bad. Water availability is important in drier areas. Cannabis can be quite sensitive to drought, which produces stunted and lower-potency plants, not desirable for any purpose.

Cannabis prefers a pH level between 6.0 and 6.5, which is to say, mildly acidic. If the pH gets much below 6 or above 7, it will compromise the plant's ability to absorb nutrients, and signs of mixed nutrient deficiency may be seen (yellowing leaves from the bottom up – short of nitrogen; leaf edges curling upwards – magnesium deficiency; dark colouration between the veins – potassium deficiency). Droopy leaves in addition to one or more symptom suggest that the plant is being overwatered; allow to dry, and if that does not help, check for root rot (roots are brown and slimy. Cut away affected parts and replant in clean soil).

The ideal fertilizer provides a balance of nitrogen, phosphorus, and potassium, with a strong emphasis on nitrogen during the seedling and vegetative phases, phosphorus and potassium during flowering and fruiting stages. In real life, these fertilizers are available at any garden centre. After the Catastrophe – or indeed, before it or in real life if you want to find out how it works and/or avoid artificially-produced fertilizers – a mixture of fish, blood, and bone-meal, with a good quantity of well-aged horse or cow manure, should be worked into the soil before planting. This will suffice for the first months; supplemental fertilizers should be added every two weeks or so after the plant (assuming it is a standard; the dwarves aren't nearly as much use for fibre) has reached a height in the general neighborhood of 3 feet/1 metre.

Cannabis grows very fast in the vegetative stage and needs lots of nitrogen. One of the best options for a liquid fertilizer after the Catastrophe will be a water-based infusion in which aged manure and comfrey leaves (and you should be growing lots and lots of comfrey, given its immense valuable in speeding the healing of bruises, sprains, and broken bones, none of which will be in short supply after the Catastrophe) have been left to soak in the sun for a week or two. Dip the water out and sprinkle it around the roots. The urine-supplementation method I describe in Appendix I may also prove a good nitrogen source or enhancer for the manure/comfrey tea. Do be aware, however, that some strains need less fertilizer than others, particularly many of the pure "sativas".

If the tips of the leaves start curling into "claws", it's time to stop fertilizing for a while and give the plants plenty of clean water. When flowering commences, the nitrogen level of supplemental fertilizers should be lowered if possible. That is to say, cut down the amount of manure in the tea to less than ¼ and stop widdling in the pot. Add steamed bone meal instead to bring up the phosphorus level. If you can afford it at this time, a sugar such as molasses or honey may be added, especially if you have a way to separate your medicinal plants from your larger primarily-fibre/seed plants and thus can give the former special nurturing. Except for molasses/honey supplements, all fertilization should cease at least two weeks from harvest to allow the plant time to clear itself, though that is less of an issue with post-Catastrophe or totally organic natural fertilizers than with real-life concentrates.

Another technique recommended anecdotally to increase the bulk and quality of flowers is to add hops to the medicinal-plant fertilizer infusion, possibly throughout the plant's lifetime and certain ly from the time the first pre-flowers (described below) begin to show. The logic behind this is that the high phytoestrogen content of hops, which are the nearest relative to cannabis, will basically fem-roid up the female cannabis flowers. Hops are also notably good fertilizer in general, as discussed in Appendix I; so even if the phytoestrogens themselves have no effect, the plants will still benefit from doing this.

The only reports I have heard of hops specifically as a cannabis-fertilizer were anecdotal...the ever-popular Internet documentation of, "I tried it and it seemed to work for me"...but the logic makes relative sense, and the close botanical relationship between the two plants suggests that their preferred nutrient profiles are likely to be similar. If you have the hops to spare, it might be worth a try. Hops grow as a vine, are incredibly easy to grow, and produce a large volume of flowers (the part used both for flavouring/preserving beer and for this purpose) per plant. Some people recommend tomato juice as a fertilizer for cannabis. Don't do it. Tobacco mosaic virus. Grow the tomatoes elsewhere and eat them yourself.

Kuru was a prion disease in New Guinea, transmitted by the practice of cannibalism. Even with its long incubation period (5-50+ years, mean of 14 years, since the Foré and other New Guinea tribes stopped eating their dearly departed ca. 1960, kuru is now considered extinct. It is debated whether the last patient died in 2005 or 2009.

However, the theory is that kuru originated when one villager developed spontaneous Creutzfeldt-Jakob disease and was eaten according to proper mourning rites – and that word "spontaneous" should be a hint.

Eating sheep with scrapie or cows with BSE may also be a route of transmission to humans. There is no way to tell clinically whether someone is incubating a prion disease until they actually become symptomatic, which is why there have been cases of CJD transmitted through surgical instruments (normal sterilization doesn't destroy prions) and transplants.

Despite the many claims that have been made, suggested, or supported for the medical uses of cannabis, treating prion diseases has never been among them.

III) Spacing

The spacing of cannabis plants is also recommended to follow the example of tomatoes. In pots in a greenhouse, one 18"x18" (five-gallon) pot, the size of a large tomato pot, suffices for one standard and is ideal for a dwarf. Some hemp plants, particularly sativas and sativa-indica hybrids which have not deliberately been bred for a short bushy phenotype, can grow much larger outdoors than in a pot, and cannabis resents sharing its space. At least two feet between plants is recommended for standards grown for medicinal purposes (and after the first year's growth, you may discover that a wider spacing is required for the strain you are growing), and a foot and a half for auto-flowerers.

Hemp grown chiefly for fibre is close-sown (8-12" or even less) between plants, which shades out weeds and allows the plants to support each other against the wind. If part of your patch is focused on seed and part on fibre, the seed plants should be spaced like the medicinal plants (or just use the same plants for both, since they're all going to get pollinated by the same males in the great outdoors anyway unless the medicinals are fast-flowering dwarves) and the majority of the male plants removed to make space for the female flower/seed producers. For fibre hemp, as noted later, you have reason to keep your males longer.

IV. Pests

Birds, mice, rabbits/hares, and deer or other ungulates are all a concern from seed to flower. Mice and birds will eat seeds both between planting and sprouting, and as soon as they start to form; mice will eat seedlings until they are large enough not to be bothered. Ungulates will eat cannabis plants at any time, as will other grazing. Cat patrol is perhaps not as reliable for cannabis as it is for the majority of crops. Having seen cats on catnip lie about watching as a mouse nibbled from their food bowl ("Peace, mouse! Like, wow, have some cat crunchies!"), I would decline to vouch for the motivation and reaction time of a cat in a hemp patch.

I am also given to understand that cats have been known to help themselves to cannabis at any stage from seedling to dry flowers. Sowing the traditional four-for-one ("one for the rabbit, one for the crow, one for the weather, and one to grow") is probably the best advice. Having an armed watcher out in the hemp field ready to shoot any rabbit/hare, deer, or elk (what Europeans call the American moose) with ideas is a really good idea for most of the growing period, as these animals will compensate for taking a few nibbles by providing a quantity of good protein. The same goes for feral swine, which, as so ably detailed in S.M. Stirling's Emberverse series, are likely to be a problem after the Catastrophe ("'If you grow it, they will come'" – Dies the Fire).

To paraphrase Lazarus Long (Heinlein, Time Enough for Love)...what a sounder of swine can do to a field shouldn't happen to Sodom and Gomorrah. But they make excellent suppers.Slugs and snails are massively destructive to cannabis seedlings, but seldom a concern once the plant bursts into swift vegetative growth. The solution for these molluscs in the early stages of growth is the same as it is for poppies: a sweep at dawn and dusk, possibly with a small bounty put on them to motivate young children. Cannabis is not particularly vulnerable to micropests when growing outdoors, but greenfly, whitefly, and aphids can all be significant problems if you are trying to seclude a few medicinal plants in a greenhouse while preventing pollination from your fibre/seed strains. Tobacco should not be used on hemp as an insecticide due to the possible vulnerability of this plant to tobacco mosaic virus. A solution of 1 teaspoon of soap in one liter (or quart, close enough) of water will be the best you can get after the Catastrophe.

Do not use this less than two weeks before harvest. Because the small flowers are so tightly clustered, mould can be a significant problem in more humid areas and indoors. If you can't control the humidity, and post-Catastrophe you probably can't, watch closely and, if needed, harvest your medicinal plants early. If you live in a warm and humid area, one of your chief criteria in strain choice (assuming that you had the opportunity and foresight to make that choice before the Catastrophe) should absolutely be fungal resistance!

Training methods which favour multiple smaller budding sites rather than a huge thick central cola also reduce the odds of mould creeping in unnoticed. Mould renders cannabis flowers unsafe to either dry directly for inhalation or baking, or make into a tincture. However, the processing of water-resin extraction (described below under "Medicinal Harvest") both separates the pure resin glands while clearing their outer coats, and cleans the mould and whatever untowards chemicals it may have produced from the remaining plant materials, so that they may then at least safely be used in an alcoholic extract or a topical preparation, though lipid extracts for oral use would remain questionable at best.

As with poppies, the most dangerous post-Catastrophe macropest likely to destroy your crop of cannabis is an invasive, tool-using simian species. The chances that a raider band or warlord's scouts will fail to recognise the iconographic leaves of this plant, or the distinctive and pungent scent of a hempfield in bloom, are roughly none. The solution is perhaps regrettable, but unavoidable. As with this particular pest in regards to poppies, the remains are similarly useful in growing next year's crop, as they are rich in nitrogen, potassium, phosphorus, and protein. Do not eat them directly, they carry many nasty diseases, all of which you can readily catch. If you have no alternative, be sure to cook them very, very well, and avoid the brain and spinal tissues, as prion diseases are not destroyed by heat.

2) Cannabis Life-Cycle

The three stages of a hemp plant's life are seedling, vegetative, and flowering.

a) Seedling

The seedling stage lasts from germination until the plant has sprouted its third or fourth pair of "true leaves". These are to be distinguished from the cotelydon, the two small round leaves that appear when the seed husk falls off. The seedling phase generally lasts around two weeks. During this time, the seedling either should not be fertilized, or should be fertilized at an extremely low dilution (1/4 or less of what an adult plant would get).

b) Vegetative; Training and Pruning Methods

The vegetative phase begins when the seedling breaks into exuberant growth. This continues in standard plants until the photoperiod changes from summer to approaching equinoctical. A 12 hour light/12 hour dark period is used by most indoor growers to stimulate flowering, but in practice, it may begin when the light period drops below 14 hours. The outdoors grower is dependent on the cycles of nature; the indoor grower may choose to force flower as early as 3 or 4 weeks (some people start a 12/12 cycle from seed, but that generally loses in production what it makes up in time), or they may choose to do high-stress training of some sort and let the plant veg longer to recover.

Technically dwarf/autoflower plants do not have a vegetative stage. The flowers may not start showing for a month or so, but they are in flowering stage, in a metabolic sense, from germination onwards. When reading a strain description, be aware that "flowering time" for a standard strain is the time between photoperiod flowering activation and harvest; whereas, for an autoflowering strain, it is the period between early seedling stage and harvest. The vegetative phase is the time when the vast majority of "training" or shaping the plant takes place.

There are several methods for this, but all of them serve the purpose of breaking the apical dominance of the central shoot in order to produce a larger number of smaller colas (a cola is a heavily flower-laden branch tip). Debates rage in the growing community – sometimes quite literally rage! – as to which of these methods is best, and whether any of them actually produce a significant increase in yield, or simply make it easier to keep the plant low and open so that all buds receive roughly the same amount of light (only a factor for the indoors grower; the Sun has much greater canopy penetrance and side-lighting value than any artificial system). In areas that are prone to mould, training plants to produce more smaller colas on a more open structure is greatly preferable to letting them form one massive, dense cola where mould can easily eat a large percentage of the internal bud before it is ever noticed.

Low-Stress Training (LST)

This method is preferred for autoflowering plants and plants which are being grown 12/12 from seed or switched to the flowering photoperiod at less than 6 weeks. It does not actually injure the plant, so no recovery time is required. In LST, the main stalk is gently bent over, a bit more each day, until its tip is below the level of the other growing tops. The side branches are also tied to make them grow more horizontally away from the plant and to keep them from blocking each others' light, u.s.w. This is usually done with soft gardener's wire (fine wire with a smooth plastic coating to keep it from cutting the stalk).

High-Stress Training (HST) methods include

Topping – cutting off the stem of the plant, usually just above the fourth node or so. Causes the next node down on the truncated stalk to throw out two main stalks in place of the original. Some growers do this repeatedly to achieve a specific shape with many upper colas (see "manifolding/mainlining" below). It is fairly stressful on the plant, and may require an extra three days to a week in vegetation for the plant to fully recover. If growing outdoors, vegetation time will not be an issue; it takes longer for outdoors hemp to reach flowering unless it was planted quite late, so the plant already has veg time to spare, not to mention better lighting and, if grown in the ground, more room for its root system to develop.

Fimming – from the acronym FIM ("Fuck, I Missed!"). Immortal words said by a grower who went to top his plant and only got the upper 75% or so of the top bud, with what turned out for him to be serendipitous results. The plant's upper bud is cut as described, around ¾ of the way down. This forces the development of (usually, but numbers may vary) four main stalks. Said to be less stressful than topping; may take 2-4 days to recover. Can also be done multiple times.

Manifolding (or mainlining) – a specific sequence of toppings done to produce a symmetrical plant with the desired number of large side branches. When it has reached ca. 6 nodes total (not counting the cotelydon), the plant is topped above the 3rd node from the bottom. The shoots and foliage are also removed from nodes 1 and 2, leaving only the two side shoots on node 3 and their fan leaves. Some consider it preferable to wait a week or so between topping and cleaning the lower stem, in order to let the plant recover and put out a bit more leaf. When the two remaining stalks have reached 5-6 nodes each, repeat the process of topping above the 3rd node and either removing all foliage on the branch below it, or removing all foliage at node 2 while letting 1 and 3 grow out. Most people growing indoors consider eight stalks to be sufficient, although a large plant could well support 16 or even 32. Best when a long veg period is contemplated or when growing over the summer outdoors, since at least two recovery periods will be needed. This technique is reputed to be the best in regards to increasing both yield and evenness of growth, particularly when applied to tall sativas, the lower buds of which often do not develop well or do not ripen until two weeks or more after the top cola is ripe.

Supercropping: this is a technique aimed at producing stronger stems with a greater nutrient flow, hence, it is hoped, higher yields and more powerful medicinal effects. The logic is that a plant stem which has been severely bent or even broken (but without the outer surface being damaged...nutrients can still flow, and pathogens are not being invited in, so long as the "skin" of the stalk stays in one piece) will recover with greater strength; some even form a thick "knuckle" which serves to increase water/nutrient flow above itself. A branch is rubbed gently between the thumb and forefinger until the fibers begin to separate internally. The branch stalk becomes soft and floppy; it is possible to bend over at a 90 degree angle without snapping the stem (if the stem does snap or break, put it together with a duct tape splint and leave it be for two or three weeks. Cannabis is a very resilient plant).

Repeat as often as desired. Some people will go down a branch, starting just below the top node and making one supercrop bend between every node in succession. Recovery time is relatively short (1-4 days, depending on how severely the plant was supercropped). During vegetation, the plant's chief need is for nitrogen, although it also requires some phosphate and potassium, as well as a range of other minerals. If the soil has already been prepared with a high-nitrogen fertilizer (manure, garden wastes, fish, blood), as well as a moderate amount of potassium (banana peels, dandelions) and phosphorus (steamed bone meal, lime if your soil is also acidic), you should be well-covered.

b) Flowering

i) Preflowers

Preflowers usually begin to appear around six weeks after germination, or four weeks into the vegetative stage. They are the plant's version of showing that they are entering puberty, and ready to be put into flower whenever the grower desires. The chief importance of preflowers, however, is that they allow the grower to positively identify most female plants and probably identify male plants. Preflowers are tiny budlets which appear at the nodes (leaf/stalk junctions). Female preflowers are longer, narrower, have more elongated tips and develop a pair of white "hairs" (pistils) sprouting from their tips. Male preflowers are shorter and rounder, strongly resembling the seeds in shape and general proportions, with just the tiniest point at the terminal end; "spade" is a commonly-used description.

If the preflower is standing on a tiny stalk ("pedunculated") rather than growing directly from the internode, it is definitely male; but not all male preflowers have stalks. Note that female preflowers may not sprout pistils immediately, and in some strains the pistils are minute; a magnifying glass or jeweller's loupe (which you may also want later for evaluating the resin glands on your medical hemp plants) may be needed to see them. If in doubt, watch and wait. You will absolutely be able to tell the difference once the plant begins true flowering. Unwanted males, once definitively identified, may be removed and processed at this time, or they may be allowed to mature a little longer in the interest of increased strength. Male plants develop little resin outside of a few glands on the mature flowers and occasionally small leaves, but that does not mean they are useless.

While it has commonly been believed that any given part of a male plant will be lower in cannabinoids than the corresponding part of a female of the same strain, investigations are suggesting that this is highly variable. A Moroccan study indicated comparable levels of THC in male and female leaves, and only slightly lower levels in male flowering tops; a Thai landrace (native-grown strain without selective crossbreeding) had maximal levels of THC approaching the female minimal levels, but a 1:9 THC:CBD ratio.

Males will father the next generation of plants; they are valuable for the finer and more elastic fibre they produce (making the considerable additional effort of separating the stalks by gender for harvesting and processing worthwhile); and, even if culled before flowering, when the cannabinoid levels are lower, they are still useful in the production of infused or extracted medicinals. While they are of less value to the real-life grower who is not a breeder, and who lacks the space to use for anything that will not produce the numerous and powerful female flowers (or who lives where there is a restriction of numbers to be grown for personal use), male plants will be absolutely vital after the Catastrophe.

II) Photoperiod and Stimulating Hermaphrodites for Feminized Seed

Photoperiod

The standard cannabis plant is dependent on photoperiod to fulfill its life-cycle. When grown outdoors, or in a naturally-lit greenhouse, it is commonly planted as soon as weather permits and the days are longer than 14 hours. The longer a plant stays in vegetation, the larger it can get and the higher its cannabinoid content is likely to become. This is probably your only post-Catastrophe option for standard hemp when electric lights are no longer easy to come by and when you are growing it in larger quantities for fibre and seeds/oil as much as, and indeed probably more than, for medicine.

It grows throughout the summer, but cannot begin to flower until stimulated by the photoperiod shift moving towards the autumnal equinox. Indoor growers in real life, of course, are able to plant and harvest at their own convenience, simply by changing the lighting from a summer photoperiod (16 hours light/8 hours darkness is the most common standard) to an equinoctical one (12:12). For the dwarf varieties, photoperiod is irrelevant to life-cycle, but the optimum for production and potency is generally considered to be a 16:8 photoperiod from germination to harvest. However, in an area with warm winters, you could probably grow a dwarf crop between the time of the standard-strain harvest and the next year's standard-strain planting; then grow a second one at the same time as the standard crop and harvest it before the standards begin to bloom.

Irregularities in photoperiod are generally avoided by indoor growers, as bouncing the photoperiod around, especially after the switch from summer to equinoctical timing, is known to induce hermaphroditism in female plants. This is discouraged, as not only does it reduce the quantity of flower produced, but one male flower can seed a whole plant. Like all plants, a cannabis plant has only so much energy in total, and energy it is putting into seed production is diverted from flower bulk and resin production and quality. This is why "sinsemilla" ("without seeds") is preferred for medicinal uses, and why growers who are not dependent on producing their own seeds for next year's planting and not concerned about fibre quality generally weed out the males altogether as soon as they can be identified.

Hermaphrodites and Feminized Seeds (and colloidal silver)

Hermaphroditism is sometimes deliberately courted in real life for the specific purpose of producing "feminized" seeds: that is, all plants grown from such seeds will be female. This is likely to be of considerably less value following the Catastrophe than it is for real-life cannabis gardeners. After the Catastrophe, you will likely be growing this plant in large quantities for fibre and oil if you can, and therefore will not have to worry about wasting the limited allotment for home use/space in your growing cupboard, or about the possibility that of the ten seeds you bought, eight of them might turn out to be male after you've spent three months nurturing them lovingly through their vegetative stage.

Not as disastrous as most real-life growers think, given the manifest inaccuracy in at least some cases of the "male plants are too low-potency to bother with"; but not ideal in limited-space circumstances. If you do wish to produce and reserve some feminized seeds for a special medicinal plot of auto-flowerers or secluded greenhouse, since you can't turn the Sun on and off at night to stress your plant into hermaphroditism, your best post-Catastrophe option will be the use of colloidal silver if available. This is sprayed on a single branch daily from the time the pre-flowers appear until you start seeing the male "bananas" form on the chosen branch. Only a light misting is needed, and colloidal silver can easily be stockpiled, since it does not go off unless actively contaminated.

Colloidal Silver

Colloidal silver is a good thing to stockpile for other uses as well, specifically spraying on bandages as an anti-bacterial – particularly important if a section of skin has been removed or seriously damaged, as in a burn: antibiotics of proven strength will be hard to come by, and even a very shallow hole in the skin is like waving a big sign asking every dangerous bacterium in the area to come party in your body.

!

Colloidal silver should never be taken internally. At best it causes argyria (skin, nails, and mucous membranes turn irreversibly gray-blue); at worst it is fatal. It is suitable only for topical use and use on bandages (especially when retaining a certain degree of moisture is desirable, as with burns), and even more so after the Catastrophe after the supply of sealed sterile bandages has run out.

While topical use is safe due to low absorption, absorption through mucous membranes is high. Colloidal silver should not, therefore, ever be used for oral, anal, or vaginal disinfection, nor can it be used to sterilize tampons against toxic shock syndrome.

Colloidal or ionic copper, on the other hand, is considered quite safe to absorb through mucous membranes, also has good antimicrobial efficacy, and would serve quite well for all the latter purposes.

Even in the context of modern life, with all our superior hygiene, I once sustained a very severe infection, with a high fever and full-blown lymphangioedema (red streaks running up the affected limb – though called "blood poisoning", it is not the blood vessels showing red, but the lymphatic vessels), from a scrape that wasn't even deep enough to bleed. After the Catastrophe, the smallest breach in your number one defense against infection – your skin – has the potential to be a fatal disaster. You should remember the sad end of Orkneyinga saga hero Sigurðr Eysteinsson (Sigurðr the Mighty)...who took the head of his enemy Máel Brigte as a trophy; Máel's tooth slightly grazed Sigurðr's leg as he rode home in triumph, and Sigurðr died of the resultant infection. This is an extremely plausible tale, especially given the pit of microbial nastiness that is the human mouth. And it could happen to you when the modern range of powerful, wide-spectrum antibiotics is no longer available (or if you don't at least go to your GP when someone nips you hard enough to break the skin).

In real life, colloidal silver is sometimes used as a coating for internal medical devices where there is a high risk of bacterial biofilm formation. Ionic silver (there is some argument over whether this can or should be called "colloid silver", but that is mainly of interest to physicists; suffice it to say that, for all practical purposes, they can be considered the same thing), can be made at home with relatively little difficulty. You will need some functioning batteries (3 9-volt batteries are most commonly recommended), a power pack of some nature, electrical wire, two alligator clips, and some pure (.999) silver such as is used in bullion. Sterling silver is less pure and not suitable to the purpose. But you stocked up on at least a few bullion silver coins before the Catastrophe, didn't you? Directions are readily available on the Internet; I recommend checking and comparing several sites, because none of them come with guarantees.

The topical or bandage-treatment use of colloidal silver is, of course, awesomely unsuitable for any supernatural patients with silver sensitivities, most commonly shapeshifters. But generally that is not a major concern, as both shapeshifters and vampires tend to be highly resistant to bacterial infections and thus unlikely to require the additional prophylaxis that might save the life of a standard human. Whether a spray of colloidal silver would have a deterrent or destructive effect on a non-corporeal supernatural being probably depends on the individual being, though an iron infusion would be more effective for some Scandinavian spectres.

Some vampires are sensitive to silver, as in Laurell K. Hamilton's Anita Blake: Vampire Hunter series (Ace, Berkley; 1993 ff; the first book, Guilty Pleasures describes fatal silver nitrate injections, although she also makes it clear that this may be ineffective on older/more powerful vampires). Some are not. Know your world! Northern European fey (Sidhe, álfar, various other related species) are reputed to have no difficulties related to silver and may well have a higher tolerance for silver than humans do.

Iron is more commonly their problem, though the exact risk to these patients of anything with a high iron concentration, including food supplements, is unknown. I have been unable to find any studies relating to the question of possible iron-defiency anaemia in Northern European fey, or even to their haemoglobin/haemoglobin-equivalent composition. They are capable of ingesting red meat without difficulty, so low levels of iron do not appear to be excessively toxic to them. However, their high reported sensitivity to iron in general suggests that, if any invasive procedure from an IV upwards must be performed on such a patient, then silver or gold - or virtually any other metal or stone, e.g. obsidian, used even in real life for medical instruments on occasion due to its extreme sharpness - is far preferable to iron/steel even for needles or scalpels.

III) Breeding: Pollination and Propagation

Cannabis is wind-pollinated, and pollinates promiscuously. Allergy-provoking pollen concentrations originating in the Moroccan Rif have been identified in southern Spain when the wind blows from North Africa – a travel distance of 48 kilometres (ca. 29.8 miles). It is rumoured in cannabis-interest circles that hemp pollen can travel as far as 2000 miles, though I have not been able to find any verification of this. There just is not a field spacing that can really avoid cross-pollination unless you are working with another community at a distance that is over at least 50 miles away.

If trying to grow or preserve different strains – which you probably want to, since the tall "sativa" types that produce the best fibre are also usually very low in CBD – your best option is to have obtained dwarf/autoflower seeds for your primary medicinal use, as those, even if planted at the same time as your fibre- and probably high-THC standards, will flower and be harvested long before the standard males can pollinate them. Other than that, you will need either to keep your medicinals in a protected greenhouse and hope against hope that screening and main wind directions keep the other pollen out, or alternate strains between one year and the next. If you live anywhere in the neighborhood of a pre-Catastrophe industrial cannabis field, auto-flowering dwarves are likely to be your only real chance of maintaining a strain with a useful level of medicinal constituents. Start them as early as possible so as to avoid any risk of your neighbor's plants contaminating yours.

Male plants, including the auto-flowering varieties, usually begin to flower two to three weeks before female flowering becomes abundant. Male flowers appear in clusters which resemble bunches of grapes. The mature male flower has five white to pale green petals, much more similar in appearance to a standard "flower" than the female, and the stamens dangling from the centre resemble a bunch of tiny green grooved bananas. It was often common historically, and still is in some places where hemp is grown industrially, to harvest the male plants first while the female plants are allowed to grow on for the seed harvest.

If pollinating your medicinal cannabis in a controlled manner to produce enough seeds for the next planting, while reserving as much for the more powerful sinsemilla as possible, there are a couple of options available to you. Some growers remove all but one flowering branch of the chosen male plant, and bag that branch, shaking it every so often so that the pollen falls into the bag. If doing this before your favourite female (same general means of pre-guessing potency apply) has produced a reasonable number of flowers, pollen can be stored for a short time in an airtight container with desiccant (water kills pollen right off), preferably in a dark cool place. If commercial desiccants are not available, the pollen may be mixed with dry flour or put into a paper bag inside the airtight container with a quantity of rice.

If the female is already getting well-started by the time the male has finished flowering, the bag can be tied directly over a flowering female branch, shaken, and left on for 12-24 hours with regular gentle shaking. Now all the flowers on that branch will be as pollinated as they're going to get; remove the bag and mist gently with water to avoid sharing the pollen with the rest of the medicinal crop.

Choosing a Pollinator

While it is difficult to evaluate the medicinal qualities that a male plant may pass to his offspring without direct testing, various methods are used for a rough guesstimate in choosing the surviving pollinator. It is commonly advised to avoid the largest males and the first to show flowers: both traits are associated with lower potency. Shorter stature is also preferred in real life, especially by indoors growers, as shorter plants tend to be easier to light in an artificial system. However, if you are using the same strain for fibre and medicine and simply nurturing the medicinal part of the patch more carefully, you may want at least moderately tall males.

Height is to fibre hemp what potency is to medicinal hemp! Large and hollow stems are said to be a promising sign for male medicinal plants, while pithy stems are not. Long spacing between the leaf/stalk junctions is said to be strongly associated with low potency; look for tighter spacing for medicinal pollinators. The most reliable simple home method is to dry a couple of leaves from each male and smoke or vapourize them on successive evenings (testing more than one in closer sequence is likely to make the later-tested plants seem stronger in comparison than they actually are).

Often medical potency is directly correlated with scent intensity, as the factors that produce terpenes correlate to a reasonable degree with the factors that produce the primary constituents. Thus, some growers choose their plant sires by crushing a leaf of each between the fingers and sniffing them. Other factors such as resistance to pests and fungi may come into play as well, if you have a pest/fungus problem. The male who doesn't succumb to mould or bears a visibly lesser insect burden, even if he is not the best in terms of strength and aroma, is still one you want to breed into your lines. If you have let all your medicinal males live until the beginning of true flowering, one which has visible stalked trichomes (resin glands) on the small leaves is definitely the lad to keep.

Propagation of Female Plants

The commonly used technique of directly propagating or "cloning" female plants is a technique which will not be particularly useful after the Catastrophe unless you maintain a means of artificial lighting, or wish to produce a number of copies of a specific female over the summer. You probably could deceive the plants into believing their photoperiod has been extended by keeping them indoors by the fire or a few candles, as any more light than the full moon provides is said to interfere with photoperiod-based development. Your chief reason for trying this technique will be the preservation and propagation of special female plants, especially if you were unlucky enough to be caught by the Catastrophe when you only had a packet of feminized seeds available.

If you can bounce the photoperiod around long enough (or have some colloidal silver), hopefully at least one of your clones will go hermaphroditic and solve your lack-of-pollination problem. Some real-life growers keep a single giant "mother plant" in vegetation indefinitely and just keep cloning off her. Propagation takes place before the change of photoperiod in standard hemp plants. It cannot be done with dwarf/autoflower varieties to any useful effect, since they will fulfill their life-cycles no matter what you do with their environment. The best you can do is get a few extra small flowering plants that finish at the same time as their mother. After the plant has shown her first pre-flowers (if you have a mixed-gender bag of seeds), but before the light levels drop under 14:10, use a clean sharp knife to cut diagonally just above the second leaf-junction down on one or more of the lower branches.

If you have any hormone rooting powder left from your pre-Catastrophe stock, dip the cut end into it; then place it into a small hole in damp soil. The pot or tray should be covered, with only minute vents, in order to preserve moisture content in the clone while it roots. You may also wish to pinch off the outer half of each sub-leaflet for the same reason; it will not hurt the clone, and it will reduce water exhalation. Make sure the soil stays damp, but not saturated, until either the sprig wilts and collapses (total failure) or until it starts sprouting new leaflets (total success). Continue as if you had grown it to that size from seed, maintaining the vegetative photoperiod overwinter by keeping the plant in a lighted area at night and setting it where it can get as much benefit from the sun as possible during the day.

It is advisable to clone in batches of at least ten or twelve, to be sure that you will get some positive results. If you've survived the Catastrophe and its aftermath long enough to be worrying about planting and propagating, you probably know by good sense and experience that it is not wise to depend on a single plant, animal, or circumstance if you can possibly avoid it. In the absence of commercial cloning gel or powder, willow water and aloe gel (the gel from the inside of an aloe vera leaf) have been used successfully. Take a number of the green-barked growing tips of a willow's branches (no thicker than a pencil at maximum, down to the very tips of the thin shoots), chop them up, and soak them in warm water.

Leave to soak until the water is needed, or the willow pieces start rooting themselves, in which case, replace them with fresh pieces. Mix the willow water 50-50 with aloe gel and soak the cut end and stalk nodes for approximately 12 hours before planting. Note that willow water is more effective when made in spring or summer, when the tips are actually growing, and not so effective during winter dormancy. Honey and cinnamon may be added for their anti-bacterial/antifungal properties; it is not known whether they contribute any positive benefits to the rooting process, but keeping pathogens out of the vulnerable cut stems is vital to a successful propagation.

Aloe vera gel can also be used as a general fertilizer or foliar feed for your other plants (ca ¼ cup/gallon of water). It increases resistance to fungi and diseases, stimulates cell division, improves the ability of roots to assimilate water and nutrients, and strengthens the plant against environmental stresses.

D) The Harvest

I) Fibre for Textiles and Paper

Note that when processing large quantities of hemp (or cotton, or flax, or jute) for fiber, it is strongly advised to wear some manner of covering over nose and mouth to prevent byssinosis. This is a reactive airway disease which may be directly caused by irritation from inhaling fibre-particles, or more indirectly by bacterial endotoxins. Bronchoconstriction occurs, and may lead to airway scarring, respiratory compromise, and death. Although this disease is now rare in developed countries, it is most commonly seen in fibre-industry workers: the professions of 48.2% of byssinosis deaths in the US between 1990 and 1999 were listed as workers in yarn, thread, and fabric mills.

Cannabis stems are separated into an inner layer (pith); woody core (hurds); and long outer fibres (bast). The hurds can be used for fuel, mulch, animal bedding, and so forth. The bast is the important part of the cannabis plant for fibre. Hemp fibre provides textiles, chiefly rope and rough cloth; stable bedding (said to be superior to straw in regards to diminishing the smell of ammonia from urine), and paper.

Hemp is harvested for fibre between the period when pollen begins to shed and the time of the seed harvest (which is usually ca. 4-6 weeks after female flowering is well initiated). In mixed fibre/seed cultivation, male plants are normally harvested as soon as they have produced the desired amount of pollen, whereas female plants are left to ripen the valuable seeds. Due to both earlier harvest and growth habit, the fibres produced by the male plants are usually finer, softer, and considered more suitable for clothing and household goods, whereas the tougher female fibres are superior for rope and rough fabrics. The cannabis stalks are most commonly cut close to the ground, traditionally with a particular type of scythe called a “hemp hook”.

The hand-harvester – post-Catastrophe or in real life – may find it easier to simply use the traditional method of pulling the stalks out of the ground: the stalks are very tough, and the roots quite shallow (this also allows the option of using the roots medicinally). The stalks are bundled into armful-sized sheaves and laid on the ground. Harvested stalks are left in the field to rett for a period of time depending on temperature and humidity: this may range from one week in warm damp weather to six weeks in dry cool weather. Retting, sometimes accurately referred to as “rotting”, breaks down the binding of the fibres to allow easier extraction.

They are turned every few days to keep the moisture level even. A swifter retting process may be done in the same manner as that most commonly used for flax: the stalks are soaked underwater in ponds, streams, or tanks for ten days. Anaerobic soaking is said to yield a finer fibre than the open-field method. At the end of the retting period, the cannabis stalks are brought indoors to dry. Field-retting returns the majority of nutrients to the soil, which makes cannabis useful as a rotation crop, or allows the farmer to grow it in the same field for years without exhausting the land.

Retting is complete when: the inner stalks snap, but the bast fibres remain intact and are very difficult to break; the fibre near the base of the stem peels easily but does not break after several inches of peeling; several stems are broken at the same point together and the wood separates readily from the fibre. If the bast fibres break easily, the hemp has been over-retted. Check frequently to avoid this. Retting is a decomposition process, and your stalks (hemp, flax, or nettle) will verify this by their aroma. The stink does not mean they have gone bad; it means the retting is proceeding properly.

The retted stalks are then crushed in a breaker – a simple wooden device resembling a sawhorse with interlocking wooden blades. This is the same breaker and the same process you will use for processing your flax stalks. The object is to crush the pith and hurds; the bast fibres, being more flexible, remain intact. In the absence of a proper breaker (though it should be easy to build with simple tools and the most minimal knowledge of carpentry...that is, how to saw a few pieces of wood and use a hammer and a hand drill...), breaking can be done more slowly by hand or with a mallet. The hand-peeling of the fibres required by this method is time-consuming, but also scutches (below) while you are breaking.

» The broken stalks are then scutched: that is, the pieces of pith and hurds are separated from the long bast fibres.
» The fibres are hackled, or combed, to align them neatly and remove any last detritus. This is similar to the carding process used in preparing wool.
» The next step is roving...twisting and drawing out the fibres...which increases their strength and prepares them for spinning.

Hemp may be spun on a wheel or by a drop spindle. Usually the fibres are well-wetted prior to spinning, which increases their flexibility and the coherence of the final yarn or string. For both cannabis and flax, you will want to equip yourself with a distaff, which is essentially a stick on which the unspun fibres are wound so that they can swiftly be fed onto the wheel or drop spindle. The traditional Scandinavian distaff, in its simplest form, consisted of a pine branch with all needles removed, stripped bare of smaller twigs for three-quarters of its length, with the upper twigs bound into a sort of "cage" around the top.

A number of iron variants of this have been found in Viking Age graves, some extremely elaborate and almost certainly possessed by women of high status. If folk magic is a functional element of your post-Catastrophe life, or if you have travelled in time back to the Viking Age, it may be worth noting that there is believed to have been some overlap between the flax/hemp distaff and the magical stave of the witch or seeress. The process of spinning hemp or flax from a distaff is described, with illustrations, here; a picture of a breaker and its use are also provided: http://www.wildfibres.co.uk/html/linen_flax.html

The same processes can also be used for preparing and spinning nettle fibres, which can make a fine fabric similar to cotton. Nettle fibres were used as a cotton substitute in providing British uniforms during World War I. The nettle harvest for fibre begins in early August, when the plants are reaching their peak of height and strength. Nettles may be retted as hemp and flax are, or, if a coarser fibre is acceptable, the old stalks can be left to stand until spring ("root-retting"), at which time they may be dried, gently baked until brittle (ca. 70 F/21 C), broken, scutched, etc. The retting process renders nettles completely stingless. For the harvesting process, it is a good idea to avoid exposing your skin; and knowing the nearest patch of plantain (Plantago major or Plantago lanceolata) or having prepared yourself with some plantain ointment is also a good idea.

Nutritional profile of hemp-seeds per 100 grams:

Omega-3 and -6 polyunsaturated fats – 36% whole/44% dehulled
Protein = 25 gr whole/33 gr dehulled
Carbohydrates = 28 gr
Calories = 526 (2200 kilojoules)
Thiamine (B1) = 0.4 mg (daily recommendation 1.1-1.2 mg)
Riboflavin (B2) = 0.1 mg (daily recommendation 1.1-1.3 mg
Vitamin E = 90 mg (maximum safe dose 1000 mg)
Phosphorus = 1,160 mg (adult daily minimum 700 mg, adolescent 1250 mg
Potassium = 859 mg (adult daily recommendation 4,700 mg)
Magnesium = 483 mg (adults at least 310-420 mg; max safe dose 2500 mg
Calcium = 145 mg (pre-menopausal women 1,000-2,000 mg; pregnant/lactating women at least 1,500 mg; adult men 1,000 mg; adolescents 1,300 mg)
Iron = 14 mg (adult men min 8.7 mg, adult women 14.8 mg)
Manganese = 7 mg (adult minimum 1.8 mg women, 2.4 mg men; toxicity ca. 11 mg)
Zinc = 7 mg (recommended adult 15 mg; anaemia/copper deficiency begin at 11 mg
Copper = 2 mg (recommended adult .9 mg; upper safe limit 10 mg)

Fresh plantain can be crushed and applied to nettle stings as a poultice with reportedly excellent efficacy (plantain is also effective against insect bites). Cannabis is stronger and more resilient than flax, hence its traditional role as the preferred fibre for ropes, sails, and heavy canvas. The sturdier and coarser fibres of female plants are preferred for this purpose.

Hemp is less elastic than flax; it is generally held that it is easier to produce a finer fabric with flax or nettles, but sufficient care and preparation can produce an excellent linen-like product from cannabis, particularly male plants that have been retted underwater. As well as a spinning fibre, cannabis also makes a fine homemade paper. Instead of retting, the stems are crushed and soaked overnight (ca. 1 part stems to 3 parts water, crushed into roughly the consistency that a fine blender grind produces).

Sodium carbonate, or "soda ash" (obtained by drying and burning brown algae or kelp, saltworts, glassworts, or other plants that thrive in saline environments, then washing the ashes with water to form an alkali solution and boiling the solution dry) is blended into water in a proportion of 20% by weight to the dry weight of the fibre and brought to a boil before adding the soaked fibres.

Lye may also be used for this purpose, and is more effective at breaking fibres down; the ratio is 9% of dry fibre weight, or 1 tablespoon (ca. 15 grams) to 2 quarts (ca. 1.9 litres) of water. In either case, the caustic must be poured into the water and not the other way around; pouring water onto a caustic can cause explosions. Total soaking time in the alkaline mixture for hemp, a quite sturdy fibre. is approximately 6-8 hours.

Rubber gloves, if at all possible, should be worn for all parts of the process where your hands might come into contact with the alkaline/fibre solution, as alkali can cause nasty burns. Eye/face protection and long sleeves are also recommended. The fibre is rinsed a number of times in clean water to remove all traces of alkalinity and re-mixed with more clean water to make a slurry. A wooden frame with a screen (preferably a silkscreen if available) is passed through the slurry to achieve a thin even concentration on the whole screen.

This may be pressed between two sheets of felt or cotton under a flat piece of wood and some weights to speed drying and get a smoother result. The paper is removed before it is fully dry to prevent it sticking to the screen; it is easier to handle if the screen is also removable from the frame. The paper is usually brown, but may be lightened with hydrogen peroxide added during the soaking process. It generally is markedly more durable than wood-pulp paper.

However, despite a common rumour to that effect, the final version of the Declaration of Independence were not written on hemp paper: using parchment for the final versions of important documents was standard at that time, and Congress ordered that to be done in this case. The two earlier drafts were indeed written on paper, but whether that was hemp paper or flax paper is uncertain. Flax paper is made in the same manner as hemp paper. It has often been stated, based on a 1916 report from the USDA, that 1 acre of hemp plants can produce as much papermaking fibre as roughly 4.5 acres of trees. This does not seem to be verifiable in terms of more recent evaluations, and is likely to have changed significantly with more recent production methods for making wood-based paper.

II) Seeds

The seeds are usually harvested at the earliest maximum point of ripeness, especially if also using the female plants which grew them for fibre production. In real life, bulk seed harvesting is normally done by machines designed for the purpose. Unless you have such a machine and know how to use it, not to mention having the petrol to run it (or the ability to reconfigure it to run on ethanol), you will be reduced to a far simpler method. The benefit of the simpler method is that it preserves the flowers for medicinal use, although it is time-consuming and exhausting. After pulling each stalk, quickly hand-strip all flowers, seeds and all, into a bag. Do not be concerned about including small leaves with the flowers; they will not notably diminish the quality of the medicinal product if the flowers are used for that purpose later. Lay the stalks on the ground to be bundled into sheaves as you go; traditionally binders follow the reapers.

Spread the contents of the bag out on paper or close-woven cloth in a dry indoor place, well-protected from rodents and other forms of vermin. If you leave a cat in the room where the seeds are drying, beware of any tendencies to definitively identify the material as theirs for the benefit of other cats (feline marking will render the material effectively unusable). In other words, absolutely do not choose an intact tom, or even a tom who thinks he's intact, as your guard! But mice and rats absolutely will eat the seeds right out of the flowers, so a well-behaved feline presence is a good thing. Hempflower resin expert Robert C. Clarke described cannabis resin as "the Superglue of the plant world" (Hashish!).

Hand-stripping the flowers from the stalks is likely to leave the harvesters with their hands gloved in the stuff. It can be scraped off with the aid of butter or oil (not water-soluble), and reserved for medicinal use. Or possibly enjoyed by the harvesters as a reward for their day's work. Hand-rubbing is actually a traditional method of resin collection in many areas. Harvesters with hairy hands and forearms might be well-advised to either shave the exposed extremities beforehand or wear long rubber gloves. Mammalian shapeshifters with a furred semi-human shape are strongly advised not to use that shape for harvesting in this manner, no matter what physical advantage your half-animal form may give you. Or you'll end up having to shave your resin-matted fur off, and that would just look embarrassing, not to mention wasting good resin.

Once the flowers are dry, they may be quickly hand-crumbled and the seeds collected. If working in large quantities, the dried material may simply be threshed and the heavier seeds separated from the lighter residue. The dried flower/leaf material may then be turned over to your group's physician or equivalent to be rendered into medicine, while the seeds are ready to press into oil or store for food or next year's crop. The flower/leaf material will, due to rough handling, be inferior to that which is tended and carefully harvested for medicinal use...but if you're growing enough hemp to make a seed harvest worthwhile, you will likely find that, as Stalin observed, "Quantity has a quality all its own".

Lehman's hand-cranked oil press is a sturdy steel object which will do up to 8 cups (1.9 litres) per hour, and can press oil from any seeds with more than a 25% oil content, without needing to dehull first. One kilo (2.25 lbs) of hempseeds produces 0.3 litres (1 ¼ cup) of oil; flax seed produces a third again as much. The chief fault of hempseed oil is that it degrades easily. It must be kept, as much as possible, from exposure to light, heat, and oxygen. In addition to its excellent nutritional profile, cannabis seed protein, like that of egg whites, has a high absorption availability. Hempseed meal (post-pressing) is an excellent supplement for cattle, sheep, chickens, and other livestock.

Note, however, that most vegetable proteins, including cannabis seed, lack the essential amino acid lysine, which must be supplemented in children under ten (red meat, poultry, cheese, and eggs are all excellent sources; lentils, black beans, and soy also contain lysine). Callaway and Pate (op. cit.) cite a report from former Czechoslovakia (1955) in which children with tuberculosis showed marked improvement on clinical examination and X-ray after being treated with a diet including a porridge of oats and crushed cannabis seed. They consider the most likely explanation to be the improved nutrition from the polyunsaturated fatty acids and increased protein content provided by hempseed. When you're trying to keep your survivor group reasonably nourished and healthy, this is an account to take into serious consideration! Remember that although hemp seeds are not psychoactive (unless left in their bracts), they do contain potential allergens. Someone who is sensitive to cannabis pollen and/or smoke should avoid eating them. There has been at least one case of a patient developing major anaphylaxis after eating hempseed-encrusted seafood (the patient did not react to a subsequent seafood challenge).

III) Medicine

III A) Maturity

The best way to tell when medicinal hemp is ready to harvest is to examine the resin glands on the flowers and small leaves (trichomes). These are usually pedunculated (the glandular spheres are raised slightly on a tiny stalk), sometimes sessile (sitting directly on the leaf or flower). Initially, they are clear; then they become milky, then pale gold, and finally amber.

The clear-to-milky stage maximizes THC for the strain; the amber stage holds more CBN and perhaps CBD. A magnifying glass or jeweller's loupe may be helpful in assessing the trichomes. Another way to gauge flower maturity is to look at the pistils. When two-thirds or more have turned brown, the plant is definitely ready to harvest for medicinal use.

Depending on light access and variety, it may be desirable to harvest the plant in stages. It is not uncommon for the upper branches of a tall plant, particularly the "sativa" variety, to be fully ripe while the lower branches still have a week or even more to go. For the best medicinal cannabis, it is worth putting in the extra effort to harvest each branch or set of branches when it is ready, not before or after.

III B) Pre-Harvest Enhancement

There is a great deal of lore, some probably accurate and some not, floating around the community of medicinal hemp growers. Techniques which are probably worth considering:

--Clearing out fertilizer residue in the last two weeks before harvest. Some people flush (soaking the soil very thoroughly) at least once at this time. Some people simply switch to watering with pure water. If you have, as you will probably have been after the Catastrophe, limited to (or chosen to limit yourself to) the readily-available fertilizers processed by you from plant, animal, and sometimes mineral materials, this is not going to be nearly as necessary, though it won't hurt. If you have used more chemically refined and intensive products, such as standard tomato bloom/fruit fertilizer, then it might be a really good idea.
In any case, I would at least continue to add a spoonful of molasses or honey, to the water, and I see no reason why you shouldn't keep watering with an herbal "tea" until the end.

--Reducing water over the last two weeks before harvest, and denying it for the last 3-4 days. This will help somewhat in speeding the drying process, as your plant will already be slightly dehydrated when you cut it. The mild stress may or may not increase resin production and cannabinoid/terpene levels, which hemp does indeed produce as a reaction to stress (since they are meant, after all, to discourage insects).

--Keeping the plant in total darkness for the last 24-72 hours before harvest. This has been hotly debated, but is based on sound principles of general herb harvesting. The aerial pests which afflict cannabis are chiefly active by daytime. Therefore, like all herbs which must discourage daytime pests, hemp produces its active components most strongly overnight, with the level peaking at dawn (maximum production before the effects of increased light and warmth cause a certain amount of evaporation over the day).
A prolonged period of darkness probably does stimulate this production while also preventing the normal daytime evaporation. A study done in the Netherlands some years ago by the Stichting Institute of Medical Marijuana allegedly indicated that 72 hours of darkness just before harvest increased THC levels in some strains by up to 30% in the dried bud. CBD and CBN levels remained the same; terpenes were not evaluated at that time, but are quite likely to increase as well within the genetic parameters allowed by the plant. This study is, apparently, no longer readily available for unclear legal reasons, so it is now impossible to determine whether the Stichting Institute also tested shorter time periods (12, 24, and 48 hours).

This technique is sometimes touted as a way to achieve more trichomes, which is desirable because the resin glands contain ca. 50% of the cannabinoid/terpene content of the flowers and trim leaves, and is also obviously desired by those who intend to separate resin or live rosin for future use. While it is highly unlikely that more trichomes are produced in the short period of 72 hours, what is likely is that the smaller trichomes, nearly invisible without magnification, might be induced to swell by the increased cannabinoid and terpenoid production, producing the effect of greater coverage by more noticeable glands and increased potency/resin collection capability.

If you do not have the opportunity to, or decline to, try this technique, it is still recommended to harvest just at dawn, as you would with most herbs that are not specifically night-bloomers. Temperature control in the last week or two before harvest. Cannabis appears to respond strongly to lower temperatures, particularly in their "nighttime" period. This plant developed to flower and set seed in response to increasing darkness and lowering temperatures. The nighttime temperatures should generally go no lower than 12 C/ca. 50 F if avoidable to keep from killing the plants or at least slowing their metabolisms to inactivity, although some outdoor growers, with strains designed for outdoor growth in colder climates, have had good results even with nighttime temperatures in the mid- to upper-forties.

If growing indoors and if you have even crude methods of temperature control, however, it probably does help to get the night temperatures for the last week of flower ca. 13-15 C (55-59 F) in order to stimulate the plant into a last burst of activity. If using the pre-harvest total darkness, the temperature for that period should be brought up to ca. 15.5-18 C (60-65 F). This may convince the plant that its insect predators are more likely to be active and help its biosynthesis to maximum. Whether this knowledge is of any use to you after the Catastrophe, other than telling you that you might as well harvest straight away after a solid freeze since your plants will be dead unless they were in a very sheltered position, depends on your circumstances.

iii c) Harvesting Techniques

Harvesting medicinal hemp for maximum potency is a more complex and time-consuming process than harvesting hemp for fibre and seed. Some people cut the stem at the base or even pull the plant out by the roots and hang it in a dark place to dry (note: hanging hemp upside down does not encourage medicinal constituents to "drain into" the flowers. What is there, is there already, and is not going to move from one part of the plant to another. You might as well swing a black cat over it by the tail – which also will achieve nothing for the plant, but will annoy the cat). Pulling rather than cutting also permits the medicinal use of the roots, whether collected at the time of harvest or after the plant is fully dry.

The actual advantage of drying in this manner, if you have a suitably dry place and little to no mould risk, is that the plant will dry more slowly, which breaks down the chlorophyll to a greater degree and is said to produce a more pleasing effect for both smoking and edible purposes. However, this does make the plant more vulnerable to mould if that is a problem in your circumstances. Water curing, if desired, is done before the hemp is dried, and is said to produce a much smoother flavour; the plant is soaked in clean water for 5-8 days, changing the water daily, and then spread out thinly and thoroughly dried to avoid mould.

Honey or a favourite alcoholic beverage may be added to the water to enhance the flavour. Once dry, the fan leaves are separated (normally reserved for infusing lipids or alcohol). Stems can also be decarboxylated and used in the same manner, if not being used for fibre production. The small leaves springing from the clumps of flowers are then trimmed off and either used for the same purposes as the fan leaves directly, or utilized in resin separation first and then reunited with the fan leaves in their final processing destination. This leaves the dry flowers, which can then be processed at once or cured for smoking over the course of two weeks to 2-3 months by stacking them loosely in a glass jar kept in a dark cool place and unsealing it once or twice a day for ca. 15 minutes to allow accumulated water vapour to escape (if the buds begin to develop an ammonia-like smell, the jar should be left open for 2-3 hours to help them dry out).

The glass jar also protects retained seeds from rodent predation, and is considered to be the optimum method of storage. Some people prefer to add a bit of flavouring during the curing process by such means as wrapping fruit rinds (scooped out and briefly baked) or - for a savoury such as butter for Italian cooking, garlic - in a tight ball of cheesecloth and suspending the ball over the hempflowers inside the jar. Assuming that you're not producing all your plants as female clones from a "mother" – unlikely after the Catastrophe, as discussed – you will also have seeds.

Some of these will fall out during dry-trimming and should be carefully gathered and preserved in a dark, low-moisture environment until it is time to plant again. The rest can be collected as the flowers are utilized, as long as the rodents didn't get them while they were drying. If you harvested at the golden-to-amber stage, you could probably have collected some ripe seeds from the fresh plant directly to tuck away for the next planting. Another option is to do the main processing while the plant is fresh.

Carry out the fan-leaf separation, putting them to dry separately or straight into an extract which is to be heated long enough for decarboxylation (if you don't mind the taste of chlorophyll), The small leaves are trimmed and used in a similar manner. For resin separation of fresh material by means of water-straining (below), it is recommended to put these small, trichome-rich leaves and any flowers used for that purpose into a freezer or at least the coldest environment possible overnight.

Otherwise, the flowers are spread to dry evenly and slowly (again, try to collect the ripest of the fresh seeds, and beware of rodents chewing the rest of the seeds right out of the clumps!), and then either processed or cured as described above. It is noted to be considerably easier and less messy to separate the small leaves from the flowers in an effective manner with fresh-trimming, should that be desired. Less resin is lost in the trimming process with fresh-trimming, and the residue on trimming utensils is said to be admirably suited for rewarding the harvester with a special smoke in the traditional hand-rubbed Nepalese manner when the work is done. The great majority of reports I have read and heard, especially in the years after the advent of fresh-frozen resin separation, come down strongly in favour of fresh trimming rather than dry trimming.

III D) Resin Separation

Resin separation from fresh plants is highly favoured by most real-life hash producers, both because it is more efficient and because it produces a purer product than the traditional means of separating resin from dried plants. This method, known variously as "ice hash" or "bubble hash", requires a large bucket (ca. 5 gallons), straining bags (20-25, 70, 135-150, and 220 micron mesh; meant to separate plant material, large glands, and small glands; the crucial two bags are the 220 for plant material and ca. 20-25 to catch even the smallest free glands, but most people add at least a 70 micron bag which is said to produce the highest quality), cold water, and, if at all possible, a quantity of ice cubes and an electric mixer with paddles (not blades, which will chop the plant material rather than agitating it, and lead to more leaf or flower particles in the resin).

The finer bags are put into the bucket, with the largest size on the inside and the smallest size on the outside. Their edges should overlap the edge of the bucket sufficiently that they can be secured with a rubber band or string. Cold water is poured in; the frozen herb is put into the 220-mesh bag together with the ice cubes; that bag is put inside the 135-150 bag; and the bucket topped up with cold water to ca. 3 inches or so from the top. You then beat the herb/ice cube mixture with the electric mixer or vigorously with a large wooden spoon for 3-5 minutes; let the resin settle for approximately ten. The inner bag is lifted out and all liquid is allowed to drain. Don't squeeze it; again, that will force flower/leaf particles through.

When the bag has drained, you may want to ladle more water through it and drain again a couple of times to be sure you have rinsed out all available resin. The second bag is lifted out and allowed to drain thoroughly into the third. There should be a quantity of what looks like sludge at the bottom. This is the resin, or hashish. When that has drained, it may be scraped out with a spoon and spread on a plate to dry. Repeat the process with the third bag. Alternatively, if you have a small hand-cranked (or electrical, if you still have a power source) washing machine with a drainage hose, you can put a sealed bag of plant material and ice cubes into it with a quantity of ice and the coldest water possible. Run for two to five minutes and drain through the series of bags; scrape out the resin and repeat. Several washings may be done, though the quality will drop with each. However, if you are separating resin for convenience of use or for pressing live rosin, this is not a great concern; the only contaminant is hemp plant material.

The difference between top-quality bubble hash and medium-quality bubble hash is primarily an issue for the gourmet inhaler, though more of the medium-quality may need to be added to maintain the potency of dosage in medicinals produced from resin. The potency of live rosin will be the same regardless of the original hash quality. First-rate hash will produce more rosin per volume pressed... but some purists would advance the theory that it is blasphemous to waste full-melt hash in such a manner. The proportion of resin caught in each bag will depend on how large the glands of your particular strain were. Sativa strains are said to generally have small resin glands, sometimes as tiny as 25 microns; some indica strains, particularly those described with names like "Hash Plant", may have very large glands, up to 150 microns or even larger.

The bag holding the plant material and ice cubes should be 220 microns to make sure that all the resin passes into the collection bags. Some people use up to five or even seven bags within this range, and are very particular about the quality of resin derived from each mesh size. Unless you have the trained sensitivity of a Cannabis Cup judge or the like, however, having one collection bag that catches the large-to-medium glands and one to pick up the medium-to-small glands ought to suffice (and, as mentioned above, all you really need are the coarse plant-material bag and the fine 25 micron collection bag). While the bags are not in use for this purpose, they can also be used for straining jellies, tinctures, and so forth.

This process may be repeated several times, although the quality of resin will go down as more fragments of leaf and flower break off (it will start appearing greenish rather than golden). After the final draining, spread the plant material to dry. Although, ideally, you have removed the vast majority of the external resin glands, the remaining material still contains a fair quantity (perhaps half) of the total desired constituents, and, when dried, may be gainfully processed further by any of the means described above. Resin collected by this method is said to be the purest in the world, excepting only the concentrated "live rosin" (section 6 e) which is pressed from this resin. The term "bubble hash" refers to the propensity of the pure resin to bubble when first ignited, which is a recognized hallmark of quality.

A quantity roughly the size of an hemp seed (with which, by this point, you are undoubtedly extremely familiar) should suffice for one strong dose of smoke or oral preparation, or two doses of vapourized medication. The resin may also be dissolved into essential oil in the same manner as an alcohol, butane, or rosin concentrated extract. Assuming that you were not using this method to rescue your harvest from a mould attack, the water should be poured back onto the patch it came from, as it is rich in essential hemp-growing nutrients. If you did have a mould problem, pour the water out somewhere far away from your planting site. In the case of mould, although the main plant material should have been well-washed and beaten clean, it is wisest to use it only for an alcoholic tincture or alcohol extraction. When dry, the resin should be pressed put into an airtight, dark, cool place for storage if it is not immediately incorporated into another form of remedy. Pressing homogenizes the resin glands, and also aids in getting the last water out of the resin.

While some claim that, when properly dried, the results of this process break down into a powdery substance, and while gland "powder", at least from dry-sifting, has better storage qualities than pressed resin, other reports indicate that the extracted hashish tends to remain as sticky clumps, probably best stored in a tight-sealing glass jar which is not so large as to expose the product to any more air than necessary. Resin pressing can be done by one of the small machines sold for this purpose, or by hand. Robert Clarke's Hashish! describes these processes in detail, along with providing a great deal of other information which will be found fascinating and useful by both the Catastrophe survivor and the real-life person who is in a legal position to try this for themselves.

Dry resin separation is less efficient and produces a less pure product, as fine particles of the dry plant material will inevitably be given off along with the resin. However, it does produce that tiny-grained “kif”, which is not prone to mould and keeps better than ice hash, pressed or unpressed. A common method for small quantities is to place the plant material on a tight-stretched piece of silk or nylon of an appropriate weave size (ca. 185 microns), with a tray lined with non-porous material under it, and drumming on it to break the resin glands off so that they fall through the mesh and are collected in the tray. The efficiency is low; to get the absolute best quality may require a ratio as high as 500:1 (50 kg/111 lbs flowers = 100 g/3.33 oz hashish), but the purity is probably the highest that can be attained with a dry-processing method.

Traditionalists, however, have been known to claim that the taste of dry-separated resin is markedly smoother and the overall qualities superior to fresh-separated resin. The difference in tastes may owe something to the increased current awareness and appreciation of terpenes, which are higher in fresh-separated resin. Traditional dry-resin hashish is also notable for the high presence of an unusual terpenoid named “hashishene”. This stems from the oxidation of beta-myrcene by exposure to light (the hemp plants are traditionally dried outdoors in the sun), and is found in significant quantities, to date, only in hashish. Beta-myrcene is a common cannabis terpene, and increases blood-brain barrier penetration, as well as being analgesic, anti-inflammatory, and sedative. The specific effects of hashishene have not yet been studied, but may be responsible for differences in both flavour and perceived effect between first-rate hashish produced in a traditional manner and, for instance, full-melt bubble hash.

A metal screen may be used in place of the silk or nylon, and performs separation faster, but is likely to allow more powdered plant material through with the resin. Large quantities are traditionally processed by threshing the plant material in a sealed building or over a fine-woven carpet and scraping the residue off the walls or shaking it carefully out of the carpet. This method is obviously inefficient, and really only suited for hemp grown by full-time cannabis farmers or collectively by communities. In all cases and types of resin separation, the colder the plant material can be kept, the better. Frozen, or at least highly chilled, resin glands break off with far greater ease than do room-temperature ones. Traditional processing of large quantities was (and still is in some regions) done on the first good frosty day of winter. If at all possible, for both dry and fresh methods, the plant material should be frozen when processed, or at least as cold as you can get it. The ice cubes or chips in the fresh-processing method, assuming that you either still have a freezer or live where you can keep an ice-house through the summer, also aid in breaking the trichome heads off via increased agitation.

8. Sources and Strains of Interest

In looking for the individual strain or strains that will best suit your post-Catastrophe needs, the Internet is your best friend. No other plant, including more commonly-grown favourites such as roses and tomatoes, is likely to have such extensive reviews on the growing characteristics and constituents of every possible variety. Many reviewers and seed suppliers also list at least the maximum THC content of varietals which have been tested, and sometimes either cite or at least generally describe the THC : CBD ratio. Advice regarding susceptibility to fungi and pests may also be provided in either the seller's description or the independent reviews. Terpene analyses are becoming increasingly available.

Note that all plant constituents may vary according to individual characteristics within a strain and growing circumstances; the analysis of one particular batch of a strain is only a rough guide to what might be expected of it. It may be that, with further experimentation for both medicinal and recreational uses, ten years from now we will have a better idea of what conditions, nutrients, usw. promote the development of which cannabinoids and which terpenes. Genetic traits, however, are the predominant determinant.

Currently, the only way to affect the constituent profile of your medical hemp is to select a strain which has the potential and tendency to be stronger in the constituents you want (and weaker in those you don't want, or don't want as much of); and then to make sure the plant receives appropriate soil and water, good lighting, good nutrients appropriate to the life-cycle period, and protection from pests and pathogens.

I am including listings of a few of the best-known strains for which terpene analysis is available (these examples from the archives of Analytical 360, a scientific company which offers both commercial and private testing of hops, fibre hemp, and medicinal hemp: https://analytical360.com/cannabis-analysis) in order to give a general sense of how the different terpene profiles contribute to different effects, which is increasingly becoming a factor in appropriate strain selection. These particular strains have all been highly recommended to my attention by people of considerable experience from cannabis-legal areas whose opinions I respect, backed up by a good number of published reviews.

Blue Dream

- » THC: very high (20-25%)
- » CBD: low (0.08%)
- » Terpenes: alpha-pinene 0.843%, myrcene 0.415%, caryophyllene 0.346%, beta-pinene 0.290%, humulene 0.193%, limonene 0.07 %, linalool 0.02%. Total terpenes: 2.177%.
- » Common effects: Calm, euphoric, good analgesic qualities without being sedative. Said to be a good choice when high THC levels are medically required, but sedation is not wanted.

Harlequin

» THC: low (6.05%)
» CBD: high (10.83%)
» Terpenes: alpha-pinene 0.309%, myrcene 0.298%, caryophyllene 0.238%, beta-pinene 0.099%, humulene 0.082%, limonene 0.058%, linalool 0.01%. Total terpenes: 1.094%.
» **Common effects:** Physical and emotional relaxation with mild mental stimulation; a good painkiller without significant psychoactivity.

Northern Lights, versions from various sources. Also available as an autoflower.

» THC: very high (ca. 20-25%)
» CBD: low (0.18%)
» Terpenes: humulene 0.33%, caryophyllene 0.31%, myrcene 0.29%.
» Total terpenes: .93%.
» **Common effects:** sedative, sleep-promoting, excellently analgesic and relaxant, strong appetite stimulant. Marked "couch-lock", a term which means just what it says on the tin.

Romulan, currently from Next Generation (Canada). Reported to be one of the most effective analgesic strains around.

» THC: high (ca. 15-20%)
» CBD: low (0. 11%)
» Terpenes: caryophyllene 0.69%; humulene 0.67%; terpinolene 0.63%; myrcene 0.12%; alpha-pinene 0.02%. Total terpenes: 2.13%.
» **Common effects:** notably sedative, relaxant, and remarkably analgesic. If one is a Star Trek geek, it comes with the added bonus of the opportunity for all sorts of humour about the name.

Super Lemon Haze

» THC: moderate-high (ca. 15%)
» CBD: low (0.33%)
» Terpenes: 3.22% limonene, 1.55% caryophyllene, 1.49% linalool, 1.27% humulene, 1.2% terpinolene, 0.7% alpha-pinene, 0.5% caryophyllene oxide, 0.25% myrcene. Total terpenes: 10.18%.
» **General effects:** energetic, euphoric, uplifting. Often described as a "party strain". Limonene, the dominant terpene in this strain, is known to have stimulant and mood-elevating effects and is also responsible for the distinctive citrus flavour/aroma after which it is named.

White Widow, versions from various sources. Also available as an autoflower.

» THC: high (15-20%)
» CBD: low (0.42%)
» Terpenes: linalool 2.45%, myrcene 1.43%, alpha-pinene 0.85%, caryophyllene oxide 0.66%, caryophyllene 0.55%. Total terpenes: 5.75%
» Common effects: a light, euphoric, but powerful effect; also an excellent analgesic. Linalool is also found in lavender essential oil, and persons familiar with both have reported that the feeling of relaxed uplift is similar, though rather enhanced by the cannabinoids in White Widow. The floral aroma of some hops strains is due to linalool, which plays a small part in the relaxing effects of this plant.

Terpenes are also becoming available as separate products. Terpenes are legal everywhere, not least because they are found in a wide range of plants other than cannabis. Producers in areas where hemp itself is illegal are able to recreate specific strain profiles with terpenes derived from, for instance, lavender (linalool), pine (alpha- and beta-pinene), and so forth. These terpene combinations are used to achieve some of the benefits of particular strains of whole cannabis without issues regarding either legality or psychoactivity. They are also used to restore scent, flavour, and terpene effects to forms of medicinal hemp which may have lost their natural terpenes in processing, more likely if the whole plant is water-cured (done before drying) or an ice-water resin separation is performed.

In regards to higher CBD strain producers, I will mention CBD Crew in particular. They have been around for several years, are considered highly reputable; and, as it says on the tin, they specialize in high-CBD percentage varietals. Their seeds are available through a great many distributors, and can be found with a swift Google search. They even produce a dwarf/autoflower variety, Med-GOM 1.0, which has approximately a 1:1 THC:CBD ratio (may vary with individual plant and circumstances). In other words, less than $200 spent on seeds, alcohol, and a spray bottle could provide the MS sufferer (where it is legal or after the Catastrophe) with a year's supply of Sativex (pharmaceutical version estimated at 4500-5000 euros/year by Ireland's National Centre for Pharmacoeconomics, 2014).

Normally, using a home herbal preparation rather than a pharmaceutical one when available is strongly disrecommended – is often a remarkably bad idea - but the dosing latitude of cannabis makes that concern irrelevant. A 10% variation in a drug with a low therapeutic index could kill (either by toxicity or inefficacy); a 10% variation in a cannabis-based drug cannot, especially given the safety of upwards titration. CBD Crew have recently produced a second strain of Med-GOM with a higher CBD percentage, called, with little imagination but no possible confusion, Med-GOM CBD (4-8% THC:8-15% CBD).

The most commonly known highest CBD/lowest THC strains, notably Avidekel (from Israel), Harlequin, and Charlotte's Web, have been notoriously unavailable as seeds for some time. Elev8 now produces a feminized Harlequin (6.5% THC:9.1% CBD), and clones are reputed to have been available at some dispensaries for some time now. Avidekel is just beginning to be seen outside Israel, but seeds are not yet readily available by mail order. The producers of Charlotte's Web appear to be focusing on CBD oil; I was unable to find any references to seeds for this plant.

Fortunately, more high CBD/low THC strains are now being bred for public availability, such as Medical Marijuana Genetics' Candida CD-1 (0.3-0.9% THC:10.6-20.6% CBD), Elité Seeds' Solodiol CBD (<1% THC:20+% CBD; also available as autoflowering), and Elité Seeds' Sedativa (CBDV:CBD ratio 7:8; no THC or CBD numbers given, but stated as "low THC and high CBD"; the CBDV in this plant may make it particularly suited to treatment of seizure disorders and muscular spasms). Candida CD-1, according to the Seedsman website, produces both "sativa" (taller, with "wispier" buds and a lower per-plant yield, but also has a higher CBD count), and "indica" (short, stocky, heavier buds; not quite as potent) phenotypes.

The pre-Catastrophe character thinking that this also would be a good strain to use for fibre and seed hemp might be advised to get some of the seeds (feminized only available) and do their best to induce hermaphroditism in the tallest, rebreeding the hermaphrodite to itself and possibly the second tallest. Rinse and repeat through multiple generations, concentrating on height; and in the meantime, look for the highest CBD/lowest THC strain that is available as non-feminized seeds to offer the option of large-scale and on-going pollination after the Catastrophe. Note that, in commercial strain descriptions of medicinal hemp, the phrase "CBD-rich" simply means "above 4% CBD".

Look for specific percentages and get the complete ratio when seeking out your high-CBD seeds, whether preparing for the Catastrophe in fiction or growing where it is legal in real life! The UK supplier Seedsman (not to be confused with Seedman, the source of nearly all seeds except cannabis and some of the most toxic herbs described in the next section) is particularly good about listing both THC and CBD percentages whenever those are known, and does carry both Med-GOM CBD and Candida CD-1, among a wide range of other cannabis seeds (excepting the low-constituent "industrial fibre" strains; but a good tall rangy sativa or hybrid with a sativa-like phenotype might do as well for you as the true industrials in fibre-production terms).

They are also very good about citing estimated height range and yield whenever possible. The Seedsman website assures the customer that they ship discreetly to every country in the world, with the caveat that the customer should check their local laws to make certain that they can actually legally purchase the product. All of their products are legal to order and own in Europe and the UK – if not necessarily to actually germinate in some countries at the time of writing. UK site Seed City also comes highly recommended, and also ships internationally. If your area includes cannabis dispensaries, you – the character, the author, or the real-life grower/user/health-care professional - might do well to ask the staff any questions you have about specific strains or types of cannabis, or about guidelines and usage in general.

Dispensary staff, like general pharmacists, are expected to be both knowledgeable and helpful. If that ever proves not to be the case, you have grounds for complaint. Another advantage of dispensaries is that it is possible to purchase small amounts of different strains and learn what works best for your needs before the Catastrophe hits and while you can still purchase seeds...or at least, in real life (assuming that you can legally grow for home usage, which is not the case in all legal-use regions), before you put in the time and effort needed to grow your plants. This is a much better idea than just going on the Internet and ordering a strain by description, phytocannabinoid contents, and, possibly, enticingly creative name.

The increasing awareness of terpenes and terpenoids does mean that these components are increasingly evaluated and listed as well; and they ought not be ignored either in terms of efficacy (having medical functions and perceptual effect-distinctions of their own) or safety (it is quite possible to be allergic to specific terpenoids, but not to cannabinoids, for instance). With increasing legalization in many parts of the world, some breeders are also working on the aesthetic qualities of their hemp plants. There are several strains which, particularly in cooler weather, demonstrate deep purple leaves and/or flowers ("Ayahuasca Purple", "Purple Urkle", "Frisian Dew", and many others).

Flowers may also show visible tinges of blue, a red colour to the pistils ("Atomic Sherbert" and others), and can sometimes be really very pink ("Pink Kush", "Pink Lady", "Pink Starburst"). Some can actually be quite colourful, and well-suited to an aesthetic garden grow if you are allowed to do that where you live. The name is often an hint: "Purple Strawberry Bliss" is described as "(turning) an astonishing range of colours from deep purple through red shades, blues, and dark green" (Seedsman website). A certain degree of amusement may also be derived from scanning through a seller's website and enjoying the imagination, or possibly speculating about the quantity and quality of the plant being used by the originators, that went into some of the strain names.

Devices for Processing and Storing

A good metal grinder with a screen through which dislodged resin glands can fall and a collecting tray is the most efficient means of preparing dry plant material for any purpose, including infusions, tinctures, extractions, and smoking/vapourizing. The finer the grind, the more surface area will be exposed to the medium of your choice (or the better the material will smoke/vapourize), and the more efficient the production process will be. Grinders come in various sizes; after the Catastrophe, you will want the largest one you were able to obtain.

Large metal grinders can also, in a pinch, be used for spices and even coffee beans, assuming that someone in your survival group has strong hands. Resin presses are similarly available in a range of sizes, as are airtight and self-vacuum-sealing storage containers. The Honey Bee extractor mentioned earlier is for those who are brave (or stupid) enough to try butane extraction. All of the above are sold in various shops catering to the home processor. Growshop Alien, in the Netherlands, is a famously reliable supplier with a long history, sells a good range of all the devices mentioned, and also has an excellent seed selection.

They ship worldwide, with the usual caveat about ensuring that what you order from them is legal where you live, and politely mention the discretion of their packaging. Tracking and tracing services from Growshop Alien are only available in Europe and a few other countries, which they list on their website. As in Part I: for home quantities of food oils pressed from seeds, I can personally recommend Lehman's hand-cranked oil press.

Lehman's (lehmans.com) is informally known to many as Your Amish Supply Shop, and they carry a wide range of high-quality items which, if you didn't buy them before the Catastrophe, you'll wish you had. Sadly, this does not include flax/hemp breakers, though those really are easy to make. Another good hand-operated oil press is the Piteba (made in Holland), which can be ordered directly from www.piteba.com. Potency of dried plant material or other medicinal hemp products can be assayed at home by means of such tests as the CB Scientific Test4 Combo Detection Potency Kit (THC and CBD), available via Amazon. The California-based company SDPharmLabs (www.SDPharmLabs.com) offers testing for potency and/or gender from the time of a young plant's third leaf-pair on.

Sources which you are likely to find useful, informative, and entertaining:

Callaway, JC, and David W. Pate. "Hempseed Oil" (article revised from a book chapter; full biblio in references) is the most thorough guide to the nutritional characteristics of cannabis seeds yet written, to my knowledge. It is available and free on-line: https://www.impolankasvitila.fi/img/file.php?id=37916

Clarke, Robert C. Hashish! (Red Eye Press, 1998). As indicated above, this is pretty much the go-to book for anything related to hemp resin. History, tradition, and practicalities: Clarke researched them all most extensively (although the book pre-dates rosin extraction, and was written shortly before ice/bubble hash became a common household processing method), and presents them in a highly intriguing and entertaining manner. His

Cannabis: Evolution and Ethnobotany (U of California Press, 2016) may also be of interest, as may Hemp Diseases and Pests (John C. McPartland, Robert C. Clarke, and D.P. Watson, CABI, 2000). His Marijuana Botany (Ronin, 1993, 2nd edn) is still considered to be the best guide to the challenging task of selecting male pollinators for medicinal plants. Clarke is probably the leading expert today on cannabis agriculture, genetics, and roles in human history.

Malanca, John (host). The Sacred Plant: Healing Secrets Examined. A seven-episode video series, this is an excellent introduction for anyone who may be unfamiliar with the many indications for which medical cannabis is starting to be used, or retains excessive wariness/emotional antagonism as a result of the legal and social attitudes of the past few decades. The series is very heavy on the personal anecdotes, which are well-chosen to evoke emotional response (episode 4, which deals with hemp in cancer, is occasionally described as "heart-rending"). However, these are interspersed with health-care professionals and researchers giving wider overviews and some introduction to the science behind the particular uses; some indications of dosages and cannabinoid percentages that are considered in practice to probably be effective are also given. While the series is not by any means an objective evaluation of safety and efficacy and doesn't claim to be (the title should be something of a hint), it is a good overview of potential benefits presented in an accessible and humane manner. https://thesacredplant.com/

Richter, Gary. Natural Pet Care.

Rosenthal, Ed. Marijuana Gold: From Trash to Stash (Quick American Archives, 2002). Offers a plethora of ways to process and use medicinal (and recreational) hemp, including those parts such as the fan leaves and trim which may be ignored by some modern growers, but which the Catastrophe survivor will not want to waste.

An excellent list of clinical studies and case reports regarding cannabis can be found at: https://www.cannabis-med.org/studies/study.php

There are a great many guides to the art of growing medicinal cannabis in various circumstances, both in hard copy and on the Internet. Advice can easily be found on fine details such as training a plant to grow and flower in a specific way (multiple central clusters instead of a single one, optimal for achieving even lighting indoors); the issue of pruning and techniques for better flower yield such as topping and fimming (described above). Although, no matter what a source tells you, don't take off any more fan leaves than needed to allow light through to obscured clusters.

This is as true for cannabis as for tomatoes or roses: your plant needs those leaves to provide it with energy. If you live where you can grow medicinal hemp in the first place, gardening guides should be expected in stores that cater to the activity, and will probably be appearing swiftly on the shelves of general bookshops. Post-apocalyptic cannabis use has generally been avoided in fiction outside the odd mention of recreational and/or fibre use (and where did American characters get their fibre hemp, when even non-THC industrial strains were illegal in the US until mid-2018? From the bottom of a stash bag, that's where).

This is presumably a result of authors/publishers wishing to stay clear of controversial topics, plus the fact that the range of proven, indicated, and possible medical effects has only truly started to come to light within the past ten years or so due to the serious social prejudice induced against this plant for much of the 20th century. I have mentioned Diana Gabaldon's Outlander series and the primary heroine's observation of hemp efficacy in several regards corresponding eerily to the expansion of the knowledge base in her future. Regrettably for the characters of S.M. Stirling's Emberverse books (in which hemp is grown for fibre), his Change happened in 1998, after the most significant medical uses of the 19th and early 20th century had been forgotten, but before we knew or suspected a fraction of what is known or suspected today.

Part III: The Witch's Brew

Introduction

The herbs I talk about here are truly the ones that deserve the label "extreme herbalism". Several of them supply components still used – with due care! – in modern pharmacology; all of them are a good deal more toxic than poppies, and pretty much infinitely more toxic than hemp. After the Catastrophe, these will mostly be the "kill or cure" remedies...but correspondingly, they may be the only remedies that can save lives in certain situations. So you will want to have your (fenced and locked, child- and critter-proof) medicinal garden and your stock of these herbs ready for when you really need them.

This is not a total overview of all herbs in this category; here I am chiefly dealing with the European herbs with which I am familiar and which are still, directly or indirectly, a significant part of medicine in real life. Indeed, very few people realize how often extreme herbs or their extracts or synthetic analogues are prescribed by physicians; Stephen King once wrote a rather humourous short story playing on that point ("The Mangler" – a series of accidents including a virtuous young worker cutting her hand on the machine...and an older worker dropping a box of an over-the-counter indigestion remedy containing atropine from deadly nightshade...cause a laundromat machine to be possessed by a demon. Night Shift; Doubleday, 1978). All of these herbs can both pass the placental barrier and be secreted into breast milk. They should not be used by pregnant women or nursing mothers unless there is no possible alternative, and with the understanding that death of the fetus or baby is a highly possible outcome.

Cholinergic/Anti-cholinergic Effects

Sarin nerve gas and organophosphates are cholinergics. Their effects are known by the acronym SLUDGE: Salivation, Lacrimation, Diarrhoea, GI distress, Emesis.

The active constituents (tropane alkaloids) of henbane, deadly nightshade, and mandrake are anti-cholinergic.

The typical symptoms are "red as a beet (flushing), dry as a bone (suppresses all secretions, including saliva and sweat, and causes urinary retention), blind as a bat (blurred vision; can precipitate narrow-angle glaucoma), hot as a hare (elevated body temperature), and mad as a hatter (hallucinations, delirium, manic outbursts)."

I. Henbane (Hyoscamus niger)

a) Introduction

Henbane is one of the less poisonous herbs in this section. It is a member of the same family as deadly nightshade, potatoes, and tomatoes (Solanaceae), and has been used as an analgesic and intoxicant for at least 2000 years. It was one of the most common anaesthetic agents in the Classical world, and a bag of seeds was found in the grave of the Danish Viking Age "Fyrkat witch". Whether she was using it for magical purposes, as a medicine, as a poison, or for all three remains unknown. In parts of Germany, it was added to beer for its psychoactive effects; the well-known "Pilsner" brand is named after this herb (German Pilsenkraut or Bilsenkraut – B becomes P in some German dialects).

All parts of the henbane are poisonous, though some less so than others. Henbane is a strong analgesic and hypnotic, hence its frequent historical use in surgical treatment. It formed a part of the "soporific sponge" recipe: a sponge was soaked in henbane, hemlock, and opium, possibly together with other herbs (Nicholas of Salerno mentions mulberry, mandrake, ivy, and lettuce – probably wild lettuce, which is a mild soporific), and held over the patient's face. This allegedly induced up to 96 hours of sleep. Ayurvedic medicine uses it for treating the symptoms of Parkinson's disease, for which it probably is effective, particularly in regards to tremor and via its strong anticholinergic effects.

b) Chemical Constituents

Henbane contains hyoscyamine, scopolamine, and atropine. Hyoscyamine, the main alkaloid in henbane, is anti-cholinergic and anti-spasmodic. It is particularly used for relaxing smooth muscles, including those of the GI tract, the bladder, and the uterus. It decreases stomach acid secretion, and is sometimes used as an antacid and painful spasm-reducer for stomach ulcers, as well as diverticulitis, colic, irritable bowel syndrome, and pancreatitis. Constipation is not uncommonly seen together with the expected anti-cholinergic side effects, including urinary retention (relatively contraindicated in patients with prostate difficulties). Tachycardia and arrhythmias are also a concern.

Hyoscyamine is also used for motion sickness, hyperactive bladder, and severe allergic rhinitis (runny nose). It is sometimes used in asthma for its bronchodilatory effect and reducing mucus overproduction. After the Catastrophe, the main indicator for its use will most likely be treating a patient with kidney stones or severely painful cystitis. Kidney stones are recognised clinically by extremely severe colicky (intermittent cramping) pains in the mid-to-lower back, radiating to flanks and groin. If you and your patient are very lucky, henbane may relax the smooth muscles of the urinary tract in order to allow the stone to pass. At low doses, henbane is also a mild diuretic (at high doses it causes urinary retention), which, unless the tract is completely blocked, may be of assistance in moving the stone along.

Cannabis, particularly with a higher CBD level, can assist in this relaxation while aiding with the pain. Care, however, must be taken that the side effects of hemp (dry mouth and eyes, psychoactivity) do not mask the same effects caused by henbane. From cannabis, they are largely harmless; for henbane or other anti-cholinergics, they may be a sign of approaching a dangerous level of concentration. The pain of a kidney stone has been likened to childbirth; opiates absolutely should be given if needed, together with henbane if there is no real-life alternative, though a close watch on the patient's vitals to avoid oversedation with the combination of poppy and henbane is vital.

Scopolamine (a.k.a. hyoscine)

Scopolamine is most commonly used to treat nausea and motion sickness, usually as a transdermal patch. It is also anti-cholinergic, and many of the cautions and benefits of hyoscyamine also apply: the risk of urinary retention, bowel blockage, etc.; the use in treating smooth muscle spasms (bladder, GI tract). Sometimes it is used pre-surgically to reduce secretions, and post-surgically for nausea control, although in real life it has largely been replaced by cloperadine and ondansetron for the latter use. Scopolamine crosses the placenta and is secreted in breast milk. Plants containing this should be avoided in pregnancy and while nursing if at all possible. Scopolamine and morphine were used in the late 19th through early 20th century for surgical analgesia or "twilight sleep", like henbane, poppy extract, mandrake, and deadly nightshade previously. They have since been replaced by much safer and more effective anaesthetics.

Atropine

Henbane contains only a relatively small amount of atropine, another anti-cholinergic alkaloid which will be discussed in full under "Deadly Nightshade".

c) Dosing

Dosing with henbane is most reliable when the seeds are used. Seeds are ca. 0.5-0.6% (mostly hyoscyamine) alkaloid; the dried leaves and flowers, according to the British Pharmacoepia of Mrs. Grieves' day, vary from 0.045% to 0.14%. The roots had already passed out of medical use by the 1930s. The stems contain little alkaloid.

M. Grieves notes that "In the case of adults, twenty seeds have been proved insufficient to prove fatal, though they induced grave results". The British Pharmacoepia dosage for dried and powdered leaves which she cites ranges from 2 to 10 grains (roughly 130-650 milligrams; 1 grain = 65 milligrams). This goes higher at maximum than the amounts currently used by herbalists (those who dare to use it at all, who are very few indeed in Western herbalism), ca. 100-150 milligrams of dry leaf. The leaf is normally administered in the form of an infused tea. It may also be made into a tincture (1:10 in 70% alcohol, dosage 2-5 ml).

It was traditionally smoked to relieve toothache, and smoking may be the safest way to administer it due to the ease of titration. Leaves, flowers, and seeds can all be smoked. Either the alcoholic extract or a steeped oil may be used as a topical analgesic and anti-inflammatory. While the danger of overdose is reduced by topical use, it is no coincidence that henbane is a common ingredient in the topically-applied hallucinatory "flying ointment". The oil should be made to the same percentages as the tincture, with the same dosages, and diluted in a carrier oil if more than 2-5 ml. is required to cover the area in question.

The symptoms of a henbane overdose include hallucinations, delirium (sometimes combative), coma, respiratory paralysis, and death. Convulsions, slurred speech, dilated pupils with photophobia and blurred vision, vomiting, dry mouth, intense thirst, inability to swallow, loss of coordination, high fever, speedy heart rate, arrhythmias, urinary retention with possible backflow kidney damage, and spiking blood pressure are also seen at lower doses. Considering how difficult it is to estimate the actual level of active constituents in any whole herb...this is why you shouldn't use henbane if you have any less dangerous option. Treatment for overdose: gastric emptying, activated charcoal, and benzodiazepines (if not available, use valerian, which also activates the GABA receptors).

d) Growing

Henbane can be either annual or biennial. It is often difficult to cultivate from seed, except when you don't want it, in which case it will self-seed persistently. Seeds can lurk in the ground for up to five years before germinating. If collecting seeds, they should be planted straight away, but may not come up until spring. Henbane requires cold stratification (at least two weeks in the refrigerator, or just plant in autumn and let the herb follow its natural course). Henbane does not have much horizontal spread – it sends up a single flower stalk from a rosette of leaves – so it can be planted in clumps.

It can also be grown in pots, though it stays rather smaller than when it is grown in the ground. Due to the smell, you probably do not want to try growing it indoors – definitely not if you have small children or house animals! – but it can be grown indoors by a good window. Henbane prefers sandy or well-drained loamy soils, preferably mildly alkaline, though it will grow in mildly acidic earth. It will not stand for being waterlogged, but does need to be kept from drying out, and needs a bit more water when flowering; it is most at home in Northern Europe, and thrives in the damp temperate climate of Ireland and the UK. It often grows on waste ground or disturbed soil (fields, roadsides). Fertilizer and foliar feeding are both appreciated by this plant, but decent earth or potting soil will quite suffice it.

The most important thing to keep in mind when selecting a henbane plot is that it must not be accessible to animals, especially poultry, or to children. It is claimed that pigs are largely immune to the toxicity of the aerial parts and may seem to enjoy the effects of the plant; but this does not seem to have been tested. In any case, if you intend to eat the pig, letting it feed on henbane is probably not a good idea. The roots certainly can kill pigs. It is advised to wear gloves when harvesting henbane. If seed is desired, the pods should be covered with a bag as soon as the flowers have withered, unless you want the plant to continue self-seeding (probably the most reliable way to ensure an ongoing supply).

Visually, henbane is a very striking garden plant in a creepy sort of way when in flower. The randomly curving serpentine stalks, which may grow up to three feet high, are lined with a double row of elongated yellowish-white bell-shaped flowers with deep violet throats and sometimes violet veining (black hemlock; white hemlock is a variant with pale whitish-yellow flowers), resembling the bones of a snake's spinal column. Or, as others have observed, teeth in a jawbone, which may or may not have contributed to the folk use of this plant as an analgesic for toothache (the "Doctrine of Signatures" – the theory that a plant's appearance tells you what it's good for, or, in my opinion, the proof that you can find something in the appearance of every plant which can be made to serve as a mnemonic for its uses).

The gardener who plants henbane for aesthetic effect is probably deliberately creating either a Goth look or a visual witch's garden. If you are a witch or similar practitioner, whether fictional or in real life, you will probably want to plant henbane for magico-spiritual reasons, even if you're too sensible to use it as a psychoactive magical aid or entheogen. Henbane also has a distinctive and rather nasty scent, but whiffing too closely is not advised, as even too much of the odour is reputed to cause giddiness and dizziness.

II. Deadly Nightshade (Atropa belladonna)

a) Introduction

The most characteristic "witch's herb", this close relative of the tomato and potato looks very like a tomato plant with small purple-black fruit. It was one of the better-known poisons of Europe; the Empress Livia is said to have used it on Emperor Augustus, and there are various stories of Scots employing deadly nightshade against either English or Danish foes.

In the Renaissance and early modern periods, deadly nightshade was used cosmetically to widen women's pupils, creating a lustrous and mysterious look; hence the name "belladonna" ("beautiful woman"). Deadly nightshade is one of the herbs most commonly referred to in both recipes for surgical analgesia/anaesthesia and recipes for witch's "flying ointment", due to its narcotic and hallucinogenic qualities. It is sometimes confused with woody nightshade (Solanum dulcamara). The latter is a relative, but is not the same plant.

B) Chemical Constituents and Effects

The primary active component of deadly nightshade is atropine, named after the plant in which it was discovered. Atropine is a powerful anti-cholinergic, the first-line treatment for organophosphate poisoning and (by injection) the standard antidote against nerve gas. Symptoms of excessive atropine are the anti-cholinergic symptoms described in the sidebar above. Like henbane, deadly nightshade contains scopolamine and hyoscyamine. A common pharmaceutical use for belladonna in real life is treating gastro-intestinal disorders, particularly those involving severe cramping, pain, and diarrhoea.

In real life, it is often compounded with phenobarbitol for this purpose. After the Catastrophe, when all other methods have failed to control the problem, you will probably have to go with the earlier (and still alternate) combination of poppy extract with deadly nightshade. If you are in a situation where you must do this, remember that morphine and scopolamine interact to a high degree in producing medicinal effects, so it is better to start with less than half a dose of each. Deadly nightshade constituents are also sometimes used in treating the symptoms of Parkinson's disease, and until recently were used to relax spasming lungs and dry up mucous secretions in asthma and bronchitis.

The most common use of atropine is in extremely minute amounts to dilate the pupils for eye examinations. Extremely minute = 1/50,000 of 1 grain (65 mg/50,000) per eye; it is unlikely that any post-Catastrophe herbalist will be able to dilute the herb to this level, let alone make eye gels with it. Deadly nightshade has been used as a topical liniment to ease pain and inflammation, notably in regards to neuralgia, gout, rheumatism, and sciatica.

Side effects: anti-cholinergic effects (flushing, fever, dry mouth, dry skin, blurred vision, constipation, dizziness, dilated pupils, fast heartbeat, urinary retention), nausea and vomiting, spasms, delirium, hallucinations, convulsions, coma, and death. Long-term memory impairment after surviving large doses has been anecdotally reported, but not confirmed. Symptoms usually appear within 15 minutes of ingesting the plant, and may last for several days.

If poisoned, induce vomiting at once with a glass of warm vinegar or mustard mixed thickly into water. The real-life treatment is physostigmine (blocks the breakdown of acetylcholine, increasing the concentration and blocking the anticholinergic effects of deadly nightshade) or pilocarpine (stimulates the M3 muscarinic receptors to cause cholinergic effects).

c) Dosing

As little as half a berry can kill a child; four berries cause significant toxicity in an adult, and 10-20 can kill. The lethal amount, like the therapeutic amount, depends on the percentage of atropine and other alkaloids in the individual plant that year. The root normally contains 0.4-0.6% total alkaloids, but may go up to 1%. Dried leaves contain 0.3-0.7% total alkaloids. Dosages according to Mrs Grieve are:

aPowdered leaves: 1-2 grains

aPowdered root: 1-5 grains.

She does not give the details for liniment, that having been available as a British Pharmaceutical preparation with directions in her era; but one can take it that the amount in a dose of liniment ought not exceed the oral dose, and lower is probably better. Start with a minimum dose, or better yet, half or a quarter of the minimum dose, on the basis that lack of effect is, in the vast majority of cases with this herb, better than active poisoning. The only exception to this would be nerve gas exposure...if it happened when you were in the right place, while the plant had berries, and you had an empty syringe and lived long enough to draw the juice out of a berry or three and shoot it into yourself. In such circumstances, you're going to die anyway, but you might at least die trying.

d) Growing

Deadly nightshade is a perennial, which dies down in the autumn and resprouts in mid- to late-spring. Reports of which livestock can safely eat deadly nightshade and which can't vary. Horses have been reported to have eaten it without harm, and to have been poisoned by it. Poisoning in pigs is said to be rare. Cattle and rabbits are alleged to be able to eat deadly nightshade safely. However, the high risk of toxic contamination of meat and/or milk if the animal has been eating deadly nightshade suggests that all livestock should be firmly kept away from this plant. Dogs and cats are certainly vulnerable to it. The berries are said to be extremely sweet, which makes keeping children (and dogs) away from the plant particularly important. Children should be told strictly that if they eat deadly nightshade, it will kill them.

Soil and Siting

Deadly nightshade prefers rich and damp, but not saturated/boggy soil, and grows well in shade to partial sun. It is fairly acid-tolerant, and can take a pH anywhere from 4.5 (very acid) to 7.5 (mildly alkaline). It grows best on chalk or limestone. Despite its love of moisture, I have seen it growing vigorously in the wild in the San Diego area; the fogs appear to suffice when rain and moisture-holding soil are lacking.

The seeds require striation and soaking (two weeks to a month in water in the refrigerator, or plant in the autumn for spring germination and make sure the site stays wet from at least the end of the last frost). For a spring sowing, they should be planted in May, preferably after a heavy rain or good watering. Seeds are difficult to germinate indoors even with striation; gibberellic acid treatment is said to be helpful. Deadly nightshade can also be propagated by root division.

Seedlings should start at 18" (ca. 46 cm) apart; as they die down in autumn of their first year, they should be thinned to 30-36" (76-91.5 cm) apart to allow sufficient room to spread. As long as deadly nightshade is not devoured to the ground by slimy gastropods (are there non-slimy gastropods?) or allowed to dry out too much, it is a strong, fast-growing plant which can quickly recover from traumas.

Pests

Snails and slugs love deadly nightshade more passionately than one can imagine. I have, more than once, come out in the morning to find a thriving young plant (not a seedling, a plant!) eaten down to a few stalks. Fortunately they did manage to resprout from their roots. Deadly nightshade is vulnerable to anything that can attack tomatoes or potatoes, including tomato mosaic virus, potato blight, and wireworms.

The Ornamental Garden

Deadly nightshade is quite an attractive garden plant, especially when flowering and fruiting. It grows as a thinly-branched bush, and can reach ca 6 ½"/2 metres tall. The leaves are a strong green, smooth and shiny, oval tapering to a point at the outer end. The flowers are a dull dark lavender to purple colour with a faint greenish tint, shaped like elongated bells; the outer end of the throat is often darker than the outside of the flower, while the inner depths of the throat are yellowish-green. The berries, as mentioned, look very much like tiny black cherry tomatoes, very shiny and potentially fatally attractive. When choosing where to plant this herb, I repeat: Be very careful that neither children nor animals can reach it.

III. Woody Nightshade (Solanum dulcamara)

a) Introduction

Woody nightshade is not the same plant as Deadly Nightshade, though the two are in the same family and are sometimes confused.

b) Chemical Constituents

Woody nightshade produces solanine (in unripe fruits), solasodine (from flowers) and beta-solamarine (from roots). Both solanine and solasodine inhibit E. coli (a Gram-negative bacterium) and S. aureus (a Gram-positive bacterium. This plant also produces dulcamarine, which is similar to atropine in structure and effect.

c) Uses and Effects

Woody nightshade stem has been approved in Germany as an adjunct for chronic eczema. The whole aerial plant is also used topically for skin inflammation and abrasions. The fruits have narcotic effects. Woody nightshade may be effective in treating ringworm. Side effects: vomiting, convulsions, vertigo, cyanosis, diarrhoea, dilated pupils, difficulty speaking or swallowing, headache, stomach cramps, subnormal temperature, paralysis, death. Woody nightshade causes haemolytic and haemorrhagic damage to the GI tract; symptoms may not manifest for several hours, and can be mistaken for bacterial gastro-enteritis. The unripe fruit appear to be more toxic than fully ripened fruit, and the leaves are also markedly poisonous. Children are considerably more vulnerable to woody nightshade's poisons than are adults; the quantity of a dangerous dose in adults varies widely, from as few as six berries to as many as 200. This plant's alkaloids have documented teratogenic effects. It should not be used in pregnancy or when pregnancy is a possibility.

d) Dosage

Stems are given at 1-3 grams/day, as a decoction or infusion in 250 ml of water.

e) Growing

Woody nightshade is a very hardy and successful climbing perennial. It thrives in a wide range of soils and situations, but prefers damp, rich ground, partial shade, and high nitrogen levels. The flowers are purple and five-petalled, with a bright yellow, prominent cone of fused stamens in the centre, and grow in loose clusters; the berries, when ripe (September through November), are bright red ovoids, resembling small pear tomatoes.

Fatal poisoning from this plant is relatively rare, but the attractive fruit make it a danger to small children, household animals, and livestock. Birds, however, can eat the fruit without taking any harm, and the European thrush commonly propagates the plant from seed in this manner. Woody nightshade cuttings are easily rooted, and the plant can be grown in pots as well as directly in the ground. It appears to die back in the autumn, but will recover in the spring with no difficulty.

Like its relatives, woody nightshade is notably vulnerable to slugs, snails, and the diseases to which its family is prone (tobacco mosaic virus, potato blight, etc.). Woody nightshade can be supported on stakes or against a wall, or left to form a low ground-covering thicket. The vines have been reported to reach a length of 9 metres (29.5 feet) or greater. It grows readily from seed as well as propagating through suckers, and is considered an invasive weed in North America.

IV. Mandrake (Mandragora officinalis/autumnalis)

a) Introduction

The European or true mandrake should not be confused with the "American mandrake" or may-apple (Podophyllum peltatum). The two are not even remotely related, nor do they have any medical (or toxic) effects in common. If looking for mandrake for any purpose, always be sure to get the Latin name! It is not uncommon for herbal and seed suppliers, particularly in the States, to say "mandrake" when they mean "may-apple". No plant has been the object of as many magico-cultural beliefs as the mandrake. The early Hebrews associated it with fertility: Genesis 30:13-18 describes Rachel and Leah using it for this purpose, and it is also referred to in the Song of Songs (7:13) as one of the plants producing a scent conducive to romantic activity.

A variety of beliefs surrounded the digging and aftercare of the mandrake root; the most famous belief, that the uprooted plant would let out a deadly shriek, was recently repopularized in Harry Potter and the Chamber of Secrets (J.K. Rowling, Bloomsbury, 1998). Mandrake roots were made into, or treated as, luck-bringing homunculi, to such an extent that carved bryony roots were often sold to the gullible as mandrake roots. Mandrake has considerable scope for attraction to most persons of a supernatural character. Being strongly associated with death and the dead, it should be expected to have an effect on vampires and ghosts, and to be prized by necromancers in particular and a wide range of magical practitioners in general.

Romano-Jewish historian Flavius Josephus, writing in the first century C.E., informs us that "(the mandrake) is only valuable on account of one virtue it hath, that if it be only brought to the sick persons, it quickly drives away those called demons, which are no other than the spirits of the wicked, that enter into men that are alive, and kill them; unless they can obtain some help against them." In Germany and Britain, it was believed that mandrake would be found growing under a gallows, springing from the urine/semen/tears of a hanged man (sometimes with more specifics: an innocent man who was hanged unjustly, a virgin, a murderer, u.s.w.). The German folk name Galgenmaennlein ("little gallows man") and the Icelandic thjófarót ("thief's root") may both stem from this belief-complex.

The alternative "natural" growing site in Welsh folklore was a crossroads, particularly if someone who had committed suicide were buried there. Simoons also cites the 17th-century German poet Rist describing a mandrake that had been kept carefully by one family for over an hundred years, housed in a coffin which was covered with a cloth showing the image of a thief on the gallows and a mandrake growing beneath him; the youngest son traditionally inherited his father's mandrake, but also bore the responsibility of putting money and bread in his father's coffin. The traditional descriptions of lycanthropes as suffering from constant thirst, with dryness of the mouth and eyes as well as impaired vision, may reasonably suggest the possibility of the use of mandrake (or one of its close hallucinatory and anticholinergic relatives such as henbane or deadly nightshade) to induce the psychiatric condition of lycanthropy. In a fictional world, of course, this could easily be translated into genuine shapeshifting.

b) Chemical Constituents

Mandrake contains the same tropane alkaloids (hyoscyamine, atropine, and scopolamine) that henbane and deadly nightshade do. Its medicinal uses and side effects are very similar to those of deadly nightshade: hypnotic, narcotic, anaesthetic, hallucinogenic, and producing the full range of anti-cholinergic effects. The results of mandrake poisoning are also very similar to those of poisoning with deadly nightshade. The roots contain the greatest quantity of alkaloids, followed by the leaves and then the fruit. The root was the part most commonly used for surgical anaesthesia. The duration of the effects may be as short as four hours (for a small dose) and as long as 36 or 48 hours (for a large one), with some residual visual effects lingering for days.

c) Dosage

Mandrake has a very low therapeutic index; which is to say, there is not much difference between the efficacious dose and the highly toxic dose. One gram of the dried root is considered quite sufficient for most purposes. It may be administered as a tea, or taken directly as a powder in a capsule or pill. Most commonly, the bark of the root was used in surgical anaesthesia. The alkaloids are water-soluble, which means that an extract can be made with water, beer, wine, or spirits. The leaves can be dried and smoked – probably the least unsafe way to use this plant - or chewed fresh. Again, a gram should be the maximum amount for an adult dose under most circumstances.

The fruit can also be eaten, although not more than one at a dose. Although they are the least toxic part of the plant, ten fruits were nearly fatal in an adult male; the observing physicians note that his survival was probably due to the early induction of vomiting (plus prostigmine injections). The fifteenth-century Turkish physician Serafeddin Sabuncuoglu, in his book Cerrahiyet'ül Haniye (Imperial Surgery), recommends, as a surgical anaesthetic: "Take and cut the fresh parts of Luffah (mandragora), pound and mix it with almond oil and let it stay for a day and night. Then, the surgeon who wants to use it must give one drachm of it to be eaten before meal.

A little later you'll see that the patient will lie down and fall asleep without perceiving you. Then, practice whatever treatment you want to do. Give one drachm (dirhem = dram = 4 g) of it to the adult, but administer only the amount needed for children, so that no malpractice occurs. This is the narcotic I used all through my life and did not need any other anaesthetic medicine." Unfortunately, he did not give the proportions of almond oil to mandrake that he used; but it seems plausible that it was a 1:1 mixture, with a total mandrake content (fresh root – less concentrated than dried root) of 2 grams for rendering the patient entirely unconscious for surgery.

d) Growing

Mandrake is notoriously slow to germinate – some have reported it taking as long as a year to sprout - but is usually reliable over the course of time. I have found that wrapping the seeds in moist paper towelling and leaving them, making sure they don't dry out, is the most effective means of getting them to sprout. Mandrakes sprout best if they are planted fresh in the autumn. Some people recommend cold stratification (ca. 2 weeks in the refrigerator, wrapped in a moist paper towel inside a plastic bag), but I have regularly gotten good results without it. Mandrakes prefer full sun and slightly sandy soil with good drainage. Despite their southerly origins, they can be surprisingly cold-hardy; the finest specimen I have ever seen, several years old and loaded with fruit, was growing in Gotland's Krusemynta herb garden. The root of a mature mandrake can get as long as four feet (well over a metre).

Nonetheless, mandrakes can be grown in smaller pots, in which case the roots will tend to coil in interesting and rather Lovecraftian ways, though the plant may always be somewhat stunted. The leaves are large and dark green, spreading out from the top of the root and tending to lie along or just above the ground. The flowers are either white (officinalis) or purple (autumnalis), star-shaped, and quite attractive in a quiet sort of way. The fruit bear a close resemblance to small yellow tomatoes when fully ripe.

It normally takes a year or so for the plant to bear its first flowers, and may be another year or two before it starts setting fruit. Be patient. Mandrakes should be planted where you want to keep them. They bitterly resent being transplanted; they may not actually scream, but they will sulk and go dormant for long periods of time. They should not be grown where children or animals can get at them. I have read that mandrakes can be propagated by root division, but I have never managed to make this work myself.

Mandrakes dislike having their roots disturbed so intensely that it seems an implausible means of propagation to me. Mandrakes are absolute magnets for slugs and snails. They are also prone to being infested by wireworm. The best way to deal with wireworm is to cut a raw potato into chunks, then put a bamboo skewer or similar through each chunk and bury them around the mandrake. The injured potato will draw the wireworms away from the mandrake root; you have only to pull up the skewer and dispose of the worms. Mandrakes are vulnerable to everything that can attack potatoes or tomatoes, and require spraying for potato blight in warm humid summers.

V. Thornapple (Datura stramonium – Jimsonweed, moonflower, Devil's Trumpet) and other Datura species

a) Introduction

The Datura family is found worldwide, particularly in warm regions, although these plants also grow copiously in North America and Southern Russia, and can be cultivated without much difficulty in Ireland and Britain, growing wild occasionally. D. stramonium is, or was, the most commonly used for medicinal purposes. Daturas are members of the same family as henbane, deadly nightshade, and so forth (Solanaceae). Mrs. Grieves mentions that the Jamestown settlers ate, and experienced untowards physical and psychological effects from, the leaves of this herb, naming it "Devil's Apple"; and that it is also known as "Jamestown Weed" (or Jimsonweed) from this association (p. 804).

She does not vouch for the accuracy of this tale; probably a more correct version is Berkeley's account (1705) of the effects of the herb on British soldiers attempting to subdue Bacon's Rebellion (1676), who were variously delirious, delusional, and effectively clinically insane for roughly eleven days after eating the fresh young green leaves as a boiled salad. Datura species have been used as an entheogen by a number of peoples; in Haiti, they are called "zombi cucumber", and E. Wade Davis (author of The Serpent and the Rainbow) noted that, subsequent to the application of tetrodotoxin and the apparent "death" of the victim, he would be given a Datura mixture to induce a state of psychosis in which he could be more completely convinced of his death and exhumation as a zombie.

B) Chemical constituents

D. stramonium (and other daturas) contain hyoscyamine, hyoscine (scopolamine), and atropine. They are anti-cholinergic and hallucinogenic, having the same side effects and signs of toxicity as deadly nightshade, etc.

C) Dosage

The seeds are more powerful than the leaves, but more difficult to extract alkaloids from; the leaves are generally the part used for medical purposes, and are strongest when fresh. Mrs. Grieve observes that the strength and actions of thornapple and deadly nightshade are so similar, that they might almost be considered the same plant, except that thornapple does not appear to have the constipating effects of belladonna. The relevant dosage given by Grieve is 1/10 to 5 grains of powdered leaves (the other means of administration she lists are dependent on BP or other established formulations, so dosages are not usable without knowing the precise details).

It should be noted that there is more difference between individual plants of the same Datura sp. than in general between the different Datura spp.: D. stramonium can vary fivefold in strength between two given plants, and drastically between different harvest years of the same plant, based on fertilizer and weather. As well as being a sedative and analgesic, dry thornapple leaves were also smoked for asthma relief (the atropine effect on relieving bronchial spasming and drying up secretions); topically, it was used in analgesic ointments or plasters (no formulation given) for severe arthritis, neuralgia, and other inflammatory conditions (Grieve, pp. 802 ff).

D) Growing

Thornapple grows well enough from seed, but may require scarification (gently rub down a piece of fine sandpaper) and 24 hours of a warm-water soak. Germination may take 3-8 weeks. The seeds or young sprouts should be planted after the last danger of frost, ca. 3 ft to 1 metre apart; it likes a rich and slightly chalky soil or sandy loam, and a situation in full sunlight. An increase in nitrogen is noted to increase the alkaloid content. Once established, it is hardy and swift-growing, reaching between two and five feet tall. It is noted for a rather unpleasant odour, and animals tend to avoid it. The flowers are large, with a wide-flared "trumpet" shape, and usually either white or purple, though yellow or red are seen occasionally. The seed capsules are very spiky, splitting at maturity to release a number of small black seeds.

Leaves are harvested and dried once the plant has come into full bloom, usually in late summer, though it may be significantly earlier in warmer regions. While seeds germinate readily, they can also lurk in the ground for years, a characteristic which does not endear the plant to agricultural agents or people who like to know where and when very poisonous plants might be inclined to sprout. Once established, thornapple can be quite invasive – it is classed as a "weed" in many places – but it can also be grown in a pot, or even indoors if it can get enough sunlight.

VI. Ephedra (Ephedra sinica, Ephedra equisentena, Ephedra intermedia; Ma Huang)

A) Introduction

Chief concerns about post-Catastrophe medical care include the problems of potentially fatal-level allergies and asthma. When there are no more pharmaceutical sympathetic-agonist drugs available, herbal medication will be the only option; and E. sinica is one of the most powerful herbal stimulants available. Having said that: the FDA had a very good reason to ban this herb, starting with a number of sudden cardiac deaths and toxicity effects requiring critical-care hospitalization in healthy young people using ephedra-containing supplements as directed. However, the risk is less than that of dying when anaphylaxis or a major asthma attack has fully set in.

B) Chemical constituents

The three species of oriental ephedra contain ephedrine, pseudo-ephedrine, norephedrine, and norpseudoephedrine. Ephedrine is the primary constituent. It is a mixed sympathomimetic, similar in action to adrenaline, activating both the alpha and beta receptors of the sympathetic nervous system. Ephedrine raises blood pressure, increases heart rate, dilates the bronchi and other smooth muscles, and reduces the swelling of mucous membranes in much the same manner as the first-line pharmaceutical treatments for asthma and anaphylaxis (beta-agonists and adrenaline). As a pharmaceutical drug, ephedrine is normally used in the contexts of the emergency room and intensive care.

Because ephedrine is a powerful stimulant, its use carries significant risks. It should not be administered outside of a physician's guidance if there is a choice. The elevated blood pressure and heart rate, and increased likelihood of arrhythmias, significantly increase the risk of stroke and heart attack, particularly in vulnerable patients (existing cardiovascular problems; seizure disorders; glaucoma; diabetes; liver abnormalities; thyroid abnormalities, especially hyperactivity; pregnant or nursing mothers; children under 18). As always with a whole herb displaying a certain degree of toxicity, there will be no way in the post-Catastrophe world to find out how strong each year's harvest is without someone (or at least a rodent or two) personally testing it.

Other side effects of ephedra include: anxiety, headache, abdominal pain, vomiting, hyperthermia, tremor, sleeplessness, loss of appetite, and irritability. Under non-emergency circumstances, ephedrine should not be taken together with any other stimulant (including caffeine); any cardiac drug; any drug which affects the autonomic nervous system such as the beta-agonists often prescribed for asthma. It should not be used with cannabis, especially not high-THC strains, due to the compounded risk of stroke and cardiac complications. It should be used only with caution and under supervision for patients who are receiving MAOI anti-depressant, anti-diabetic, or anti-convulsant medication, including herbs used for these purposes. Ephedrine, pseudo-ephedrine, norephedrine, and norpseudoephedrine are all used in cold medications to reduce mucous membrane swelling and secretions.

c) Use in anaphylaxis and asthma

Intramuscular injection of ephedrine is recommended for anaphylaxis where the symptoms are primarily cardiovascular, but remain below the level of full cardiac or circulatory arrest. The ideal first-line treatment is IM adrenaline injection, but adrenaline is unlikely to be available after the Catastrophe unless you managed to stockpile a hoard of Epi-Pens. Assuming that you planned ahead while you still had the opportunity and planted some ephedra of the correct species ("Mormon tea", Ephedra nevadensis, is an ephedra, but contains no ephedrine; none of the American ephedras do), ephedra will probably be your only option, or close to it. If necessary, caffeine can be used as an adjunct. To reference Diana Gabaldon again (An Echo In The Bone): to treat an imminently fatal asthma attack in the late eighteenth century, her doctor uses "jointfir" along with strong coffee (caffeine plus a small amount of theophylline; synergistic effects with ephedrine), followed up by cannabis (smooth muscle relaxant, among its many other functions); and mentions the Oriental origin of her "jointfir" (a generic for Ephedra spp.) a bit later in the book. Ephedrine is antispasmodic as well as causing bronchodilation.

d) Dosage

The maximum dosage for E. sinica is 9 grams (ca. 1 ¾ teaspoon) dry herb in divided doses over the course of a day; the minimum is ca. 1.5 grams (a smidgen over a quarter-teaspoon); but except in an extreme emergency, the higher doses should be avoided, considering once again the considerable variability of active constituents in any whole natural herb. The quantity of ephedrine in ephedra may be as variable as from 1.1 to 15.3 mg/dose. In an extreme emergency, you may need to inject a dose of tincture (or a water extract, if you have time to make it) intramuscularly. Ephedrine is highly soluble in water; Mrs. Grieve describes it as "shining white crystals". The dose of ephedrine she recommends is .5-1 grains (32-65 mg).

The parts of the plant used are leaves and stems. Ephedrine and its associated alkaloids are most effectively derived from the dry plant material by ethanol extraction, although prolonged boiling (2 hours) in water produced 0.902% of alkaloids, comparable to the expected 1-2% found in a high grade of E. sinica; the ephedrine proportion of total alkaloids ranges from 30-90%. This is obviously a matter of concern with a potential medication that has a comparatively low therapeutic index.

If there is any choice, as always, it is better to start at minimal doses and titrate up with great care. Toxicity from this plant would ideally be mitigated with sympathetic blockers, but after the Catastrophe, your best option is likely to be valerian, a non- or minimal-THC strain of cannabis (or CBD extract derived from the same), and/or chamomile (German, Matricaria chamomila, is more potent than Roman, Chamaemelum nobilis). Hawthorn's moderating effect on the heart may also prove to be helpful in controlling cardiovascular symptoms of ephedra overdose.

E) Growing

Ephedra is a dioecious plant, which means that it is not self-fertile: to reproduce by seed, it is necessary to have a male and a female parent. It is an evergreen shrub, may grow a foot and a half tall or so (ca. 1.4-1.5 metres), and flowers from May to June. The common name "jointfir" accurately describes the habitus of this plant: the leaves are hardly visible, and the plant resembles a collection of green twigs with slightly enlarged brown "joints" at the nodes, or a small and apparently leafless bamboo. The pale yellow pistillate flowers (female) grow in small clusters semi-enclosed by two larger petals; the staminate flowers (male) hang as catkins; and the berries, which last into September, are bright red. Ephedra requires full sunlight, and a light or loamy soil. It often grows wild in dry waste places. It is quite tolerant of drought and at least moderately tolerant of cold once it is established, but should be kept in a pot indoors or in a warm sheltered area during its first winter. Ephedra does not thrive well in damper climates in general, but has, with careful tending, been successfully grown in Britain. Seed can be sown in a greenhouse in the autumn or outdoors in spring. Ephedra can also be propagated through root division and layering (bending a sprig or branch down and covering part of it with earth to encourage new root formation.

VII. Foxglove (Digitalis purpurea)

A) Introduction

Foxglove is famed among orthodox doctors and herbalists alike for being the plant that bridged the gap between folk herbalism and official medicine, and was thus responsible for making much of modern pharmacology possible. In the early 1780s, one Dr. William Withering observed a patient recovering from "dropsy" (lower limb oedema and ascites – the swelling of lower limbs and belly due to fluid effusion and collection, a common symptom of severe congestive heart failure) thanks to a folk remedy. Withering identified the foxglove plant as the active component of the remedy, performed a number of clinical trials, and, in 1785, published An Account of the Foxglove and some of its Medical Uses, discussing both the efficacy and the toxicity of the herb. He has also been credited as perhaps the first physician to rely on clinical trials and dismiss the "Doctrine of Signatures" as the utter nonsense it is.

B) Chemical Constituents

Digitalin and digoxin, the drugs derived from foxglove, are used less in real life today than was formerly the case, due to the development of more efficacious and safer cardiac drugs. They are still a valuable part of the pharmacopeia, however. The crucial use of digitalin and digioxin (and hence foxglove) is as cardiac strengtheners and stimulants. Foxglove increases cardiac muscle contraction, causing an initial spike in blood pressure; increases blood flow in general; and at the same time works upon the heart's "pacemaker" (sino-atrial node), slowing the heartbeat and rendering it more regular; hence its value as an anti-arrhythmic.

The digitalis drugs are particularly used to treat atrial fibrillation and congestive heart failure. Digitalis is also a powerful diuretic, which is important in ridding the body of accumulated fluid in the patient with congestive heart failure (who may also be suffering from electrolyte imbalance. Do not give them salt, which will exacerbate the fluid buildup; help them get rid of the water). Because of its cardiac effects, its diuretic effects are relevant only to the congestive heart failure patient.

Digitalis is also used as an antidote to aconite poisoning.

It takes approximately six hours for digitalin to distribute itself through the body, and may be twelve hours or longer before any therapeutic effect is seen. This means: do not increase the patient's dose because they do not immediately appear to be responding. Give them at least a day before you consider it. Foxglove is not an emergency treatment; it is an ongoing tonic.Once the appropriate dosage for a patient has been established, it is essential to continue monitoring them. Plasma levels of the drug can slowly rise to toxic levels, particularly in older patients who may have reduced metabolic and/or organ functions; so what has been a well-tolerated dosage can gradually begin to cause difficulties.

A wide range of drugs inhibit digitalin metabolism, including many other cardiac drugs (amiodarone, amiloride, beta-blockers, calcium-channel blockers), diuretics (hydrochlorothiazide, furosemide a.k.a. Lasix, spironolactone), macrolide and tetracycline antibiotics, and benzodiazepines, among others; all of these can contribute to developing digitalis toxicity. While little or no work has been done on herbal equivalents re digitalis metabolism, it is probably safer to avoid prescribing additional herbs which fall into any of the above classes together with digitalis if possible.

Side effects of digitalin treatment may include erectile dysfunction and gynecomastia, photophobia, nausea, diarrhea, a generalized tingling sensation, headache, and rash or hives. These are not necessarily signs of clinical toxicity, but may indicate that the drug is not well-tolerated by the patient. Histamine reactions (rash, hives) should be viewed very seriously, particularly if they appear to worsen, as that may suggest that the patient is developing a potentially dangerous immune reaction to the drug. Symptoms of digitalis toxicity include visual disturbances, specifically a general yellow or green cast to the vision and haloes, often blue, around lights. It has been theorized that Van Gogh's "Yellow Period" was the result of building toxicity from digitalis being prescribed, as it was at the time, for epilepsy.

His blurred stars also suggest digitalin poisoning. Nausea, vomiting, and diarrhoea can occur, along with arrhythmias, abnormal heart speed (usually very slow, but sometimes very fast), and cardiac collapse; the patient may feel dizzy or weak, or suffer tremors, seizures, and abdominal pain. Pupils are dilated. A high plasma level of digitalin, especially from acute ingestion, may cause hallucinations and delirium. Digitalis toxicity, either from acute or unmonitored chronic ingestion, can be fatal; and after the Catastrophe (or before modern forensics were developed), it will be exceedingly difficult to prove murder by digitalis if the victim was already known to have heart trouble.

Atropine has been used to counteract digitalis poisoning, and is likely to be your only option after the Catastrophe. In real life, the use of digoxin-specific antibody fragments is preferred. The first-line treatment, especially for acute ingestion, is repeated dosing with activated charcoal; inducing vomiting or stomach-pumping is not done because that stimulates the vagus nerve, which can induce or exacerbate arrhythmias. Electrolyte imbalance is virtually inevitable: hyperkalaemia (excess potassium) or hypokalaemia (insufficient potassium) and hypomagnesaemia (low magnesium) are characteristically seen. Unfortunately for the post-Catastrophe patient, the judgement on electrolyte status will probably have to be clinical, d.h., "a guess", and the symptoms of potassium imbalance are virtually identical on both ends of the scale: arrhythmias, depressed deep tendon reflexes, nausea, vomiting. The main difference is that hyperkalaemia causes diarrhoea, whereas hypokalaemia causes constipation. Hyperkalaemia is characterized by atrio-ventricular block, and hypokalaemia by premature atrial and ventricular complexes.

c) Dosing

Dosage for the herb has been estimated at ca. 1.5 grams of dry leaf per day, divided into two doses. Foxglove is often administered as an infusion (boiling water, steeped for ca. 15 minutes). Grieve, however, recommends 0.03-0.13 grams powdered leaf (p. 326); and Alstead, writing in 1936, reported that 2 grains (0.13 grams) was efficacious in increasing cardiac reserve in ca. 75% of patients, and one grain in 50%. It is advisable to start with the lower dose, especially with a drug that is notorious for increasing plasma levels with chronic use.

The name "foxglove" has been suggested to derive from "Folk's glove", referring to the Good Folk/Little Folk/whatever similar name you call the fey when you don't want to piss them off by calling them "faeries". Here in Ireland, even in real life, we are traditionally cautious about that sort of thing. If the etymology is true, then one can safely take it that this plant is attractive to the fey. It should, however, be noted that the Anglo-Saxon name is unambiguously "fox's glove", and in Norway it is also called Revbielde ("foxbell"). The Irish "Dead Man's Thimbles" may refer to the poisonous character of the plant. (Grieve, p. 323).

It is within the realm of possibility, or at least imagination, that the cardiostimulant effects of foxglove might briefly induce a heartbeat or two in a vampire, assuming that a proper method of administration could be found. Due to the toxicity, the classic "drinking the blood of someone who has partaken" is unlikely to work for this plant.

D) Growing

Foxglove is a biennial plant, forming a rosette of leaves in the first year and sending up its flower stalk in the second. When sold in garden centres, as it commonly is for ornamental purposes, the plants you buy will all be second-year. Foxgloves can thrive in anything from full sun to full shade, depending on the heat. In Northern Europe, they are more commonly seen in sunny or partially shaded locations, though they also occur as a woodland plant; they may require full shade in warmer regions. They grow best in rich, well-drained soil.

Foxgloves should be planted about 18"(ca. 45 cm.) apart. If the flower heads are left to themselves, they will reseed without difficulty. Foxgloves do not appear to be unduly attractive to pests. The main danger is accidental consumption in mistake for comfrey or elecampane, particularly in the first year when the characteristic flower-stalk has not arisen. The leaves of foxglove are bright green and more softly haired, whereas comfrey leaves are deep green and bristled; foxglove leaves bear a closer resemblance to those of elecampane, though the flowers cannot be mistaken.

As with all poisonous plants, it is best to keep children and animals away from foxgloves; but the risk is not so high as with most of the other plants in this section. The flower stalk usually reaches ca. 2-4 feet tall. It grows its characteristic bell-shaped flowers on all sides. The wild foxglove flowers are pink with a purplish tinge and spotted throats. Of the cultivated varieties, pure white is the most popular, but it can be gotten in a range of colours, including yellow and red. Foxglove is highly popular as an ornamental flower, adding bright colour and vertical interest to the garden design.

VIII. Aconite (monkshood, Tyr's Helm – Aconitum napellus and other sub-species of Aconitum, including wolfsbane)

a) Introduction

Professor Snape actually ought to have lost points for a Herbology Fail in Harry Potter and the Philosopher's Stone (Bloomsbury, 1997), where he seems to think that monkshood and wolfsbane are exactly the same plant (and you, too, Hermione!). Monkshood is Aconitum napellus, and has deep purple flowers. Wolfsbane is Aconitum lycoctonum, and has yellow flowers. Now, medicinally they are pretty much identical, and this may be the same in potion-making in J.K. Rowling's world...but still: ten points from Slytherin, Severus!

Aconite is the second most poisonous plant in Northern Europe. One gram of the plant is quite sufficient to kill an adult human; even touching it can numb the skin, and gardening with it bare-handed is enough to cause clinical toxicity. Aconite has been used in the past for nerve pain, joint pain, gout, inflammation, and cardiac conditions. In the earlier British Pharmacoepia, it was available as a liniment (oil-based preparation) for neuralgia, rheumatism, and gout; and as a tincture for the above-mentioned conditions. Mrs. Grieve notes that "the only reliable means of standardizing the potency of any of the Aconite preparations is by a physiological method: the lethal dose for the guinea-pig being considered to be the most convenient and satisfactory method. Tinctures vary enormously as to strength, some proving seven times as powerful as others" (p. 8).

b) Dosing.

The paediatric dose above 5 years for a guinea-pig-standardized tincture of aconite was 0.06-0.12 ml (0.012-0.024 tsp); the adult dose was 0.12-0.3 ml (0.024-0.06 tsp) 3x/day. Though aconite is seldom if ever used in Western medicine in real life now, the existing recommendation is 60 mg of root/dose, or approximately 1 grain. However, the variability of individual roots is as high now as it was in Mrs. Grieve's day, so it should be assumed that 1/7th of that is more appropriate until the specific root has been tested on a guinea pig.

Since guinea pigs are not likely to be common after the Catastrophe, a rat would probably be the most readily available option. Given the ease with which aconite can be absorbed through the skin, topical doses should not exceed oral doses. The folk use of aconite root continues in Slovenia to the current day. There, an alcoholic extract is made from the roots, with various recipes, as per Tables 2 and 3 from Povšnar et al: Preparation of ethanolic extracts from the roots of Aconitum spp. and their medicinal use, as reported by 5 informants who knew the preparation well, described it precisely and had prepared it themselves.

MED MEDICINAL USE, VET VETERINARY USE

[a]The first flow of the second distillation of fruit brandy

TABLE 3

Preparation of ethanolic extracts from the roots of Aconitum spp. and their medicinal use as reported by 7 informants who were somewhat uncertain in describing the preparation; they knew the ethanolic extract from the narration of their parents, grandparents, or acquaintances or they had observed the preparation as children.

INFORMANT	PREPATION OF THE EXTRACT	DOSAGE	USE	INTERESTING FEATURES
N (WOMAN, 75 YEARS OLD)	1 TABLESPOON OF SLICED ROOTS WAS PLACED INTO 2 DL OF SCHNAPPS	A FEW DROPS WERE PLACED IN WATER AND DRUNK	MED: FEVER VET: FOR WEAKENED ANIMALS	THE INFORMANT DID NOT PREPARE THE EXTRACT; HER MOTHER ADVISED HER TO PREPARE IT.
G (WOMAN, 87 YEARS OLD)	2 DL OF ROOTS WAS PLACED INTO A LARGE HALF-LITER BOTTLE OF SCHNAPPS AND LEFT TO SOAK FOR 14 DAYS	ADULTS: NOT MORE THAN 5 DROPS CHILDREN: JUST A SMALL AMOUNT	MED: SEVERE ILLNESSES, FEVER, AND INFLAMMATION	-----
A (WOMAN, 82 YEARS OLD)	2 TO 3 ROOTS WERE PLACED INTO HALF A LITER OF SCHNAPPS; THE ROOTS FILLED ALMOST HALF THE BOTTLE; THE SOAKING TIME WAS SHORT	ADULTS: 9 DROPS CHILDREN: 3 DROPS DROPS WERE PLACED IN WATER AND DRUNK	MED: PREVENTION OF DISEASES, FEVER, INFLUENZA, TREATMENT OF HEADACHE (LUBRICATION OF THE FOREHEAD); "GOOD FOR EVERYTHING"	THE LAST TIME THE INFORMANT USED THE EXTRACT WAS 50 TO 60 YEARS AGO; SHE PREPARED IT HERSELF.

MED medicinal use, VET veterinary use--Povšnar et al report that, though Aconitum poisoning occurred at times in the region, there were no cases of it related to the use of the traditional medicinal extracts.

INFORMANT	PREPATION OF THE EXTRACT	DOSAGE	USE	INTERESTING FEATURES
B (WOMAN, INTERVIEWED IN LUČE, 88 YEARS OLD)	1 ROOT WAS MACERATED IN 250 ML OF SCHNAPPS	HORSES: 10 DROPS ON BREAD	VET: HIVED AND COLD IN HORSES	THE IN-FORMAT'S HUSBANDED PREPARED THE EXTRACT FROR HORSES
C (MAN, 64 YEARS OLD)	ROTTS WERE MACERATED IN A LARGE HALF-LITER BOTTLE	ADULTS: 5-10 DROPS CHILDREN: NOT MORE THAN 3 DROPS	MED: FEVER AND COUGH	THE INFOR-MANT DE-SCRIBED THE PREPARA-TION AFTER NARRATION OF A WOMAN WHO WAS REQUESTING ACONITE.
K (WOMAN, 78 YEARS OLD)	2 ROOTS THE SIZE OF A FINGER WERE SOAKED IN 1 L OF SCHAPPS	ADULT: 3 DROPS CHILDREN: 2 DROPS	MED: FEVER	THE INFOR-MANT DID NOT PREPARE THE EXTRACT BY HERSELF
L (WOMAN, 73 YEARS OLD)	3 CM OF A ROOT WAS SOAKED IN 1 DL OF SCHAPPS AND PLACED IN A DARK ROOM FOR 3 WEEKS	ADULTS: 5 TO 7 DROPS DROPS WERE PLACED IN WATER. IT WAS NOT GOOOD IF DROPS WERE PLACED IN TISANE	MED: FEVER, FOR (PHYSICAL) STRENGTH (CHRONIC USE)	THE INFOR-MANT DID NOT PREPARE THE EXTRACT BY HERSELF. HER PARENTS HAD IT AT THEIR HOME.
M (WOMAN, 69 YEARS OLD)	A ROOT THAT WAS LONG AS LITTLE FINGER WAS MACERATED IN A LARGE HALF-LITER BOTTLE SCHNAPPS	ADULTS: 2 TO 3 DROPS CHILDREN: A DROP LESS THAN FOR ADULTS	MED: FEVER VET: INDIGESTION IN LIVESTOCK AND STRENGTH IN LIVESTOCK	IN THE INFORMANT'S CHILDHOOD, HER MOTHER PREPARED THE EXTRACT.
INFORMANT	PREPATION OF THE EXTRACT	DOSAGE	USE	INTERESTING FEATURES
N (WOMAN, 75 YEARS OLD)	1 tablespoon of sliced roots was placed into 2 dl of schnapps	A few drops were placed in water and drunk	MED: fever VET: for weakened animals	The informant did not prepare the extract; her mother advised her to prepare it.

G (woman, 87 years old)	2 dl of roots was placed into a large half-liter bottle of schnapps and left to soak for 14 days	Adults: not more than 5 drops Children: just a small amount	MED: severe illnesses, fever, and inflammation	-----
A (woman, 82 years old)	2 to 3 roots were placed into half a liter of schnapps; the roots filled almost half the bottle; the soaking time was short	Adults: 9 drops Children: 3 drops Drops were placed in water and drunk	MED: prevention of diseases, fever, influenza, treatment of headache (lubrication of the forehead); "good for everything"	The last time the informant used the extract was 50 to 60 years ago; she prepared it herself.

c) Aconite poisoning

Aconite poisoning is characterized by numbness and tingling of the tongue, hypersalivation, nausea, vomiting, and diarrhoea, following within hours of ingestion. The toxins of aconite attack the heart causing conduction problems and arrhythmias, notably sinus bradycardia and the highly dangerous ventricular tachycardia, which may lead into ventricular fibrillation, which, if it continues for more than three minutes or so, leads to death), with the option of cardiovascular collapse. Respiratory paralysis, paraesthesia (unusual skin sensations...tingling, prickling, numbing, u.s.w.), and convulsions may occur. If the dose is fatal, death may occur at any time from almost immediately after ingestion (with very high doses) to around six hours after ingestion.

The first step in treatment is gastric emptying (induced vomiting and/or pump and lavage) and activated charcoal. Digitalis (foxglove) and atropine (chiefly from deadly nightshade) have both been used as antidotes to aconite poisoning; Grieve recommends 1.2 ml (roughly 1/4 tsp) of digitalis tincture. Anti-arrhythmic drugs are also used for this purpose; there is one case report of high-dose magnesium sulphate (Epsom salt – maximum paediatric dosage is IV 50 mg/kg/hour up to a total of 8000 mg/4 hours; upper level of adult dosage for arrhythmia may be as high as 3-4 g IV over 30 seconds) successfully restoring normal rhythm. In real life, patients with aconite poisoning are monitored in hospital for at least 24 hours due to the potential need for defibrillation; after the Catastrophe, CPR is likely to be the only hope of restoring normal heart rhythm.

Respiratory assistance may be required. IV fluid and electrolyte support is recommended, particularly as vomiting and diarrhoea can cause dehydration, electrolyte imbalances, and hypotension; potassium supplementation should, however, be avoided due to the high risk of cardiac catastrophe.

D) Aconite and Supernatural Persons

The relationship between wolfsbane and werewolves is debated. The name suggests that werewolves would be more sensitive to the effects of A. lycoctonum than ordinary humans, and there are many recent references to wolfsbane as secondary only to silver in terms of harming werewolves. However, since the release of The Wolf Man (1941), with its catchy invented "folk rhyme", "Even a man who is pure in heart, and says his prayers by night; / May become a wolf when the wolfbane blooms and the autumn moon is bright", there has been an ongoing trope indicating a positive interaction.

Various suggestions include: werewolves are attracted to/gain something special from the plant; the scent or pollen of the plant either provokes or reverses transformation; it is an element of becoming a werewolf by magical means; or it may cure or aid in curing lycanthropy. It should be noted, though, that the plant in the earlier film Werewolf of London (1936) does not seem to be any sort of Aconitum, but is identified as "mariphasa", with rather iris-like long bladed leaves, a flower with six narrow radiating petals, and a pod resembling that of a slender poppy. At any rate, until further studies have been done, or unless your werewolf patient has previous experiences with wolfsbane to draw on, it is best not to expose werewolves to A. lycocotum or any of its relatives. This may hold true for other shapeshifters as well.

Other types of supernatural persons seem to have no special interactions with the aconites, and treatment should be regarded as for any poison. If vampires cannot be poisoned by, for instance, strychnine, then they cannot be poisoned by aconites, although it is equally unlikely that the herb will do them any good. As the name "wolfsbane" suggest, aconites have in fact been used to kill both potentially dangerous predators and pests such as foxes. Just make sure that the creature you want to kill is the only one that can get at the aconite-infused bait! Smearing aconite juice on a blade is also an option. I do not know whether aconite juice on a bullet would survive being fired, though if it can, it might be a good way to avoid getting killed by a seriously-wounded and very angry large animal. As long as you don't plan to eat said animal afterwards.

E) Growing

A. napellus is commonly sold as a decorative herb in garden centres, often with no warnings regarding its severe toxicity. Aconite likes a rich, slightly damp loam, and prefers shade. It is, for all practical purposes, a perennial. The primary root gives off several "daughter" roots every year and dies back, while the following year's plants spring from the "daughter" roots. While it can be grown from seed, propagation is usually done by separating the "daughter" roots in the autumn at the time of harvest (note well: roots are almost always strongest in the autumn, and weakest in the earlier part of the spring) and replanting. One aconite plant quickly becomes a clump of aconite. It does not self-seed with any particular enthusiasm, so seed control is not a concern. Most people who do not buy their aconite at the garden centre get roots or extra plants from a friend who is thinning a clump; and once established in a good location, it requires no care whatsoever.

I have several aconites acquired from a friend's father's thinnings, which have been growing enthusiastically in place for over ten years now without any special tending. When doing anything with your aconites, it is crucial to wear gloves and long sleeves. Getting the juice in a cut, or even over-handling this plant bare-handed, can have catastrophic consequences. Monkshood is an extraordinarily beautiful plant, with a stalk of dark purple flowers rising two feet or so above rich green deep-fronded foliage. The flowers are the source of most of the folk-names such as "monkshood", "Auld Wife's Hood", and "Tyr's Helm"; a ridged "hood" or "helm" shelters the lower petals. Wolfsbane is similar in appearance, except that the flowers are yellow.

If you do not have child or animal issues, this plant is splendid for decorative gardening. In fact, the tall spikes of flowers make it an excellent companion to poppies, providing vertical colour against the silvery-green poppy foliage. If you do have children or animals, make sure they cannot come into contact with these plants. The friend who provided my aconites told me that his mother always shouted at his brother and himself when they would play too near to the aconite clumps, and he had never believed that they were any danger as long as one didn't actually eat them. He was quite shocked to learn his mother had been right all along about not even touching them. The gods protect fools and children – but one shouldn't rely on their protection when good sense can do as well.

INFROMANT	I (WOMAN, 78 YEARS)	H (WOMAN, 82 YEARS OLD)
AMOUNT OF ACCONITUM SPP. ROOT	HALF A BOTTLE THINLY SLICED ROOT	HALF A BOTTLE OF SLICED ROOTS
PREPERATION	THE ROOTS HAD TO BE FRESH	-0.1 L; IT IS WASHED AND SLICED ROOTS; THICKER ROOTS ARE OLDER AND THEREFOR STRONGER
TYPE OF SOLVENT	VERY STORNG SPIRIT; THE BEST WAS CYET	HOME FRUIT BRANDY USUALLY MADE FROM ROWAN BERRIES (SORBUS AUCUPARIA); STONG SPIRITS MAKE THE FINAL EXTRACT MORE EFFECTIVE
AMOUNT OF PREPARED EXTRACT/ CONTAINER	-APPROX. 0.1 L -A SMALL BOTTLE	GOOD THAT THE FRUIT BRANDY IS AT LEAST 1 COM ABOVE THE SLICED ROOTS -A BOTTLE
DURATION OF MACERATION	3 WEEKS	IT IS GOOD TO LEAVE THE EXTRACT STANDING FOR APPROXIMATELY ONE MONTH
INTERESTING FEATURES	AT THE END OF MACERATION, THE ROOTS WERE FILTERED	THE EXTRACT COULD BE USED FOR 50 YEARS OR MORE.

DOSAGE	THE INFORMANT DID NOT REMEMBER THE EXACT NUMBER OF DROPS	ADULTS: 3 TO 4 DROPS CHILDREN OLDER THAN 3 YEAR: 1 DROP THE EXTRACT WAS PLACED ON SUGAR OR MIXED INTO WATER BEFORE INGESTION; MILK WAS CONSUMED WITH THE EXTRACT TO PREVENT POISONING CATTLE: 10 TO 15 DROPS WERE PLACED ON BREAD
MEDICAL USE	MED: FEVER	MED: PNEUMONIA, INFLUENZA, COLD, SPANISH DISEAS (SHAKING, FEVER, NAUSEA, AND SORE FEET) VET: FOR INCREASED STRENGTH IN HORSES

INFROMANT	J (WOMAN, 89 YEARS OLD)	90 (YEARS OLD)
AMOUNT OF ACCONITUM SPP. ROOT	10 CM OF SLICED ROOTS; THE AMOUNT OF ROOT WAS APPROXIMATELY ONE FINGER HIGH IN A 1 L BOOTTLE	WAS AS THICK AS A WATER PIPE
PREPERATION	CLEAN AND FRESHLY COLLECTED ROOTS; IT DOES NOT MATTER WHETHER YOU USE OLD OR YOUNG ROOTS; THEY USED TO SAY THAT THICKER ROOTS WERE OLDER AND STRONGER AND YOU HAD TO USE FEWER	FLOWERING OF THE PLANT; ROOTS WERE COLLECTED AS SOON AS THE PLANTS STARTED TO GROW AND COULD BE IDENTIFIED, THE ROOTS WERE WASHED AND SLICED
TYPE OF SOLVENT	HOMEMADE FRUIT BRANDY MADE FROM PEARS OR PLUMBS	USUALLY MADE FROM PEARS
AMOUNT OF PREPARED EXTRACT/ CONTAINER	-1L -A BOTTLE	OF THE EXTRACT; WAS WELL HIDDEN (BURIED); THE EXTRACT WAS USED FOR APPROXIMATELY 2 YEARS
DURATION OF MACERATION	SOME TIME BUT NOT LONG; THE ROOTS QUICKLY RELEASE THE ESSENCE	---
INTERESTING FEATURES	THE EXTRACT WAS USED FOR A LONG TIME (MORE THAN ONE YEAR); THE EXTRACT WAS PREPARED SIMILARLY TO OTHER EXTRACTS	---
DOSAGE	A FEW DROPS WERE TAKEN; THE INFORMANT DID NOT REMEMBER THE EXACT NUMBER OF DROPS	CHILDREN: 2 DROPS THE EXTRACT WAS PLACED ON SUGAR OR MIXED INTO WATER BEFOR INGESTION

MEDICAL USE	MED: FEVER; COLD; EXTERNAL USE FOR TOOTHACHE AND INFLAMMATIONM GOOD FOR EVERYTHIN; IN THE WAR, IT WAS USED FOR PAIN AND INFLAMMATION	(TOOTHACHE), INFLAMMATION

IX. Hemlock (Conium maculatum)

a) Introduction

When the band of raiders captures your town and enslaves you, this and aconite are the herbs you will want for taking care of the problem. Just be sure everyone you care about knows not to eat, or even touch, that stew with what look like the little bits of chopped celery floating in it. Hemlock is so poisonous that children have died from blowing on whistles or peashooters made from the hollow stalks; people have died after eating gamebirds that had eaten hemlock seeds. It is exceedingly well-suited for the application advised by Leslie Fish for such post-Catastrophe circumstances:

"That evenin' everyone in town showed up, all bringin' the food an' beer.
Boss Jones, he sat at the head of the table, and all his boys sat near.
Oh, they ate 'n drank 'n bragged no end 'bout what they were gonna do
While they scarfed up rhododendron honey and amanita stew."

b) Former Uses and Hemlock Poisoning

Hemlock is a strong narcotic and sedative, which, despite its extreme toxicity, has been used for treating breathing problems, bladder and skin infections, neuromuscular disorders, and pain, as well as an ingredient in the anaesthetic "soporific sponge". None of these have been studied a great deal in the modern era, due to the plethora of safer options available. And after the Catastrophe, if plant life in general survives and you aren't completely hopeless at identifying plant species, you, too, are likely to have a plethora of safer options. In fact, it's harder to find an option that isn't safer. Traditionally, hemlock was used topically on tumours, particularly ulcerating ones, as both an analgesic and a hopeful cure.

It has been demonstrated that hemlock does have the potential to treat cancer by inducing apoptosis (natural death) in certain proliferating tumour cells (the study used cervical cancer cells from the HeLa line), as well as reducing proliferation and inhibiting colony-forming ability, so there may even be something to this. It would not be your first choice for treating cancer after the Catastrophe; that would have to be cannabis, which, even though we do not quite know enough yet to incorporate it into current treatment regimes as more than a promoter of quality of life in varying ways, shows a good deal of promise in regards to inhibiting virtually every aspect of carcinogenesis. Nonetheless, should you find yourself treating a palliative-care patient with a painful ulcerating cancer, it might be good to know that there is something else you can try in addition to, or, if necessary, instead of hemp. Hemlock serves as an antidote to strychnine poisoning.

It has also been used for the extreme spasms of tetanus and rabies (and may be the kindest treatment available for rabies after the Catatrophe); but cannabis is a far safer and preferable alternative in these cases. Symptoms of hemlock ingestion include hypersalivation, drowsiness, vomiting, muscle pain, loss of speech, speeder heartbeat followed by slowed heartbeat, paralysis, unconsciousness, total kidney, liver and heart failure, and death. Hemlock poisoning is not excessively swift, and has been described by the victims (before they got to the "loss of speech" and "unconsciousness" stages, obviously) as a feeling of cold numbness with paralysis rising from the feet; death commonly occurs as a result of asphyxia when the paralysis reaches the chest. The victim remains clear-headed to the end and may remain lucid.

The Greeks notoriously used hemlock as a supposedly relatively humane method of execution which allowed the condemned to say his last words at his leisure, the death of Socrates being the best-known example; although Socrates died without pain and death by hemlock can be quite painful. But it is possible that Socrates' dose contained other analgesics; that Plato was romanticizing the account a bit and just left out the drooling and vomiting as an inappropriate element of what he wanted to present as a dignified example of a Good Death; or that the analgesic and narcotic properties of hemlock may mitigate pain in some, but not all, cases of hemlock poisoning.

c) Dosing

The only safe dosage for hemlock is homeopathic, because it's really hard to poison yourself (or anyone else) with .999% or better pure distilled water. Can't do any good with it, except in a magical sense via the Law of Contagion (that water was once in contact with a tiny bit of water that was once in contact with a tiny bit of water, etc., that was in contact once upon a time with a wee bit of hemlock). But at least homeopathic remedies are safe, unless you're using them in place of a real treatment of some sort.

Mrs. Grieve cites 1-3 grains (0.065-0.194 grams) of powdered leaves as the pharmaceutical dose (p.394). In the event of strychnine poisoning, this would be the quantity to use, with the option of minute up-titration should the alternative be the patient's certain death in any case. I should also draw attention to her remark that "since...(1760) the plant has been much employed, though it has lost some of its reputation due to the uncertain nature of the preparations made from it" (p. 392; italics mine). No specific dosage is given for topical use, but it is probably as safe as anyone will get with this plant, which basically isn't, to go with the oral dosage applied with a carrier oil or ointment. There is no actual antidote to hemlock. Treatment includes induced vomiting/gastric lavage; airway securing and assisted breathing if necessary; antiseizure medication if convulsions occur; and IV fluid maintenance.

d) Growing

The same cautions apply to hemlock as to henbane, deadly nightshade, and so forth: it must be grown in an area which cannot be accessed by animals or children. Hemlock prefers a damp rich soil in a sheltered, but sunny, area, being vulnerable to high winds. Seed should be sown as soon as it is ripe in late summer for autumn germination. The plant is a biennial, producing flowers only in its second year. Hemlock is a relatively tall plant, with frondy foliage on a central stalk that is usually around a metre or ca. 4 feet tall, but, Mrs. Grieve assures us, can sometimes double that height in sheltered areas. It looks quite a bit like wild carrot and somewhat like angelica, or most of the other Umbelliferae, for that matter. The stalk is perfectly smooth, bright green with irregular purple-to-reddish spots, sometimes covered with a sort of white "bloom" or dusting which rubs off easily. The key distinguishing feature is the irregular purple spots on the stalk (hence the name Conium maculatum). But be warned: the spots may not appear when the plant is young, or may be difficult to distinguish.

Be extremely cautious about eating any wild plant that looks even slightly like hemlock. EXTREMELY CAUTIOUS. In fact, just don't do it unless you are an experienced specialist in the field. If you were desperate or stupid enough to ignore this advice, and feel a burn as it goes down or shortly thereafter, induce vomiting at once and take whatever stimulants you have available. Hemlock does not always cause a burning sensation in the digestive tract, but it frequently does (you might want to add a few chilis to that Invader Control Stew). The roots resemble parsnips, and have been mistakenly eaten as a result, with the inevitable tragic consequences.

The flowers are small, white, and form in smallish flat umbels. Hemlock self-seeds with enthusiasm; if growing the plant in your garden, remove and safely dispose of the umbels as they form, before they can make seed. Hemlock seeds are not usually the long-term lurkers that henbane seeds are- most of the Umbelliferae do not remain viable for over six to eight months– but has been known to surprise people. If you need seed, secure a plastic bag over the smallest of the umbels and remove whole when seeds are ripe. Wear gloves and a face mask to do this. You seriously cannot – literally cannot– overestimate just how poisonous this herb is!

Hemlock is a biennial, with that long pale parsnip-like taproot. I do not know if it can be grown indoors, because, basically, no one has ever been stupid enough to try it. Its toxins can and do volatilize into the air. Do not burn any part of hemlock. Those volatile toxins? Burning releases them, as can transplanting or otherwise messing with the plant. For disposal, bury deep and leave the site alone afterward. Aesthetically, hemlock is quite an elegant and attractive plant. However, most people consider that the non-poisonous look-alikes are preferable for garden design.

X. Resources

Absolutely the most valuable single book any survival herbalist can own is Mrs. M. Grieve's A Modern Herbal. If you have to run for your life and can only bring one book with you – this is the one. Grieves was writing in a time when the British pharmacopeia largely consisted of herbal and directly herb-derived medications, but well after the advent of pharmacology as we know it. She gives dosages for herbs that most modern herbalists will not even talk about. One thing to keep in mind: her dosages are the old pharmacological standard of grains, drachms, u.s.w.: you would do well to obtain a conversion chart before the Catastrophe and attach it to your copy of the book. She is not necessarily the final word on all things – modern research has found, and is constantly finding, more uses for plant constituents than were known in the 1930's. Hemp is not the only example of this by any means, though it is the most dramatic. Likewise, there are reasons to be cautious about ingesting large amounts of some herbs her age took for granted, such as coltsfoot and comfrey (both contain pyrrolidizine alkaloids, which can cause liver damage). Nonetheless, she is seldom if ever outright wrong: her work was based on the experience and studies of a great many physicians who prescribed herbal preparations just as we prescribe more refined or synthesized pharmaceuticals today.

Seeds and Plants

Seeds for all of these species can be ordered from:

» Kykeon Plants (https://kykeonplants.mysimplestore.com/)
» Magic Garden (https://www.magicgardenseeds.ch/Ethnobotanik-Samen/Magische-Heilpflanzen-Samen-T.107-/).
» Nicky's Nursery (https://www.nickys-nursery.co.uk/index.php/seeds-herb-seeds-c-6_65)

Live foxgloves (second-year) and aconite are commonly sold in garden centres. Specialty herb shops carry deadly nightshade and mandrakes intermittently; deadly nightshade is not disturbed by being shipped and transplanted, but I don't recommend it for mandrakes, due to the massive sulk factor. However, since mandrakes, though slow to germinate, are pretty reliable about doing it... eventually...(as in, I've grown both officinalis and autumnalis fairly often, and never gotten less than a 90% success rate without doing anything except keeping them moist and leaving them pretty much alone) seeds are generally a good option.

The only place I have ever found that sold live henbane or hemlock plants was Arne Herbs in the UK (mainland UK shipping only), and Anthony, who ran it, seems to have retired now. Because of their toxicity and tendency to be invasive once they do get established, selling live plants of these species is pretty firmly discouraged, and cultivating them may actually be illegal in some areas (although I doubt that anyone has ever gone to jail for it. If the logic of "fine for cultivating hugely deadly plant vs jail time for cultivating the world's least toxic plant" makes no sense to you – well, you're increasingly not alone).

Part IV: And If the Catastrophe Were a Plague...

I. Introduction

A massive global pandemic is one of the scenarios that frequently appears in post-apocalyptic (and sometimes just in apocalyptic) novels. With possible causes including natural pathogen evolution, biological warfare (by states and, increasingly possible, terrorist groups), and even pathogens from space...and with several potential or suspected-potential pandemics that may have been headed off by international action within our own lifetimes...this is something that is frequently on the minds of anyone who thinks about potential society-destroying catastrophes, whether in fiction, theory, or real life. The most effective way not to die in a pandemic is not to be exposed.

From extensive clinical experience, Hippocrates himself gave us the word on that topic, most commonly rendered in Latin translation. "Cito, longe, tarde" – leave quickly, stay away a long time, and come back slowly! The vast majority of pandemics through human history have been airborne. Bubonic plague (Yersinia pestis) is the main exception, with epidemics usually starting via very common rodents in endemic areas. Its most immediately contagious and virulent form is the airborne "pneumonic plague", but pneumonic plague is fast-acting and 100% fatal without antibiotic treatment, so tends to burn itself out quickly.

Whereas the insect-transmitted version – at least in conditions typical for the vast majority of humanity throughout the vast majority of history – had all the requirements for pandemic transmission. Cholera is the other exception, because, in the absence of modern hygiene, it can easily be transmitted between humans, and also is able to taint a whole area's water supply. The person or group attempting to survive a pandemic should probably focus chiefly on the prevention of airborne disease - ideally by means of going far, far away and not letting anyone onto the property until the pandemic has burned out quite thoroughly – but not forget the possibility of transmission through other methods, especially since some diseases do have more than one mode of transmission. (A favourite authorial gimmick, from Earth Abides to The Stand, is for the survivors simply to be those who are naturally immune to the plague. And there probably always will be a few. Even a "slate-wiper" is unlikely to have much more than a 90% kill rate.

A specific mutation in the CCR5-delta-32 gene allowed a number of Scandinavians to survive the Black Death, which was particularly virulent in the Northern environment – that mutation was only recognised recently because it eventually turned out to also confer significant resistance [heterogenous carrier, one mutated copy and one normal one] or even immunity [homogenous, two mutated copies] to HIV infection. So it's a legitimate authorial call, if not something on which the would-be survivor might want to depend).

II. What it Takes to Become a Pandemic

For a pathogen to become a pandemic requires firstly that it must be easily transmitted and not dependent on local factors. The mode of transmission generally determines the ease and potential range of transmission. Diseases with a faecal-oral spread can become epidemics through contaminating local water supplies, but very rarely pandemics. Cholera is the only exception, and the solution is as simple as washing your hands well and frequently, and boiling your water at a rolling boil for 20 minutes. Diseases spread by insects are also less likely to become pandemics: unless the insect in question is worldwide and common (fleas and body lice, bubonic plague), the disease can easily enough become a major epidemic (i.e., malaria) or a frequent-killer endemic disease (malaria again), but it is limited to the range of the insect in question.

Even a vector as common as body lice (vector for typhus, Rickettsia prowazekii) may cause epidemics under certain circumstances (war used to be the typical breeding ground for typhus, given the limited opportunities for hygiene in the field), but is less likely to cause a true pandemic. Bubonic plague is the only exception to that rule. Current theory, incidentally, indicates that the European spread in the 1348-51 pandemic was more via human transmission (human-to-human, human fleas and body lice) than through rats, though rats on shipboard probably did their share.

Physical contact is the means by which most viruses are spread, and by definition, those viruses are generally limited to physical contact. Someone harbouring a rotavirus (severe GI distress) on a plane may pass it on their hands to a seatmate or the host/ess who takes their plate; or, if they throw up in the airplane toilet, even to those who use the toilet subsequently until it has been disinfected at the destination port. They won't pass it to everyone breathing the plane's air. Pathogens found in the soil (tetanus, botulism, gas gangrene, anthrax spores, many parasites, Histoplasma, Cryptococcus neoformans, Coccidioides immitis) are endemic and nearly impossible to genuinely eradicate, and might become local epidemics under the wrong circumstances; but are seldom if ever passed directly person-to-person, and have never yet produced a pandemic.

Anthrax can be contracted by inhalation, making it a significant danger in regards to biological warfare dispersal, but cannot be passed person-to-person, which means that an anthrax pandemic would require close to simultaneous physical dispersal worldwide. Airborne transmittable diseases, on the other hand, have the potential to spread far and fast without physical contact, especially given the nature of modern transport. Whether passed on through aerosolized droplets (especially through coughing) or as smaller particles (as with the smallpox virus), transmitting an airborne disease only requires that the source be or recently have been in the area. Secondly, the longer the pre-symptomatic (or pre-major symptom) contagious period is, the more people a patient is likely to affect, and the higher the chances of the disease reaching pandemic proportions.

HIV, being difficult to transmit, only became the worldwide killer it did because of its incredibly long latent contagious period: by the time enough people were showing consistent major symptoms for epidemiologists even to figure out that there might be a problem, a vast number more were already infected by a disease for which, at the time, there was no working treatment. Smallpox only becomes contagious once the fever develops; but in the initial stages of fever, muscle aches, and vomiting, it can easily be mistaken for the flu or other diseases such as typhoid fever, and the ease with which it is transmitted makes it a major threat in this regard – or would, if a strain resistant to the current vaccines were developed for biological warfare, unearthed in a cold dry tomb in the Himalayas, or whatever.

Thirdly, however high the final fatality rate, the pathogen cannot kill its hosts off too quickly, or there will be no opportunities for transmission beyond the immediate area. Ebola and its less-deadly relation Marburg have never become pandemics partially because of the fast rate of population burn-out (combined with the need for fluid transmission, which forms a significant brake on disease spread. If Ebola Reston, which can indeed be airborne or at least aerosolized in spittle and the like, affected humans in the same way as the other filoviruses, recent human history might have taken a somewhat different course). A list of the major pandemics of human history include: cholera (repeated pandemics), various strains of influenza (majority of pandemics), bubonic plague (the Plague of Justinian and the 1894 pandemic, as well as the better-known Black Death of the mid-14th century), the Antonine Plague (best guesses from the descriptions of the time are smallpox or measles), and HIV. Of these, only cholera and bubonic plague are bacterial; only cholera and HIV cannot be spread through the air; and only bubonic plague includes insect transmission.

Most diseases with pandemic potential are species-jumpers like bird flu and swine flu; bubonic plague probably originated in marmots and is typically zoonotic with rodents as its most common host; HIV is thought to have begun as a monkey disease that then developed the ability to affect another primate species (us); and evaluation of the smallpox genome indicates that it probably originated as a disease of rodents, which crossed into humans around the time that the development of agriculture both increased frequent rodent-human contact and made it possible for humans to live in a density that could support the virus when it could no longer inhabit the original rodent hosts.

The Johns Hopkins Centre for Health Security identified a similar list of traits in potential society-disrupting pandemics: airborne; contagious during incubation period (maximum spread); virgin-field for most of the human race (no previous exposure, no developed immunity); and a "low but significant" fatality rate – high enough to cause massive social disruption between deaths and incapacitation, but low enough that the disease can continue to perpetuate itself and spread. Their estimation is that the next pandemic will likely be an RNA virus (genetic material comprised only of RNA) with an airborne spread. RNA viruses include rabies, SARS, Ebola and other filoviruses, influenza, hepatitis C, the various "cold" viruses, Zika, dengue, yellow fever, West Nile, and many others. If the method of transmission is not known – and if the disease is a new one or a mutation of a previous strain, it may not be – assume airborne in small particles first and foremost, but also take all possible precautions against faecal-oral or waterborne pathogens and insect or animal vectors.

III. Barrier Protection

The real question for the survivor is: if physical long-term self-quarantine for you and your family/survival group is not immediately possible, how do you protect yourself? Unless you are a microbiology specialist, epidemiologist, or health-care professional working in the hospital where an early patient has landed, the favoured methods such as pressure locks and various degrees of barrier shielding up to full Haz-Mat suiting are unlikely to be relevant to you. Correctly used, facemasks plus handwashing can reduce the chances of influenza infection even among close contacts (family members) by 70% to 80%. The devil in that particular detail is "correctly used". Filter facemasks are often incorrectly configured for the individual (they're very difficult to use effectively indeed if you have a beard), and non-health-care professionals are rarely even advised on the fine details of putting them on; unlike the N95 respirator (discussed below), there is no way to check the seal.

The SecureFit Ultra surgical mask is somewhat superior to the regular model, but the N95 is better than either, particularly when sealed with Vaseline. With both the facemask and the N95, you can use Vaseline/petroleum jelly around the edges to improve the seal, but that also has the chance of becoming a reservoir for trapped viral or bacterial particles; removal and disinfection must be done with the greatest caution. A 70-80% reduction in your chances of contracting a fatal disease is a great deal better than nothing. Even the considerably lesser improvement of a poorly fitted facemask is better than nothing. But at best, those are not the kind of odds on which you'd want to bet your life or those of your loved ones if you had a choice.

A significant improvement in facemask effectiveness was recently discovered by Hyo-Jick Choi (University of Alberta, Dept. of Chemical and Mechanical Engineering), who established that a solution of table salt could be applied to the surgical mask filter in order to kill at least the influenza virus (and has received a provisional patent on the method of salt-crystallization in formulating virus deactivation systems). This works because the salt coating is dissolved by the liquid component of aerosolized particles, then swiftly recrystallizes, which kills the viruses (the authors of the original report note that less safe/readily available salts such as ammonium chloride, potassium chloride, and potassium sulfate could also be used, possibly for specialized purposes in the future).

It was achieved by: removing the outer and inner layers of a standard three-ply surgical mask; dissolving table salt (sodium chloride, NaCl) in distilled water (stirring at 400 rmp, 90 C/194 F) and adding a non-ionic detergent (Tween 20 was used; the Triton series, used in many household detergents among other things, would also serve the same purpose) to reach a final concentration of 29.03 weight/volume percentage of salt and 1% volume of detergent. Choi and his team pre-wet the bare middle filters overnight in coating solution at room temperature, then put them into the desired remaining volume of coating solution (the trial used various quantities from 0-1200 microlitres for this step; the most effective volume was 1200 microlitres/filter, but higher amounts would be unlikely to diminish the effect) and dried them in an oven at 37 C/98.6 F for one day.

This method proved highly effective on mice (100% survival with no weight loss and minimal to undetectable virus titres in the lungs, in marked contrast to the untreated-filter group). It was also not strain-specific. This suggests that when that killer drug-resistant influenza strain with no vaccine developed comes along, the salt-treated surgical masks are still likely to work. Regular surgical masks are expected to prevent the passage of Staphylococcus aureus bacteria; influenza viruses are ca. 1/10th the size of S. aureus bacteria. The crystallization filter has not been tested against other viruses, and might or might not work against, for instance, poxvirus (although both are enveloped viruses, so there is at least a reasonable chance that the pox envelope would not protect it); but since an influenza strain is a fairly good contender for the agent of the Catastrophe,

The efficacy of a facemask might also be improved by an upgrade to a technique popular in the early Renaissance. Every Swede, at least, has grown up seeing "plague doctor" masks in museums: rather frightening leather masks with long beaklike cones over the nose and mouth, which were stuffed with aromatic herbs such as lavender as a prophylactic against the Black Death. This would not have helped with insect or body-fluid transmission (such as you get when you don't scrub and disinfect after draining a bubo, for instance), but it might have offered at least a little protection against the airborne pneumonic form. Antimicrobial essential oils are more effective than whole herbs, due to concentrating the relevant constituents; a combination including various essential oils such as clove, thyme, tea tree, cinnamon, basil, rosemary, ginger, etc. on the inside of the mask might well aid in neutralizing bacteria that make it through the mask.

Also, if you're surrounded by people who are dying, or have recently died, horribly...you'll appreciate the aromatic relief. Especially if the pathogen involves bowel issues. Many otherwise keen and not overly squeamish medical students have been completely put off a career as GI specialists by taking one whiff of the "air" inside the ward in question; and that's without the special aroma of advancing decomposition added to the mixture. The N95 respirator is the standard for filtering small particles. It fits more closely than a facemask, and has a finer filter. It cannot be used by children (wrong size) or people with facial hair (can't get the edges to seal); and because air has to be sucked in, it may be problematic for people with heart or lung problems affecting breathing/oxygenation. The N95 is a single-use, disposable item which is generally considered to require at least minimal training/practice to put on correctly, although it is fairly straightforwards.

It should be checked for both negative pressure and positive pressure security. For a negative pressure check: place both hands over the mask and breathe in sharply. It should pull in against your face, with no leaks felt. For a positive pressure check: put your hands over the mask and breathe out sharply. No air should leak (if it has a valve, you need to cover the valve for this check). If you have leakage, readjust the strap and nosepiece. An N95 cannot be cleaned, disinfected, or used after it has gotten either wet or dirty. This means that the adjuncts which improve, or may improve, safety with a surgical mask cannot be used with the N95. N95 respirators suitable for healthcare professional use are labelled "For Occupational Use".

IV. Likeliest Pandemic Disease-Types (and possible treatments)

a) Influenza

If the pandemic pathogen is a strain of influenza virus (especially if there is a worldwide shortage of medications such as oseltamivir - which totally did happen in 2005 during the bird flu outbreak - or if the virus has evolved resistance to that drug; and it should be said that oseltamivir [and the similar neuraminidase inhibitor zanamivir] appears to have been considerably overrated in terms of both efficacy and safety in any case), , echinacea may actually be a viable option. It may not be overwhelmingly effective in preventing infections in general, but, as mentioned above, it is probably effective in halting or mitigating them at an early stage of infection.

An ethanol extract of this herb can be used to clean your exposed skin and any items which have come within aerosol distance or touched a possibly-contagious person (note that aerosolized particles can hang in the air where someone has, for instance, sneezed for varying times after they have left). Hand cleansing – thorough and often – is especially important, as one of the main routes of transmission even of "airborne" viruses is mucous membrane/droplet contact with hands which then contact either another person, or an item that is contacted by another person; and echinacea extract is well-suited to disinfection of influenza viruses on this route (the 65% ethanol content of a product like Echinaforce doesn't hurt either, though you might want to use a hand cream afterwards to prevent excessive drying/ chapping).

It has recently been determined that the killing mechanism of the 1918 flu pandemic was probably the massive immune over-response ("cytokine storm") it evoked. One would think that immunosuppression would help to control this sort of thing, but in practice, it just doesn't work that way. Possibly if the right dose (which we don't know) of the right drug (ditto) were given at exactly the right time in the process (which we also don't know), it might help to head off the reaction. However, immune over-reaction tends to be followed in the late stages by immune burnout, as in septic reactions – leaving the patient additionally vulnerable to bacterial infections on top of the damage done by the initial pathogen and the hyper-activated immune mechanisms.

B) Pox

Smallpox, natural or modified, is another pandemic option, especially since vaccines are no longer given population-wide. Aside from being extremely contagious and pervasively airborne, and a favourite nightmare of people who worry about biological warfare/terrorism, smallpox also has the capability to remain viability for very long periods of time, especially when protected by scab material (hence the infamous "gifts" of smallpox-infected bedding to Native Americans). Actually we don't really know quite how long smallpox can remain viable under the right circumstances (very dry, cold, and dark), except for professional scientific freezers, where we know it can remain viable indefinitely. Or at least think it can. Hopefully no one has opened those two freezers in the US and Russia to check how the (we would like to think) last live smallpox viruses in the world are doing.

And I assure the aspiring author – if you can't imagine at least three scenarios that could have led to someone getting hold of samples from one of those freezers, or preserving a cache from before the eradication, then maybe you shouldn't imagine quitting your day job, either. Also, in 2014, personnel just...sort of found...vials of live smallpox in an unused storage room at an FDA laboratory, an occurrence described by one journalist as resembling, "a plot twist in a bad Syfy network movie". This does not inspire great confidence in the assertion that Atlanta and Moscow have the only remaining live samples. Especially when one considers that the effective dose of variola to cause infection is one particle, at least in the more virulent strains.

Salmonella, in contrast, requires 105 to 1010 bacteria to achieve infection in humans. Smallpox vaccinations, unfortunately, wear off with time. Someone who was vaccinated in the 1970s is very unlikely to retain immunity to the present day. These vaccinations are no longer given to the general public, although they are still given to, for instance, some members of the US and other militaries (against the event of biological warfare); so if the smallpox of your Catastrophe has not been deliberately modified or naturally mutated to evade the protection of vaccinations, current and recently ex-military characters may well be protected. The ease of smallpox transmission can hardly be overestimated. In Demon in the Freezer, Preston cites the case of "Peter Los", where one smallpox patient infected patients on the floors above him by opening his window, as well as at least one patient who put his face near the slightly open door of the isolation corridor outside Los' room [pp. 29 ff; see also the 1970 report written on the incident].

Preston also mentions the laboratory infection of Janet Parker in 1978 – by, it is believed, a few particles that drifted into a room beside the actual laboratory, got sucked into the air vent, and travelled through several more rooms [p. 95]. The smallpox virus diffuses like smoke, can go quite a long way...and, as mentioned above, one particle is enough to initiate a deadly infection. Smallpox comes, or (hopefully past tense) came in two strains, Variola major and Variola minor. Their virulence levels are/were just what they say on the tin. The disease starts with a probably non-contagious incubation period of 7-19 days from infection (10-14 days is the norm). The initial symptoms, at which point the patient has become contagious, last 2-4 days and resemble a dose of the flu: fever, headache, muscle aches, sometimes vomiting (remember that "Vomiting Larry" video I footnoted above?

Now watch it and imagine the fluorescent stuff Larry spews is contaminated with live – persistent, long-lasting – smallpox virus. Now imagine this in, say, a public toilet. Have I put you off your supper yet?). This is the stage at which the pandemic will really get going, because no one tests for smallpox any more without a clear reason to suspect it, so patients are likely to be treated as if they had the flu. The inadequate response at Presbyterian Hospital, Dallas (2014) when Thomas Duncan presented with Ebola (initially sent home with a prescription for antibiotics; protective measures employed by staff after his Ebola diagnosis also proved insufficient to protect them) is one model for how a smallpox or smallpox-like pandemic could get a firm start before anyone realized it was happening.

Without laboratory testing, the first sign that the patient actually has smallpox rather than a dose of the flu is the emergence of a rash. The initial rash, which lasts around four days, starts as red spots on the tongue and the inside of the mouth, which break down and become sores producing large amounts of live virus in the mouth and throat; spittle, including droplets aerosolized by coughing, is highly contagious. The fever continues. As the oral sores break down, the rash starts on the face, spreading down the arms and legs to the hands and feet, usually covering the whole body within 24 hours. The fever may drop and the patient begin to feel briefly better at this point. By the fourth day, the rash pustules have filled with thick opaque fluid (awesomely contagious), often showing a dimple in the centre; and at this point you absolutely know it's smallpox, but it's probably too late for anyone who had contact with the patient. The fever rises again as the pustules fill.

After about five days, the pustules scab over. The smallpox scab is the most persistent means of transmission, and can keep the virus alive for quite long periods of time in, for instance, clothing or bedding. This regrettably suits it to low-tech biological warfare, although deliberately giving smallpox blankets to a population you want to eradicate horribly is the sort of thing that only a totally unbelievable caricature of a complete inhumane bast...Oh, wait. That was British commander Jeffrey Amherst and his cronies Ecuyer, Boquet, and Trent, ca. 1763 (regrettably, Amherst, in spite of also being a crap military leader by most accounts, kept his post, got promoted to Field Marshal eventually, and died peacefully in his own bed at home, rather than being subjected to the worst tortures that the fertile minds of his victims could devise. But perhaps your author will see fit to redress this injustice at least in fiction).

Within six days of formation, the scabs begin to fall off. Full sloughing usually takes 4-6 weeks, and severe scarring is common. The patient is still contagious until all scabs have fallen off. They may suffer blindness from corneal scarring, encephalitis, osteomyelitis, infertility (men), or, if pregnant at the time of infection, stillbirths or spontaneous abortions. This outlines the course of disease if the patient is lucky. If the patient is not lucky, the skin lesions remain relatively flat, are velvety-textured, and merge together (confluence) with a rather crepelike effect over the whole body. This is probably the result of a deficient immune response to the virus, and the large majority of patients with confluent smallpox die, even with modern medical care (as of the 1970s, anyway). If the patient lives, the lesions gradually diminish without forming the characteristic pustules and scabs, and fade away. The most fatal form – inevitably, even with the best possible hospital support available when we still had smallpox patients! – is haemorrhagic smallpox.

This is more common in adults, especially pregnant women, but we don't know why. Prior vaccination diminishes the incidence and severity of flat smallpox, but not the haemorrhagic type. The incubation period is shorter; the first-stage symptoms are more intense, often including abdominal pain as well as fever/headache/muscle aches/maybe vomiting; and the patient develops a generalized dusky flush. They may die of multi-organ failure before the rash fully develops; or they may last long enough to show bleeding into the pustules and generalized haemorrhage; but this patient is going to die. Because a huge amount of our knowledge and development of antiviral drugs dates from after the eradication of smallpox in the wild, there are no drugs that have been tested against smallpox in clinical studies. Tecovirimat, brincidofovir, and cidofovir are recommended by the CDC for use in a smallpox emergency.

Tecovirimat was originally developed as an anti-smallpox agent, but never clinically tested; cidofovir is used for cytomegalovirus retinitis (most commonly seen in late-stage HIV patients); brincidofovir is a similar drug with a better safety profile (does not seem to carry the same risk of severe kidney toxicity that cidofovir does). All of these have been shown effective by in vitro studies and animal testing, but have not been tested against smallpox in human clinical studies; even the data on using tecovirimat to counteract severe reactions to the smallpox vaccination (vaccinia, a related pathogen which is similar enough to smallpox to evoke an adequate immune reaction to the latter) is limited. Smallpox was the inspiration for the entire concept of vaccination, developed by Dr. Edward Jenner in the 1790s.

Having observed the low incidence of smallpox among people who worked with cattle (milkmaids were proverbially famed for their clear and beautiful skin in an era where many people were horribly scarred by smallpox), he introduced a drop of cowpox pus into a boy's arm by scratching, then performed the same procedure on the boy with pus from a smallpox patient some months later (protocols for human experimentation in his day were, to say the least, a lot looser than they are now!). When the boy didn't catch smallpox, Jenner knew he was on to something good. Vaccinia virus, from which the very term "vaccination" stems, was probably originally a form of cowpox or horsepox, though its genetic structure now differs slightly from both. Cowpox, should you ever have need to use it for a vaccination, is actually rare in cattle today, but is endemic in Europe (particularly Great Britain) and Asia, where the most common hosts are woodland voles and other forest rodents.

Cats occasionally contract it from their prey, and may show lesions on the face, neck, forelegs, and paws. Humans can contract it from any of these animals, but human cases are very rare in the modern world. Neither cowpox, vaccinia, nor horsepox is found in the wild in the Americas; early vaccination stocks, which might be based on any of these, had to be imported from Europe. There is one plant, the purple or Northern pitcher plant (Sarracena purpurea) which was used for treating smallpox by the Micmac (survivor backstory options could include: is Micmac/knows Micmacs/has studied Micmac culture), and was recently re-evaluated in vitro regarding efficacy against the variola viral family. It works by inhibiting mRNA synthesis, without which the virus cannot produce the proteins required for replication. S. purpurea was effective only against orthopox viruses (which include smallpox, cowpox, and monkey pox); other herbs with more general antiviral effects (echinacea [Angustifolia], astragalus, and the mushroom turkey-tail [Coriolus or Trametes versicolor]) proved ineffective against the orthopox family.

Obviously the researchers could not test it directly against smallpox, since the people in charge of the surviving virus samples keep pretty tight controls on who they allow to mess with them for any reason; but the odds are good that, at least in vitro and hopefully in vivo in humans, S. purpurea would be as effective against smallpox as it is against other orthopoxes. The method used for producing the extract used was gently grinding cleaned whole fresh plant in a steel blender together with 95% ethanol/distilled water/vegetable glycerine at 63-32-5%. The product was sealed in an amber glass container and kept at room temperature for 48 days, after which the liquid was pressed out, filtered (unbleached paper filters), and bottled in amber glass bottles.

The amber glass is standard for preserving herbal products of any sort to limit light-related degradation; the study authors do not mention keeping their extract in the dark, but as a general principle with herbs and their extracts, you should. S. purpurea is native to Canada, the US from the Great Lakes to the Cast Coast, and all the way down the Eastern seaboard. It grows well in sphagnum moss/peat moss mixed 1:1 with perlite or lime-free horticultural sand; it prefers full sun, but can get along with 2-4 hours of direct sunlight/day. This is a bog plant, and it likes being waterlogged during summer and damp in winter, but cannot tolerate any high-mineral water (rainwater, distilled water, or reverse-osmosis filtered water are all good options, and fertilizer should absolutely be avoided. This plant is a carnivore, and gets all its nutrients from its prey).

As might be expected from its habitat, can tolerate both hot summers and cold winters; in fact, it requires a dormant winter period (November-February, at the least) at cold, often sub-freezing temperatures (an unheated greenhouse or conservatory is often recommended), and thrives in Northern Europe; it was introduced to Irish bogs in the 1980s and does very well indeed here; in fact, it is considered an invasive plant in Northern Europe up through Sweden. It can be grown from seed; propagation is by root division at the end of the winter dormant period, and is are usually sold either as a growing plant or as a bare rhizome in the dormant period. If kept outdoors, purple pitcher plants will feed themselves, often quite aggressively (FEED ME, SEYMOUR!). If kept indoors, toss them a dried insect or two every couple of weeks. They are reputed to be quite fond of dead crickets.

In regards to smallpox escape and spread after the Catastrophe: with the current strains, epidemiologists estimate that (given that smallpox as we know it now does not have an animal host) a population of ca. 200,000 within 14 days travel is required to keep an outbreak going (Preston, Demon, p. 66). This, of course, could change if the virus were to develop, for instance, a longer incubation period. Monkeypox, considered an "emerging disease" (probably emerging now because of the waning immunity from pre-1980 smallpox vaccinations, and perhaps previously also confused with smallpox due to the similarity of presentation), also has the potential to evolve (or be manipulated) into the new smallpox. Despite the name, it is primarily a disease of rodents (including captive prairie dogs, which have been known to catch the disease from imported Gambian pouched rats and pass it on to each other or humans – the cause of the sole American outbreak), but infects primates including humans.

There are two strains: the more virulent Central African, which has a higher mortality rate and is readily transmitted person-to-person; and the West African, in which person-to-person spread is limited. The symptoms are similar enough to smallpox to evoke considerable worry on clinical examination (I know I'd be highly alarmed if I saw a patient with that particular rash), but far milder, with a maximum death rate of ca. 10% in Gambia where it is endemic, and 0% among the 71 cases in the US outbreak. The main clinical difference is that patients with monkeypox show swollen lymph nodes, and patients with smallpox generally don't. Smallpox vaccination is thought, but not proven, to also provide protection against monkeypox. Two small mutations in monkeypox – as small as the protein production and single amino acid shift that turned Y. pestis first into a dangerous pathogen, and then into a rapidly invasive pandemic-causer – could make monkeypox into the next smallpox...possibly with the added problem of retaining animal hosts, which would make relative eradication impossible. This potential also exists in other poxviruses, of which there are an huge number in mammals, reptiles, and insects (for insects, the effects are neurological, since insects don't actually develop pustules), but monkeypox is probably the likeliest to become a major danger.

c) Plague (Yersinia pestis)

The plague bacterium has been with us in its current form, barring the occasional strain variation such as the 1348-51 exceptionally pathogenic variant, at least since the Eurasian Late Neolithic/Early Bronze Age period. It is now classed as a "re-emerging disease", with global incidence on the rise since the late 1990s. The discovery of a particularly virulent early form (Gok2) in a Swedish passage grave from ca. 5000 years ago has, in fact, led to the suspicion that the first plague pandemic may have been a major cause of the late Neolithic population collapse in Northern and Western Europe. The two ways by which plague could become a pandemic again are natural mutation or biological-warfare manipulation. In either case, it would have to become antibiotic-resistant and, since fleas and body lice are not a major issue in much of the world today, more easily transmissible person-to-person; but these changes are by no means beyond possibility.

It only took two small changes for the mild GI pathogen Yersinia pseudotuberculosis to become pandemic-capable Yersinia pestis (the first being the development of the PLA protease gene; the second being a single amino acid shift in that gene); and four minor shifts to turn it into a disease that could be carried and transmitted by fleas and lice. The PLA protease gene may have arisen between 5000-7000 years ago; the oldest example of the Y. pestis genome which has the arthropod-transmission adaptations (inactivation of ureD, PDE2, PDE3, and rcsA by substitution or single-nucleotide insertion/deletion of a base, in case you care) tested so far dates from approximately 3800 years ago. Since then, it has remained relatively stable due to a low number of strains making shared mutations less likely than is the case with, for instance, the influenzas. Plague, which has a range of animal hosts and can be transmitted by many parasitic insects, is endemic in many parts of the world, including the American West, particularly the Southwest and coastal regions. As S.M.

Stirling presents matters in Dies the Fire: even if a mutated Y. pestis is not the cause of the Catastrophe, Y. pestis as we know it has the potential to become a serious problem afterwards, when fleas and body lice are likely to become a good deal more common than they are for most people in much of the world today. All known bubonic plague pandemics, and the vast majority of significant outbreaks, started with unusual flooding in Asia, which drove rodents out of their usual haunts and into closer contact with humans. Asia has been the origin of plague pandemics affecting Europe, but one could begin in any area where plague is endemic, including the American Southwest and West Coast. If the Catastrophe is extreme weather-related or followed by extreme weather in the wrong place or places, it absolutely will happen – and modern means of travel are not required for worldwide spread. Sailing ships, horses, and feet have been demonstrated to do the job quite effectively, although improved methods of ship construction and trans-oceanic navigation help it travel much further and faster, as S.M. Stirling ably and realistically presents in the second and third Nantucket trilogy books, Against the Tide of Years and On the Oceans of Eternity.

Diagnosis of plague is done by clinical suspicion, confirmed by Gram, Giemsa, Wright, or Wayson staining and microscopic examination of lymph node aspirate (samples from an affected lymph node may often show the bacteria even without culturing); blood testing (if the patient has the septicaemic form, bacteria may show well. Early in the disease, they are unlikely to show without culturing – no matter what characters in S.M. Stirling's Dies the Fire may have done, in real life you can't just take a plain blood smear, stick it under the microscope, and say whether an apparently healthy person is infected or not. That only works for active malaria. And you can't confirm deer meat as not being human meat that way either, unless that's meant to be another point where Stirling's world differs from ours); or sputum (pneumonic patients). The Y. pestis bacterium is Gram-negative (shows up red under Gram staining) and ovoid.

A Wayson stain - fuschin and methylene blue in an alcohol-phenol base (phenol is a weak acid, also known as carbolic acid, and was one of the earliest medical and post-surgical antiseptics; it is still used in many products, and is the podiatrists first-line treatment for permanently ingrown nails. Undiluted, it can cause skin burns and is quite toxic to ingest, 1 gram being the lethal dose for an adult human) reveals bipolar-staining, yielding an appearance like a closed safety pin with darker areas at each pole. In real life, PCR may be used for an earlier confirmation. Regardless of the microbiological investigation, if there is a clinical suspicion (usually including living in or having recently travelled to an endemic area, especially if contact with animals was known or possible), empirical treatment is initiated immediately: the patient cannot afford to wait.

Death commonly occurs at ca. 3-5 days from infection with bubonic plague, and may happen within 24 hours with pneumonic plague. Something crucial for the survivor who wishes to continue surviving to know about the plague, whether it is the agent of the Catastrophe or a local outbreak afterwards: you absolutely can catch it from the dead body of a human or animal. The 2007 death of wildlife biologist Eric Young from primary pneumonic plague, which he is believed to have contracted by inhaling aerosolized bacteria from a mountain lion corpse on which he was performing a post-mortem (in his garage, without personal protective equipment), is a grim reminder of how dangerous the plague-dead can still be. Young broke with fever and haemoptysis (coughing blood) three days after the necropsy, and was found dead in his home ca. 6 days after the initial exposure. Testing confirmed that he and the mountain lion had the same strain of Y. pestis.

Cases in North America over the past few decades have also confirmed that it is quite possible to contract plague from being scratched by an infected animal or an animal who has been fighting with an infected one – usually a cat, as felines of all sizes seem to be particularly vulnerable to this disease. Ca. 20% US plague cases have been contracted via direct contact with an infected mammal (the large majority are still via insect transmission), with house cats playing a significant part. The plague bacillus can survive for weeks in water, moist meal, or grain; for months to years at near-freezing temperatures (which may explain why it was so particularly devastating in the Northern countries of Europe); and is viable in, among other things, dried sputum, flea faeces, and buried bodies. It can be killed by several hours in direct sunlight, or heating at 72 C/161.6 F for fifteen minutes.

Burning the bodies of the dead, their clothing, and their bedding is strongly recommended; but if you are in a situation where you can't burn clothing and bedding, boil it thoroughly and hang it to dry in the sunlight, turning occasionally to make sure that there are no protected/shadowed areas. Wear personal protection while doing this. If all else fails, soak a fine-woven kerchief in salt water, let it dry, and tie it across your nose and mouth – it's not a salt-filter mask, but at least it's something – and be sure to disinfect your hands and all exposed areas with whatever you have. Plague develops rapidly from the time of infection. Symptoms may begin to show within hours (pneumonic); the bubonic form usually takes ca. 2-3 days to manifest, although it can be as long as 6 days. Once the patient is symptomatic, the disease can progress extremely quickly. There are accounts from the various historical outbreaks of families going to bed apparently healthy in the evening, and all being dead by morning. It is now established that the pneumonic form of the plague can kill within 18-24 hours. Antibiotics should be given within 24 hours of suspected infection if possible.

Signs and symptoms:

Bubonic form – fever, chills, headache, weakness; one or more painful, hard, tender lymph nodes which may be grossly swollen, turn black, abscess, and hopefully drain (buboes). Usually contracted from flea/louse bites, sometimes from contact with infected mammals. 1-15% death rate with modern treatment; ca. 50% without. It was common back in the day for those who stuck around to tend the sick to encourage buboes to ripen and drain. Moist heat can help to achieve this, and may have been the reason that (on those occasions when it was actually tried in practice rather than just being discussed in theory) the fabled "Chicken's Butt Cure" was actually considered helpful. You pluck the feathers from around the chicken's cloacal opening, see, and apply the live chicken rear-first to the bubo...A hot moist poultice of onion/garlic/other possibly effective herbs sounds like a better option, especially for the chicken.

Septicaemic form – fever, chills, extreme weakness, abdominal pain, shock, bleeding into skin/internal organs, black skin necrosis seen especially on extremities and nose. The skin bleeding and necrosis may have been the origin of the name "Black Death", although buboes may also turn black. Usually from an insect bite or handling an infected animal (or, presumably, person). This can either be the initial presentation, or develop from the bubonic form at a later stage. 40% death rate with modern treatment, 100% without.

Pneumonic form – fever, headache, weakness, rapidly-developing pneumonia (sputum may be bloody or watery); shock, respiratory failure. From inhaling infective droplets, or if the bacteria from bubonic or septicaemic (if the septicaemic patient lives that long) spread into the lungs. Effectively 100% fatal, usually within 24 hours of showing symptoms (sometimes within 24 hours of infection), no matter what you do.

Current treatment for Y. pestis is antibiotic. Post-exposure prophylaxis may be initiated within seven days of suspected exposure, although the best results are achieved if antibiotics are started in the first 24 hours. Pre-exposure prophylaxis is used in high-risk situations (close contact with infected animals/carrier insects/humans is unavoidable). Treatment continues for 10-14 days or up to two days after fever drops, whichever comes later; prophylaxis continues for 7 days. The effectiveness of penicillin-drugs and first- and second-generation cephalosporins (such as cephalexin, brand-name Keflex, or cefuroxime) against plague is considered low to non-existent. Third-generation cephalosporins such as ceftriaxone and cefotaxime appear to be clinically effective, with ceftriaxone being preferred.

They are, however, inferior to streptomycin and the other antibiotics which have replaced it as the treatment of choice, so are not recommended if those are available. Amoxicillin/ampicillin, given within 24 hours of infection in mice, did show significant efficacy (85% survival rate; streptomycin and ciprofloxacin had a 100% survival rate). However, in one phase of the experiment, the mice given ampicillin at 42 hours died more quickly than the untreated controls. This is suspected to be due to the release of endotoxins as a result of the beta-lactam mechanism of action in this antibiotic (beta-lactams affect the bacterial cell membrane. Beta-lactam antibiotics include the penicillin drugs, the carbapenems, the cephalosporins, and aztreonam).

The antibiotics used, according to the CDC, are:

Streptomycin (first-line) – adult dose 1 gr 2x/day. Child dose – 15 mg/kg 2x daily, up to 2 gr/day total. Intramuscular injection. Not recommended in pregnancy (though consider risk/benefit; better to lose the baby than to lose both mother and baby). Not normally used for post-exposure prophylaxis (probably a lot better than nothing if it's what you have). The official shelf life of the crystalline form is 12 months from the date of manufacture. FDA-approved, but described as "not widely available in the US." Streptomycin used to be the gold standard for treating Y. pestis, but further studies have led to its general replacement with more effective antibiotics such as gentamicin and ciprofloxacin.

Ciprofloxacin (first-line) – adult/pregnancy treatment dose 400 mg 2-3x/day, IV; adult post-exposure prophylaxis dose 500 mg/dose 2x/day. Child treatment dose – IV, 15 mg/kg/dose, up to a maximum 400 mg/dose; oral, 20 mg/kg/dose, up to a maximum 500 mg dose. Child post-exposure prophylactic dose: 20 mg/kg/day up to a maximum of 1 gr/day, oral.

Gentamicin (first-line) – adult/pregnancy dose 5 mg/kg 1x/day or loading dose of 2 mg/kg followed by 8-hourly doses of 1.7 mg/kg. IM or IV injection. Child dose – 2.5 mg/kg dose every 8 hours. Not normally used for post-exposure prophylaxis. Solutions are stable at room temperature for 5 days, 30 days at 2-8 C/35.6-48.4 F, longer term requires keeping at -20 C/-4 F. Gentamicin sulfate powder is stable for 48 months at 2-8 C. Not FDA-approved, but considered an effective alternative. Poor penetration of abscesses; if the patient manifests the bubonic form, use another antibiotic in combination.

Chloramphenicol (first-line) – adult treatment dose 25 mg/kg every 6 hours IV; child treatment dose (> 2 years old) 25 mg/kg, maximum daily dose 4 gr, IV. Not used for post-exposure prophylaxis. Chloramphenicol is low-cost and relatively easy to store [the crystalline form is stable for ca. 5 years; water-based solutions degenerate by 50% at 37 C/98.6 F, but are stable below 5 C/41 F for ca. 2 years; ethanol-based solutions need to be kept at -20 C/-4 F after being made up, though solubility is better in ethanol]. Not readily available in the US, chloramphenicol is rarely used in the developed world.

It can have more untowards side effects than most antibiotics, sometimes including dangerous bone marrow suppression and more rarely aplastic anaemia; but it is considered a working alternative in many developing countries. Chloramphenicol crosses the blood-brain barrier, so, despite its dangerous side effects, it has been considered the antibiotic to use if the plague patient is also showing any indication of meningitis (ca. 6%), which may develop either together with the more typical plague symptoms, or appear up to two weeks later after the antibiotic course is finished. The dose for plague meningitis is 50 mg/kg 4x/day, IV, for ten days.

Doxycycline (second-line) – adult/pregnancy dose 100 mg 2x/day or 200 mg 1x/day IV or oral for treatment, 100 mg 2x/day oral for post-exposure prophylaxis. Child doses for both treatment and post-exposure: 2x/day; > 45 kg = same as adult; < 45 kg = 2.2 mg/kg up to a max of 200 mg/day. Bacteriostatic (prevents replication) rather than bacteriocidal (kills outright), but adequately effective compared to gentamicin. Storage: powder – 1 year from receipt at 4 C/39.2 F in the dark; solutions – 4 weeks at 4 C, 3 months at -20 C/-4 F. FDA approved.

No tooth staining from multiple short courses. Note that older sources recommend against doxycycline and the tetracyclines in children under eight due to the risk of permanent tooth staining and failure of dental enamel to develop fully, but this has recently been proved largely unfounded in regards to doxycycline (though still valid re tetracyclines), so it is considered safe for use in younger children now. Doxycycline is also effective against malaria.

Levofloxacin (second-line) – adult treatment dose 500 mg 1x/day, IV or oral; may go up to 750 mg 1x/day if needed). Child dose (under 50 kg and 6 months or older): 8 mg/kg/dose every 12 hours, up to 250 mg/dose, IV or oral. Not recommended for pregnant women. Not normally used for post-exposure prophylaxis.

Both ciprofloxacin and levofloxacin are bacteriocidal, FDA-approved and effective in animal studies. Clinical testing in humans for both has been fairly limited, but the data so far is sufficient that this class of antibiotic (fluroquinolone) is considered to be one of the best choices for treating plague. Trimethopram-sulfamethoxazole was formerly recommended for post-exposure prophylaxis in children < 9 (CDC as of 1996). The above-listed represent current guidelines as of 2018, but if trimethoprim-sulfamethoxazole is the antibiotic you have, then you are not wasting it in treating or preventing plague with it.

Plague in pregnant women notoriously causes stillbirths or spontaneous abortion. Ziegler cites Jennings' report of 1903, describing 14 cases of plague in pregnancy. Four mothers survived; 13 of the 14 women, including all the survivors, suffered stillbirths or miscarriages. In contrast, she mentions the case of a Navajo woman in her ninth month, who was induced after streptomycin was started in response to her baby's heart-rate shooting up to 200/min (a sign of foetal distress). The child was delivered safely, and no evidence of infection was present in his umbilical cord blood; he remained healthy. Ziegler adds that in the few other recorded antibiotic-era cases, the antibiotic treatments rescued the pregnancy; but that immediate induction is recommended >36 weeks if there are any signs of foetal distress (the heartbeat is the easiest to measure with simple clinical tools).

The original plague vaccination was given to researchers who work with the bacterium, people in endemic areas whose job brings them into frequent contact with possibly-infective animals, and people in endemic or outbreak areas where fleas and rodents are unavoidable. It was withdrawn after it was demonstrated that the vaccine was effective against the bubonic form, but not the pneumonic form, which is the main concern regarding biowarfare/terrorism, as the bacterium would most likely be released as an aerosol. As of 2018, a vaccine offering dual protection against anthrax and plague had just been developed, and is being considered for stockpiling in case of biowarfare/terrorism.

Possible Herbal Treatments for Plague

Little or no research has been done specifically testing herbs or herbal components against Y. pestis. It is a sufficiently difficult disease, especially in the pneumonic and septicaemic forms, that the focus has entirely been on pharmaceutical antibiotic efficacy and safety. However, its close relative Yersinia enterocolitica (causes mild to moderate gastric distress) has been the object of a number of tests due to its much greater current prevalence. Y. enterocolitica is generally treated by the same antibiotics used for pestis, and is probably vulnerable to much the same mechanisms of antibiotic action. This does not make up for direct testing on the species of concern, let alone for actual clinical studies. But in the absence of better information now, and better drugs after the Catastrophe (or during it, if it's caused by a plague outbreak and the antibiotics run short), these herbs may at least offer an improved chance of survival if initiated in time.

Arjuna (Terminalia arjuna) bark water extract (15 gr powdered herb in 150 ml distilled water, boiled at 100 C/212 F for 6 hours, filtered, filtrate dried by evaporation in water bath at 100 C) showed significant effects in vitro against Yersinia enterocolitica. The arjuna was not as effective as gentamicin, but was more effective than the tetracyclines. It is reasonably probable that arjuna bark would also have some efficacy against Yersinia pestis. Arjuna is a tree native to India. It prefers daytime temperatures of ca. 20-33 C/68-91.4 F, dies if the temperature drops below -1 C/30.2 F, and needs full sun. It is fast growing, and can reach a height of 30 M (neighbourhood of 100 ft) within a few years. The bark is normally harvested from the 10th year on, taken in vertical strips to avoid killing the tree by girdling it (if you cut the bark all the way around the trunk, that tree is a dead tree).

Cloves and other ground spices (4.1 to 4.7% weight/volume preparations) also showed bacteriostatic (preventing multiplication) effects against Y. enterocolitica in vitro. The most effective spices for this purpose were cloves and allspice (both contain eugenol, suspected to be the active constituent).

At concentrations of 2000 parts per million, ethanolic clove extract showed bacteriocidal activity and prevented viable bacteria from recovering within 1 minute. Sage, cinnamon, rosemary, and oregano were the next on the list in terms of efficacy against Y. enterocolitica. The essential oils of oregano and thyme were demonstrated in an in vitro study to have a greater efficacy against Y. enterocolitica (and Staphylococcus aureus, E. coli, Salmonella typhimuria, Enterococcus faecalis, and Listeria monocytogenes) than chloramphenicol. In this study, clove essential oil also proved more effective against Y. enterocolitica and typhoid fever bacteria (S. typhimuria) than chloramphenicol.

A selection of herbs and spices that were shown to be in vitro effective against a range of Yersinia spp (Y. pestis was not included), included: lemongrass (Cymbopogon citrate), clove basil (Ocimum gratissimum), Key lime fruit (Citrus aurantifolia), papaya seeds (Carica papaya), coffee leaves (Coffea arabica), processed coffee (Nescafe brand instant), unprocessed honey, and processed honey. All of these proved to have an in vitro efficacy comparable to that of standard antibiotics against the non-plague Yersinia, except for the processed honey, which was pretty much useless. Both ethanol and water extracts were tested; the ethanol extracts were slightly more effective than the water extracts, but the researchers noted that, for those who cannot tolerate ethanol-based medications, hot-water extracts would be valid treatments for yersinial infection.

For the Key lime, the juice was used at 50% dilution with distilled water; the processed and unprocessed honeys were also diluted at 50%. The Nescafe processed coffee was prepared by diluting 1 gr 1:100% weight/volume, then further diluted to ½ concentration. The other plants were prepared by air-drying, grinding to powder, steeping in a solution of either distilled water or 95% ethanol, with occasional stirring, for 24 hours at ca. 28 C/82.4 F (room temperature where the testing took place); then filtered and concentrated to dryness by evaporation in a 40 C/104 F water bath, and diluted to a 50% concentration.

"Thieves' Vinegar" – There is a persistent legend that groups of thieves who specialized in stealing from houses where people either had just died, or were dying, of plague remained remarkably unaffected; this was attributed to their use of a vinegar infused with herbs typically including (various extant versions of the recipe) rosemary, cloves, citrus, and large amounts of garlic.

An allegedly original recipe from Marseille (said to have been posted on walls during the outbreak) called for 3 pints strong white wine vinegar; a handful of each of wormwood, meadowsweet, wild marjoram, and sage; fifty cloves; two ounces of campanula roots, two ounces of angelica, rosemary and horehound; and three large measures of camphor. This was steeped for fifteen days, strained, and bottled, with the recommendation that it be rubbed repeatedly on hands, ears, and temples when approaching a plague victim. Dubious as this sounds, the antiseptic vinegar wash on the hands alone would probably have helped to reduce transmission to quite a significant degree in comparison with the non-vinegar-washed majority.

As noted, cloves have been shown to be effective against the very similar Y. enterocolitica bacterium, as is the essential oil of oregano (nearly identical to marjoram; basil and coriander essential oils also did well against this bacterium in vitro, but oregano was the most effective) and rosemary and angelica, as well as the garlic not mentioned in the Marsaille recipe, certainly do have potential antimicrobial properties.

I wouldn't choose Thieves' Vinegar over modern methods of personal protection and antibiotic prophylaxis by any means...but if I didn't have anything better, or if I lived in an endemic area and were just generally concerned on a low-level daily basis, I would use a mixture of this general nature. A similar compound could be made from essential oils (3-10% total strength) and used topically. Clove oil can also be used directly in the mouth – it is a common remedy for toothache – and angelica, rosemary, and marjoram essential oils are safe to take orally in tiny amounts (ca. 1-3 drops each/day), although sage essential oil has a high percentage of thujone.

Appendix IV, section V lists several antimicrobial mechanisms of action, together with the corresponding antibiotics and herbs that have the same mechanism as the antibiotics. I wouldn't risk my life deliberately on the chance that I could stumble on the right dose of a herb that worked in vivo in humans for the plague, just based on the fact that in vitro it works like an antibiotic that is known to be effective... but it might at least be a chance. There are some possible methods of flea reduction that would still be available long after the Catastrophe.

None of these suggestions have been objectively tested, and it is unlikely that any of them are in any way comparable to commercial products in terms of efficacy - especially if you live somewhere that doesn't freeze in the winter and therefore is especially prone to high flea populations - but at least they might help to some degree. They include: bowls of water mixed with soap set out at night in rooms where there is a lot of flea activity, replaced nightly (it's like the flea version of flypaper); a household spray compounded of 4 litres or quarts of vinegar, 2 of water, ½ of lemon juice, and ¼ of witch hazel (if you can't get lemon juice or witch hazel, just go with the vinegar); baking soda or salt sprinkled on the floor and left to sit for a day before sweeping (or vacuuming, if your vacuum still works – if you have a flea-harbouring carpet, just sprinkle the stuff in and clean it up as best you can, both are non-toxic anyway); and flea-repelling herbs such as rosemary, pennyroyal, lavender, and spearmint kept with bedding and clothes or ground and sprinkled around the house.

For animals, a 50-50 mixture of cider vinegar and water used for bathing or at least combed through the fur if you have a cat that won't tolerate regular baths is safe and effective. Treatments need to be repeated every week or two: if you have fleas, you will constantly have hatching fleas (it is estimated that for every 2 adult fleas in the house, there are 18 eggs, larvae, and pupae), and even the strongest commercial flea bombs can't penetrate pupal shells. Some recommend a drop of essential oil (geranium, cedarwood, rosemary, thyme; or expressed garlic oil) mixed with a teaspoon (5 ml) of plain vodka on the animal's collar. Whether this is effective or not is completely unknown.

It is probably safe even for cats. Cats are sensitive to essential oils, lacking the liver enzymes for processing many of their constituents (tea tree, nutmeg, and especially pennyroyal essential oils are particularly toxic to them; 4.5 ml of topical pennyroyal oil is quite sufficient to kill a cat, though Tisserand reports dripping a single drop of tea tree oil into an abscess after draining with good results, and notes that dried, crushed pennyroyal leaves, a common flea deterrent, are probably safe). However, diffusion exposure and small doses (no more than 3 drops/dose topically; never used orally) of the vast majority of oils are unlikely to harm them, particularly if there is good ventilation.

Dogs have a better tolerance for essential oils, but are still more sensitive to them than humans; and certain essential oils (cinnamon, citrus, pennyroyal, pine, sweet birch, tea tree, and ylang ylang) are actively toxic to dogs in both topical and oral forms. The garlic in low doses is probably fine for either, though higher doses can be toxic to dogs or cats. The method could also be used quite safely on humans for insect-repelling purposes (whether it would work on humans or not is likewise unknown), as could an essential oil whole-body rub (3% essential oil content at maximum; probably would help to discourage insects to some degree, though if I were somewhere like the Northern woods in summertime, I'd use Deepwoods Off by preference). I have also heard the theory that one reason Jewish communities tended to resist plague better than their Christian neighbours was their considerably better personal hygiene (ritual hand-washing), household hygiene (a complete sweep of the house, with a special eye to removing crumbs of grain products, once a year; and overall focus on cleanliness which discouraged rodent presence as well as lessening the risk of personal bacterial transmission.

Not that it helped in the long run, since their Christian neighbors were keen to make up the differential death rates in their own favour by means of mass murder... The one essential oil which has shown flea-killing capability is California pepper tree (Schinus molle), the source of pink "peppercorns" (not actually even a pepper, but that doesn't matter to cooks in general). Fruit and leaf essential oils were both 100% effective against cat fleas, but did not deal with the eggs; and remember the whole "cat sensitivity to essential oils" thing, especially since this is not a common oil and its effects on cats have not been evaluated at all!

This plant is not especially toxic, so a water extract combed through the fur would probably be relatively safe, but it should not be given to pregnant mammals of any sort, as it has been shown that its close relative the Brazilian pepper tree (Schinus terebinthifolius) can induce foetal bone malformations and possibly other problems. It is likeliest that the above methods will somewhat reduce, but not eradicate, the household flea burden; and that combining methods will be more effective than using a single one. Like most of your post-Catastrophe makeshifts, reduction of risk may be the best you can do, and is better than not doing anything at all.

D) Cholera

Although cholera is the source of several past pandemics, and is still a scourge anywhere that people lack clean water for drinking and washing, it is unlikely to become a pandemic today under current conditions. The fact that it is not fatal if fluid/electrolyte replacement can be carried out at sufficient volume (which an untrained person can do with relative ease in primitive circumstances; see section I) also makes it less of a concern, though mutations are always an option. After the Catastrophe has happened, however, the odds of cholera becoming either a worldwide pandemic or a local epidemic will be much greater. Changes in social circumstances may also present it as an option even before the Catastrophe itself strikes (or if it comes as a combination of social-breakdown factors). The Flint water crisis of 2014 onwards, which included a spike in Legionnaires' disease (87 cases in one year; 14 deaths.

Legionella bacteria are water-borne, and sources of contagion include contaminated air-conditioning systems, showers, or any other source of aspirated water droplets), is an example of how social failures can lead to contaminated and/or insufficient public water supplies. Insufficiency will, of course, be an even bigger problem in all those population centres that were never meant to support large populations, and survive by pumping huge amounts of water in from elsewhere. Wash your hands (with soap or a disinfectant), early and often, following hospital handwashing techniques and protocols. Make sure everyone involved in food collection and preparation does the same. Boil your water for 20 minutes. And stockpile those cheap, simple, and well-keeping packets of rehydration salts. Even if you manage to contract cholera in spite of your other precautions, as long as you keep the rehydration and electrolyte balancing going, you will almost certainly survive.

V. Books of Interest and Sources

Preston, Richard. The Demon in the Freezer. Most of everything you ever wanted to know about smallpox, and possibly a few things you could have lived quite comfortably without knowing. Also covers anthrax, and, of particular interest to the author considering biological warfare as a cause or aspect of the Catastrophe, some important details on the practicalities of how it could happen. Preston, Richard. The Hot Zone. An account of the Ebola Reston outbreak, with considerable discussion of filoviruses in general. Preston has received some criticism for his rather sensationalist and overstated approach in this book, but there is still plenty of good stuff in there, especially if you're looking at a mutated filovirus as an agent for Catastrophe by pandemic.

Preston pretty much made his name as an author of what might best be described as (largely) non-fictional disease horror with The Hot Zone. If the frequency and severity of bubonic plague outbreaks continues to rise as it has been doing since the late nineties, I shan't be surprised to see him doing a similar book on the plague any time now. As well as being an informative author, he's pretty entertaining, so if he does write that plague book, I know I will buy it. One of the best ways to evaluate what might happen now in a time of plague (regardless of the actual pathogen) is to look at what happened in the past.

The Black Death in Europe (various waves from the fourteenth century onwards) was particularly well-chronicled by contemporary writers, not only in terms of the disease itself, but in human responses to it and the mass breakdown of social order and general standards of humanity in many places, particularly cities. Bocaccio's Decameron gives a fairly clear description in this regard (the frame story, set up in "Day the First", is a group of young nobles who have retired from the city in order to escape contagion, or at least distract and enjoy themselves before they die). A translation is available on-line from Project Gutenberg: https://www.gutenberg.org/files/23700/23700-h/23700-h.htm

Other good Black Death texts include:

Gasquet, Frances Aidan. The Black Death of 1348 and 1349 (London: George Bell and Sons, 1908). Focuses strongly on primary sources. Full text available on-line at https://archive.org/stream/blackdeathand00gasqgoog/blackdeathand00gasqgoog_djvu.txt

Horrox, Rosemary. The Black Death (Manchester: Manchester University Press, 1994).

Knighton, Henry. Henry Knighton's Chronicle 1337-1396. G.H. Martin, ed, trans. (Oxford: Clarendon Press). One of the most frequently cited primary sources on the Black Death, written by an eyewitness. Look for it in your local library (or get them to order it), because, like many academic works from Clarendon Press, this edition is grossly overpriced.

If looking for purple pitcher plant: US - https://www.californiacarnivores.com/products/sarracenia-rhizome-bare-root. If you live in the UK or Europe and can't be bothered going bog-hunting for your own purple pitcher plant, look up Triffid Nurseries at http://www.triffidnurseries.co.uk/browse_products_in_cat.php?pt_id=2&cid=2).

Appendix I: Post-Catastrophe Gardening: Fertilizing and Pest Control

I. Fertilizers

Natural fertilizers are best either made into compost or dug into the ground in autumn for a spring planting, particularly those such as manure which need a little while to break down. Plants generally prefer more nitrogen in the growing stage before they flower, and more potassium and phosphate during the flowering/fruiting/seed-development stage.

a) Soil pH: Acid or Alkaline?

To be sure your plant is able to use the nutrients in its soil, pH testing is important; too acidic (low pH) or too alkaline (high pH) will impair absorption. In real life, most garden centres sell pH testing kits. After the Catastrophe, you can only test roughly, as thus:

Take two large spoonfuls of soil from your garden. Pour a spoonful of vinegar on one. Mix the other with water until it is mud, and put a teaspoon of baking soda in. See which, if either, fizzes. If the vinegar fizzes, your soil is alkaline (above pH 7, which only particular plants like). If the baking soda fizzes, your soil is acid (probably in the pH 5-6 range, a bit too low for anything but bog plants such as blueberries and cranberries, or other acid-lovers such as acacia).

b) Vermicomposting and Wormery-Making

If you were wise enough to set up a wormery before the Catastrophe happened, then you are sitting well in regards to excellent fertilizer. Worms break garden trash down into high-nitrogen worm castings, generally considered one of the best fertilizers available. Worm castings may be mixed 1 part to 3-4 parts with other soil for potted plants and bed preparation, used as a top dressing around the roots of established plants, or made into a liquid fertilizer or foliar spray (1 cup/gallon, or 1:16, left to steep for a week). They can be used on their own, or added into other forms of compost tea.

If you didn't think to set up a wormery pre-Catastrophe, be aware that the common earthworm (Lumbricus terrestris) does not thrive in composter/wormeries. Earthworms are solitary deep-burrowers. The worms you want are tiger worms (brandlings, California red earthworm, redworm, red wriggler, usw – Eisenia fetida; or its close relative Eisenia andrei. The difference between the two is relevant only to vermologists, if that's a word). They can readily be obtained from many bait-supply shops and nearly all wormery suppliers. Tiger worms live in rotting compost, manure, and vegetation; they are not really soil-burrowers.

They are native to Europe, but commonly sold in North America, though their living requirements mean that there is little chance of finding feral escapees in your garden there. The other worm that goes by the name "redworm" is Lumbricus rubella (red earthworm). Native to Europe, Britain, and Ireland, but spread worldwide now; this worm is also a good composter, and might be found as a garden invader in North America. The Dendrobaena ("European nightcrawler") is also a popular fishing worm that does well in the compost bin. Dendrobaena can be kept in the same wormery as tiger worms.

They cannot interbreed. Compost worms are generally popular as live-bait because of the same traits that make them good composters. Unlike the common earthworm, they stay close to the surface, are easy to keep happy in bins, and require garden weeds or green trash and manure, which makes them easy to cultivate and sell to fishers. This means that if the Catastrophe hit without warning, but you have a local live-bait shop or pass one on your way to your refuge, you still have a fair chance of stocking your wormery. Compost worms are fast reproducers, particularly the tiger worm. A tiger worm is able to reproduce 6 weeks from hatching; each adult worm (since they're hermaphroditic) can produce 2-3 cocoons per week; each cocoon produces 2-3 wormlings; and cocoons hatch in ca. 28 days.

The figure often quoted is "doubling your worms within 90 days", but in fact, unless there is excesive mortality, tiger worms can multiply faster than that – a lot faster under the right conditions (60-75 F/15-24 C; good airflow in the bin; plenty of space and feeding). Their reproduction does slow when the population becomes too dense, so you can keep multiplying your wormeries. Like aloe vera, they are the survival gift that keeps on giving (with proper care, anyway). Lacking the opportunity for any of the above, your next option is to dig a compost trench or make a heap directly on the ground, and let your native earthworms assist in the composting process. They can deal with meat and dairy products, but those will attract rats and flies, so generally people don't.

A handful of grit every week or so helps their digestion; pulverized egg shells are excellent both for worm health and for adding a bit of calcium, phosphorus, and magnesium to what they eventually produce.

Making the Wormery

To make your own wormery, you require (1) a rubbish bin (plastic or wood) with a good lid; (2) a saw and a drill with a wide drill bit; (3) a heap of old leaves, well-aged non-carnivore manure, or vegetable kitchen scraps (excepting citrus peels, which worms can't digest easily; spicy chilis and the like; and allium – onion, leek, garlic – scraps, which they also dislike); and (4) worms from one of the recommended species. Drill holes around the bottom edge of the bin, here and there on the sides, and in the lid - the more the better - to allow air circulation. Don't worry about escapees; worms may be unlikely to write the next great American novel, but they are not stupid enough to leave a comfortable place with plenty of food.

Cut out a rectangular piece ca. ¼ diameter of the bin and ca. 1/5th its height, starting 1" or so above the bottom. Drill two holes in each vertical side and two corresponding holes in the bin. Hinge and latch as a door, or just tie it back on. This is important, because your good compost collects at the bottom. You don't want to have to dig through all the fresher stuff to get to it.

The worms also tend to hang out more in the upper layers, so collecting from the bottom up means less sifting your compost to recover your precious little wiggly friends. Layer ca. 2" gravel or small stones in the bottom of the bin. Cover with a sheet of heavy perforated plastic. This is for drainage. Make a bed ca. 1' deep out of dead leaves, grass clippings (assuming no pesticides), and similar moist worm-friendly things.

Cardboard (untreated, undyed) is highly thought of by compost worms; get it nice and damp, but not sopping. Chuck in some aged livestock manure if you have it.

Maggot Therapy

The maggots used for medicinal purposes in real life are the larvae of the common green blowfly or bottle fly (Lucilia sericata), or of the bluebottle (Northern blowfly, blue-arsed fly). These are found in rotting meat; scraps may be left out and the maggots collected, breeding them afterwards in an enclosed terrarium with a screen on top to keep the adult fiies from escaping.

Wash maggots in warm soapy water (don't drown them; but they need to be clean) and apply to wound. Maggots of these types eat only dead flesh, secrete effective antibacterial compounds, and debride better than a laser scalpel. They are not painful to the patient, and will cocoon and remove themselves within 3-5 days. In real life maggot therapy is particularly used to treat antibiotic-resistant wound infections and chronic exudative (wet and manky) ulcers, particularly diabetic and venous ulcers of the feet and lower legs. They will not help with dry gangrene; there, all you can do is debride and do your best to restore circulation.

> If maggots are taken out of a wound on a live animal (or person), look at them under 50x magnification or as close as you can get. Screwworms, which eat live flesh, generally have 2 or 3 stripes down their backs.
>
> 1-Screwworms of bot the Old and New Worlds can only live on living flesh; they are not found in carrion, dungheaps, or compost piles. Both types are found in unfortunante animals or people who have sustained a wound, possibly a very small one. They may form large pockets in the flesh even after the primary wound has largely healed; only a small scar with a pore in the centre may be seen on top of a large swelling.
>
> Screwworm infections can easily be mistaken for abcesses or sebaceous cysts. Treatmeant: cover the airhold with a thick layer of petroleum jelly and wait for the worms to emerge in search of air; use turpentine and/or ethanol and/or sulphur ointments to kill the worms; and, if available, cutaneous and/ or oral ivermectin, an anti-parasitic drug used on humans and animals alike often available over-the-counter at farm/pet stores. Avoid the turpentine and sulphur on animals who lick themselves unless you can keep a Cone of Same ("Elizabethan Collar") on the animal.

Obtain your worms. Dig a hole about 6" deep in the bedding and put the worms in. Leave them alone to acclimatize for a few days (the bedding also provides food for them), then start putting in your compostables. Note well: "compostable" bin bags are still plastic.

Not only do they not degrade as well as the package says they do, but even if they did, they would not be good for the worms' digestion. Do not put them in your wormery. Make sure worms do not either freeze in the winter or fry in the summer. Keep in a sheltered spot or outbuilding. When it gets very cold, an old quilt or the like thrown over the wormery will help preserve the natural heat of the composting process, and thus your worms. Do not leave the bin in direct sunlight in summer, even in temperate climates such as Northern Europe. Tiger worms require a temperature between 54-77 F (12-25 F); die when the temperature gets up to around 84-85 F (39 C) or below 32 F (0 C); and go totally dormant under 46 F (8 C). Dendrobaena species are more freeze-resistant; red earthworms (Lumbricius rubella) will die at freezing temperatures, but their cocoons survive freezing.

Insulating the bin in winter (old quilt, straw, or whatever you have) will keep the essential warmth of decomposition in and keep your worms alive and, hopefully, active (they go dormant when chilled; professional wormeries often refrigerate their worms before shipping to keep them dormant and thus minimally traumatized). Preserving them through a very hot summer is more difficult. The bin should be shaded, put in the coolest place possible; and you may wish to open the top for more airflow. Don't spray them down during the day to cool them! That will end up boiling your worms.

Wait until nightfall if more water is needed. The absolute best bin for a wormery is the large rubbish bin which we call a "wheelie bin" here in Ireland... usually between 4 and 5 ft. tall (1-1.5 metres), with two wheels in back. Compost bins get heavy fast, so being able to roll the wormery if you need to is a good thing. Wormery compost generally takes 3-6 months from starting, but once you have started it, you have a steady supply. Compost worm species breed quickly and easily. Compost worms are fast reproducers, particularly the tiger worm.

A tiger worm is able to reproduce 6 weeks from hatching; each adult worm (since they're hermaphroditic) can produce 2-3 cocoons per week; each cocoon produces 2-3 wormlings; and cocoons hatch in ca. 28 days. The figure often quoted is "doubling your worms within 60-90 days", but in fact, unless there is excesive mortality, tiger worms can multiply faster than that – a lot faster under the right conditions (60-75 F/15-24 C; good airflow in the bin; plenty of space and feeding). Their reproduction does slow when the population becomes too dense, so you can keep moving some out every 2-3 months or so when you harvest castings and multiplying your wormeries. Like aloe vera, they are the survival gift that keeps on giving (with proper care, anyway).

Thus you can multiply your wormeries as long as you have bins or can make them from wood and/or wire. A full bin holds about 3 kilos (6.6 lbs) of worms; the ideal starting quantity is 500 grams of worms (slightly over a pound; but one pound even will do fine).MM. About an inch (2.5 cm) of compost material can be added to each bin daily, because that's more or less how fast a colony of worms will eat it; they generally go through about half their weight in a 24-hour period. You probably will not see maggots, but if you do, not to worry! They present no threat to worms and are good little composters in and of themselves. Excessive food will decompose.

This is not a problem to the worms in general – they're quite happy to eat it anyway - but if the wormery is in the wrong place, there might be smell issues. As decomposition produces heat, it could also be a problem in the summer, when your object is to keep your little friends from overheating. On the other hand, it could equally be a boon in the winter, especially if you can't just plug in an electric heater any more and don't want a wormery in your drawing room by the fire.

I usually put in extra food over the winter for just this purpose; with a bit of insulation added, it keeps the worms pretty comfortable. They can eat it down in the spring, and then I keep track of how much they're going through each day in the summer and feed appropriately. Liquid may come out of the drainage holes in the bottom of the wormery. It is basically worm urine. Some people recommend collecting this in a drip tray or similar and diluting at ca. ½ cup per 2 gallons of water for fertilizer up to a maximum of 1 part worm liquid to 10 parts water.

Others observe that it makes a poor fertilizer and may have excessive salt and/ or harmful micro-organism buildup. At least three studies showed positive results from using diluted worm leachate on plants (tomatoes in two, corn in one), though. In any case, a lot of leachate probably indicates that your bin is too wet, which is not good for the worms, and you should throw in some dry cardboard or the like to take up the extra moisture. Worm castings (the stuff you take out of the bottom of the wormery) may be used directly at 1 lb/sq foot, up to 50-50 in a pot, or made into a "tea" in the same manner as plant fertilizer and fish.

They provide nitrogen, phosphorus, and potassium, as well as a range of trace minerals and beneficient bacteria. Another way to harvest castings and separate worms is to put the contents of your bin in a few mounds on a tarp or such in a place that is well-lit, but not in direct sunlight. Worms dislike light and will dig down to avoid it. Scrape off the first few inches of the mounds (until you start seeing worms); give them fifteen minutes or so to get away from the light. Repeat until you are down to a mass of worms in not very much compost. Put the worms and any remaining material back onto a fresh foot-deep (ca. 30 cm) layer of bedding, feed them, and enjoy your lovely worm castings.

c) Non-worm Composting

Compost can be put to break down in the same sort of bin as you were using for a wormery, heaped in a distant corner of the garden, or thrown into a pit. While meat scraps and the like can be composted, you may not want to do that if animals – rats, mice, cats, dogs, foxes, etc. – are a concern, as the rotting meat-smell will attract them. Fish is better composted in a bucket with a tight lid, as described below. A tight and secure lid will generally discourage rodents and the like, but to keep raccoons out requires something more on the order of a time-locked bank safe. Best not to invite them in the first place. Also, if you have bears in your area, you definitely want to take that into consideration when siting and going out to a compost bin that includes animal products. Either that, or consider it an opportunity to shoot over bait (don't do this before the Catastrophe unless it's legal where you live and also the proper season, you have a license, u.s.w.).

Hops

Hops, like cannabis, are dioecious: each plant is either male or female. Male hops plants are only for making seed. Hops can be seedlessly propagated in the same manner as cloning cannabis.

Pollinated seeds are undesirable for brewing, and probably for medicinal usage; hops are wind-pollinated, so breeders should be kept well away from the production field. Hops is a hardy plant, but can be vulnerable to fungal infections; do make that set of insurance seeds every year! Hops is a vine with hanging flower-bunches. It needs trellising.

Hops plants area fast-growing. Unlike cannabis, hops is perennial. Hops are chiefly known as a brewing flavouring/preservative (some anti-microbial effect). They also have sedative effects; the terpene profile is similar to many cannabis strains (humulene is named for its high presence in hops; myrcene and caryophyllene are also strongly present, and linalool is seen).

High phytoestrogens are leading to investigation of possible use in female hormone replacement therapy. They are also being considered as a replacement for antibiotics as growth enhancers in ruminants (Flythe et al.), and as alternative antimicrobials against Gram-positive bacteria in humans (Rozalski et al.). No clinical tests have yet been done.

D) Major Nutrients and Sources

1) General fertilizers

Your main concern with fertilization is the macro-nutrients nitrogen, potassium, and phosphorus (NPK). Commercial fertilizers will have the NPK ratio listed on packaging: z.B., 10-10-10 (a balanced fertilizer); 5-10-15 (a blossoming/fruiting fertilizer). In general, more nitrogen is needed for leaf production and vegetative (pre-flowering) growth; more potassium and phosphorus are needed for flowering and setting fruit.

» **Seaweed** is a valuable source of both macro- and micro-nutrients. It is probably the best single fertilizer and plant-tonic in existence. 8 cups chopped/dried seaweed to 2.5 gallons water, soaked for 3 weeks, can be diluted 1:1 with water and used directly on plants. Be sure that all the salt is out first; it may be best to soak 12 hours to desalinate before putting into fertilizer bucket. Kelp is most commonly used, but any seaweed can be made into fertilizer.

» **Chicken manure** also contains the main three fertilizer elements: nitrogen, phosphorus, and potassium (NPK), high on the nitrogen. It must be composted for 9-12 months, or will burn the plants with excess nitrogen. If using in a wormery, it should be soaked down and left to decompose for two or three weeks, and given to the worms only a shovel-full every two days to a week (depending on whether you have a lot of worms, or are just establishing your colony), due to its concentrated nature.

» **Hops flowers**, even hops that have already been used for brewing, provide one of the best all-around natural fertilizers. In large quantities, they can be dug into the field in autumn; they can be worked into the soil for smaller patches or plants of particular value; or they can be made into a fertilizer tea (warm water or long-steeping method both work) and used for watering. Many organic fertilizers include hops extracts for just this purpose. It is suspected that the close relationship between hops and cannabis means that hops flowers make a particularly good fertilizer for this plant, especially approaching and during flowering, when the phytoestrogens of the hops may help to stimulate cannabis blooming and, if desired, seed production.

2) Nitrogen

1) Animal Products

1a) Manure

This must always be used in aged form, as otherwise it will burn your plants.

» Horse or cow manure – age 6 months-1 yr outside
» Sheep manure – age 3-12 months. Good source of nitrogen and potassium.
» Rabbit manure – 0-3 months. Nitrogen and phosphorus, but levels are low enough not to burn plants (feed more often).
» Poultry manure – at least 9-12 months, preferably longer.
» Bat guano – at least 12 months. Guano from insect-eating bats is higher in nitrogen; from fruit-eating bats, it's higher in phosphorus.
» Human urine – dilute 1:10 to avoid burning plants. Do not use from donor who is ill or taking medications which may be processed out through kidneys.

This does not carry the dangers of using raw night soil: although urine is not sterile, as is often reported, a healthy person's urine is not teeming with potentially dangerous bacteria in the same way untreated faeces are. The cleanest urine is derived from healthy males; between the shorter urethra and external genital configurations, female urine tends to pick up more bacteria on the way out, and women are much more prone to urinary infections in general. In fact, alchemists and chemists back in the day often recommended "the urine of a virgin boy" for many purposes, probably because (1) male urine is usually cleaner than female, and (2) a virgin boy was least likely to have picked up anything nasty in the groinal region.

So that young lad's urine was probably a lot cleaner than anything coming out of a public water source back when, thus better suited to performing chemical processes. Do not use cat or dog manure on food or medicinal plants. Both can carry E. coli; cat manure may also carry Toxoplasma gondii. However, if you are growing hemp purely for fiber and not harvesting the seeds for food from that plant (though you'd have to be a fool to pass them up), composted pet manure may be used. Even if you have a proper composting toilet, do not use human manure on anything you are planning to consume. Only professional high-heat treatment can reliably kill off the pathogens which live in human waste. It is great for lawns, and the process of composting also discourages unsanitary build-up; but it is not suited for food or medicinal crops. And don't let your pigs eat it, either. That's one of the ways that pathogens evolve to pandemic proportions.

b) Other Animal Products

» Fish. May be buried whole or made into a liquid extraction. Cold method: as for making comfrey liquid fertilizer, only with fish; see end of chapter. Make sure lid is tight-fitting and batch is protected from pests including cats and dogs. Don't do it in the house.
» Meat, blood. As for fish. Blood is a particularly good source of nitrogen
» Eggshells. ½ tsp (2.5 gr) powdered eggshell contains 24 mg magnesium, 8 mg potassium, 8.4 mg phosphorus, and 900 mg calcium. It can be worked into the soil or steeped/boiled in water. Feeding pulverized eggshells to your composting worms is highly recommended, as they both use the nutrients themselves and pass them through into the casts, and the grittiness helps their digestion.
» Raider bodies. Bury deep enough that dogs can't dig them up. Dogs will dig them up if possible. There is a reason why the dog or wolf has been seen as a beast of death by all Indo-European cultures for thousands of years, and this is the reason: they can smell rotting meat six feet underground and will try to get to it. Even if you have reason not to respect the raiders' corpses, it isn't sanitary to have chewed human bits scattered about. Let them slowly do the plants some good. You could, of course, chop them up and put them on a hard boil for several hours to sterilize them, which should be fine unless you are so incredibly unlucky as to have been attacked by someone with latent CJD (prions are not killed by heat); the remains may be treated as fish, and the broth used directly, with the same caveats about vermin as other forms of meat.

» But then you'd have to live with the memory in your head, and, while doing interesting things with people and their parts was perfectly normal in Europe until the modern period, it is not a stressor needed by a modern person who has lived through the Catastrophe and maybe already has PTSD as a result.

» Although, if you must display raider body parts to discourage other bad people with bright ideas, the safest way to do it is to boil the bones clean and nail them up. Rotting bodies are impressive and intimidating, but awesomely insanitary, especially if they are anywhere near your water source, groundwater, or garden. Be careful while butchering anything, but especially when dealing with human bodies, as a tiny nick could easily cause a fatal infection.

» Hair, fur, and wool. All good nitrogen sources, easily broken down by natural processes (or compost worms).

» Milk and milk products. Nitrogen and calcium. Be wary of attracting pests; probably best used in a closed wormery/composter.

II B. Plant Products

- Nettles are particularly high in nitrogen and a range of micronutrients (the latter is one reason nettle tea and nettle soup make such excellent spring tonics for people who can't buy fresh fruit and veg at the supermarket year-round). If using for fibre, recycle retting water onto garden.
- Dandelions contain both nitrogen and potassium
- Comfrey has large amounts of nitrogen and protein.
- Simple lawn clippings contain nitrogen
- Hops, as described above, are one of the best all-around fertilizers. They are particularly rich in nitrogen, which should be little surprise given their extensive leafy vine growth.
- Coffee grounds have high nitrogen and moderate potassium. Although they are less acidic than coffee, unless your soil is alkaline, add ¼ tsp baking soda/2 gallons of water when using coffee grounds directly.

3) Potassium

- Wood ash. Best used in acid soil, as it is quite alkaline; do not use on acid-loving plants. Do not incorporate charcoal ash; it has to be pure wood ash. Use sparingly; no more than 1-2 lbs/100 sq foot (.5-1 kg/9.3 sq metres) or an equivalent as a maximum.
- Bananas and banana peels are high-potassium. They may be chopped and put into a bucket of water to soak for 1-2 weeks (they may ferment a bit; that's all right!), or you can finely chop the peels and dig them into the soil. Dilute banana solution 10:1 for watering.
- Seaweed (kelp, common on almost all beaches) is notably high in potassium. Prepare as described at the beginning of the section, or add to your long-brewing manure tea.
- Saltpetre (potassium nitrate) is water-soluble, a good source of potassium, provides some nitrate, and may be used as a pre-soak to encourage seeds, particularly hard-shelled ones, to germinate (not to mention that it can also be used in food preservation and for making black powder and other means of post-Catastrophe home defence, assuming that the laws of nature haven't changed in the Catastrophe). Its NPK ratio is 13-0-44. The ratio for most plants is 1 gram of saltpetre/square foot being watered, or ca. 1 teaspoon for 5 square feet. For larger areas, ca 100 kg/hectare (a hectare is 2.47 acres) may be employed; fruit trees may require 2-3 times that amount. To encourage seeds to germinate, mix ½ tsp (2.5 gr) in 1 pint (454 ml) of warm water; drop the seeds in, and screw the lid on. 4 hours usually suffices for smaller difficult seeds; larger and tougher-shelled seeds may need 24-48 hours.
- Saltpetre is something you probably want to stockpile before the Catastrophe if you're thinking ahead – but it is also something to be very careful about stockpiling, because the other people who might do that in quantity, if they're not professional butchers/meat processors, are amateur bombers. In the UK, it is officially designated as an "explosives precursor" and a Home Office license is required even to buy the stuff now, though it can still be purchased in Ireland, and is readily available at places such as Lowe's and Home Depot in the US.

Happily for the Catastrophe survivor, saltpetre can be produced in low-tech conditions, requiring nothing that is not found on a farm. If the process of purification seems intimidating, note that if simply using directly for fertilizer, the crusted crude saltpetre/rotted manure mixture can be diluted in water and applied without further effort. Purification is necessary for saltpetre that is to be used for food preservation or any other purpose. It is surprising how many authors think that their characters can make black powder by using the crystals from a manure heap or pile of bat guano directly...No, you can't, or at least you won't like the results. The best that will happen is nothing.

4) Phosphorus

Crushed bone is the primary source here. To make your own bone meal, clean all blood and fat off bones. If they are from larger animals, you may want to saw them into smaller pieces at this point (poultry and rabbit bones can easily be managed intact). Bake for 3-4 hours in an oven at ca. 200 C/392 F. This both makes the bones more brittle and kills off pathogens. The bones may then be smashed with a hammer and ground fine with a heavy mortar/pestle or sturdy grinder. The bone meal can be worked into the soil, used as a top-dressing, or soaked in water for 3 days to 2 weeks, either alone or as part of a liquid fertilizer mixture.

Eggshells, Bat guano from fruit-eating bats (usually imported from Africa or South America), Bird guano, particularly seabird, but also pigeon and others.

5) Minerals

- Blackstrap molasses (not sulphated!). A good source of many micronutrients
- Egg shells. Calcium, magnesium, phosphate, potassium, and a bit of nitrogen.
- Match heads. Magnesium.
- Epsom salts: Magnesium (but you might want to save them for human emergencies, as magnesium is a significant anticonvulsant, used in eclampsia among other things). However, magnesium is also a good stimulant for seeds that are slow to germinate. 1 tablespoon (15 gr) Epsom salts or other magnesium source/roughly 1 quart or litre can be used as a drench on soil-sown seeds; seeds can be pre-soaked in it for 4-6 hours, or a bit can be added to dampen paper towels if you are using that method.

6) Root Stimulator

The best natural root stimulator is produced by the growing tips of willows (any willows, including 'pussy willows' or 'goat-willows'. Chop a bunch of tips (green bark, no thicker than a pencil at maximum) and put in hot water. Soak between 3 days and 2 weeks, or until the willow pieces start growing roots. The water can be used to encourage seeds to germinate, to propagate clones, and early on between germination and flowering to aid root development. For the first two purposes, use undiluted; for the third, dilute 10-20:1.

7) Brewing Fertilizers

Quick fertilizer tea: Fill a 5-gallon bucket halfway full of nettles and/or other plants. Add 2 cups urine and ¼ cup of Epsom salts or 1 cup dry seaweed. Fill with water and steep for 3 days. Mix 1:1 with water and apply to plants.

Fermented Emulsion: To begin the process, fill a 55-gallon drum about one-third full with a ratio of 2 parts water and 1 part comfrey, fish waste, and/or manure.

- Allow this mixture to steep for 24 hours.
- After steeping, add more water to the drum until it is completely full.
- Cover loosely and let the drum ferment for several weeks—we usually allow about 3 weeks for fermentation. Be warned that even if comfrey is the only component, it will stink. Don't splash any on your person or clothes, or you may regret it for days.
- To use, apply the emulsion fertilizer to the soil around your plants at a rate of 3 gallons of emulsion liquid for every 100 square feet of yard or garden. Try it on a couple of plants first and give it 2-3 days to make sure the mix is not too strong (leaf tips start looking burnt, hemp leaves may claw downwards).

Manure Tea: Tie up a large shovelful of 6 month+ old manure in a piece of cloth you don't much like (a pillowcase that has seen its last useful days as bedding, for example). Immerse it in a 5-gallon bucket for 2 weeks; the ratio should be ca. 1 part manure to 2 parts water. Dilute 1:1 with water before application. If you don't use the "teabag", your tea will be ready in a week, but you'll have to strain it, which is not pleasant. Used manure can go to the wormery/compost heap.

Crunchy Revenge: Eating Gastropods

Despite the high protein content, humans should never eat raw slugs or snails. They can carry parasites such as rat lungworm, which causes fatal or crippling meningitis in humans.

If you are desperate enough to try these molluscs after the Catastrophe:

1) Snails are safer because their diet is less toxic (especially re fungi).

2) Purge for 3-5 days in a bucket with nothing but cleaned washed greenery. Change the greenery and wash the bucket thoroughly with soap at least once a day to get rid of whatever the animal exuded in slime and faeces.

3) Starve for two days to make sure intestines are clean.

4) Kill in a boiling vinegar-water mixture, remove innards, and cook very, very thoroughly.

Once purged and cooked, snails and slugs are actually safe to eat. Many Internet sites give advice on purging, desliming, and cooking them. Some people claim that deep-fried slugs, particularly banana slugs are nice. They're welcome to them.

There likely will be other options, although eating even raw slugs is probably safer (and less mentally distressing) than eating other humans, since anything a human can catch, another human can probably catch from eating them.

It is also crucial to know that people who are allergic to shellfish, are allergic to land mollusks. Fortunately, Epi-Pens are still of working strength up to 50 months after their expiration date!

II. Pest Control

Get to know your garden and your local pests now, and you won't have avoidable disasters with them after the Catastrophe. Since the first Stone Age woman (probably) realized that if she tossed some seeds on the ground, she'd find more plants she wanted there next year, agricultural peoples have suffered unavoidable disasters, up to and including nation-destroying famines; but at least try to avoid the avoidable ones.

A) Snails and Slugs

Now, the really bad news for the Catastrophe survivor or the real-life gardener who dislikes scattering poison around! According to the Royal Horticultural Society test performed in 2018, none of the "natural" remedies (crushed eggshells, copper tape, etc. – "beer traps" were the only thing they didn't try, and I am here to tell you that those are a waste of effort in a slug-rich area) actually work for slugs and snails.

Short of commercial poisons, which you won't have for long after the Catastrophe, the main solution is to go out to your garden every evening at dawn and dusk and physically remove and squish the slimy little monsters. If you have kids, you can probably get them to do this by putting a small bounty on slugs and snails.

Slugs, for reasons unknown to gods or humans, seem to love the psychoactive alkaloids that deter most pests: they are equally enthusiastic about poppies, deadly nightshade, and mandrakes. My theory is that all the rock stars that OD'd back in the day have been repeatedly reincarnated in my historical display garden and are still looking for their highs. I've probably stepped on Janice Joplin about 100 times by now (though if slugs could still sing or play instruments, I'd just let her and her colleagues have the garden).

Ducks and geese are said to eat slugs, but in some areas, you'd need a lot of ducks, and I'd worry about those big webbed feet doing more damage to my seedlings than the slugs could. I've kept ducks in gardens before, and I can't say that they made any difference to the reported quarter of a million slugs/acre found here in Ireland. Chickens do not eat slugs, though they eat many other kinds of bug; and they can also mess up a bed of seedlings something frightful by scratching.

B) Caterpillars

Every area has its own major pests, some crop-specific (such as tomato hornworms, which feed on all tomato close relatives, including tobacco). Caterpillars are a massive scourge in some areas. The treatment is similar to that of slugs and snails. Make sure you and your kids know which are problems and which are not! Caterpillars of the monarch butterfly, for instance, feed only on milkweed, and are no danger to any of your crops; and are also toxic to humans.

That Gruesome Embodiment Of All That Is Evil, the tomato hornworm, however, does what it says on the tin (goes for any of the nightshades, actually, including potatoes)...and is edible. Again, if you think you might someday be starving after the Catastrophe, find out now which edible caterpillars live in your area and which of your caterpillars are poisonous. If you are absolutely desperate: avoid any that are hairy and/or garishly coloured; they are the likeliest to be toxic. Do be aware that various insects also have a fair chance of setting off seafood allergies, due to their possession of chitin.

C) Rodents

You can bet anything you like that there will be a huge rodent explosion after the Catastrophe. Even if you've never seen a wild rodent where you live, you shall see them in large numbers then. Mice notoriously go for poppy (and all other) seeds and seedlings. I can speak from some experience as to the main post-Catastrophe means of preventing this. I have never had any sort of seeds or seedlings in the garden troubled by mice, in spite of our area's high general rodent level...due to our large crack team of Rodent Control Engineers, who are diligent in their pursuit and destruction of these menaces. The mere presence and scent of a cat, even a house-raised purebred who has never seen a rodent, will go a long, long way towards dissuading the presence of both mice and rats (we once moved our spoilt purebred cats to our new home a month before we left the original place.

We had never seen a rat in the dwelling or grounds; but a week after the cats moved, we had rats running over the bed at night). Rats can be even more devastating to your grain, growing or stored, and small dogs of certain breeds (or mixes including certain breeds) are highly skilled ratters by nature; but for mice, it's cats you want – and you will want them, not just to keep your garden safe, but to protect all your stored food. Traps work too, but are less effective. Be aware: cats hunt for fun, not for food, if given any choice. Cats who are getting food, assuming the humans have any to spare, are healthier and much better and more effective hunters, because they are fit enough to run faster, leap higher, and have the energy to spend whole days finding and playing with their little squeaky toys.

After the Catastrophe, they will be full working members of your survival team, and should be treated as such. And, if you're desperate enough...you know how cats will bring you those special mangled presents as their way of saying, "You're a crap hunter, but I love you anyway, and I will keep feeding you until you learn how to catch your own"? Yeah. That. Cook them carefully, but watch out for the fleas, especially if you live in the West or Southwest of the United States! S.M. Stirling's description of a bubonic plague outbreak following his version of the Catastrophe (Dies the Fire) was not overselling the likelihood of something of that nature happening. Melodi Grundy's The Happy Barn Cat is an excellent guide to caring for your working cat in order to get maximum rodent control from it (and keep the cat happy as well; remember that they also make very good small personal heaters on a cold winter's night if properly cared for and encouraged to be affectionate).

d) Bug Spray

For various micropests such as aphids, spider mites, etc: hot-steep 1 cup dry tobacco leaves/1 gallon (ca. 3.8 litres) of water/1 tablespoon (15 ml) dissolved soap; put in a sprayer and mist the plants. Warning: do not spray this on anything related to tobacco, such as tomatoes or potatoes: there is that risk of spreading tobacco mosaic virus. Cannabis may or may not be vulnerable to this virus, but it is considered possible. Use the soap alone in a spray for these plants; it is not as effective, but much better than nothing.

III. Resources

a) Worms and Wormeries

A few sources for composting worms and wormeries include:

» Canada – Cathy's Crawly Composters (https://www.cathyscomposters.com/products.htm#order)

» Ireland - https://www.originalorganics.ie/tiger-worms-for-wormery.html

» UK - https://yorkshire-worms.co.uk/product-category/compost-worms/, https://www.wormery.co.uk/wormery-accessories.html

» US – https://unclejimswormfarm.com/, http://www.thewormfarm.net/store/products/1284/Worms

» Australia - https://www.kookaburrawormfarms.com.au/compost-worms/, https://www.wormtech.com.au/live-compost-worms/

» Or check your local live-bait shop.

Note that suppliers of live worms generally do not ship outside their own country, on the basis that it is desirable to have the worms arrive alive. Some worm suppliers, especially in places with extreme temperatures, only offer mixtures of worm species. This is quite all right, and may be to your benefit, as the species have different levels of temperature hardiness and will not interfere with each other in the bin (they don't cross-breed, either). As mentioned above, worms are often chilled and shipped dormant.

I got quite a nasty shock with my first package, since I didn't know this; all I knew was that the worms were barely moving if at all when prodded, and, oh gods, are my worms dead or dying? No, the nice seller reassured me that they were just sleeping for transport, and indeed they perked up a treat and set to making more worms within a day or two of being installed into their cozy wormery. Wormeries range from the complex (and expensive) multi-tray models to the homemade version I describe above in the chapter. It just depends on how much time, effort, and resources you have, or maybe how squeamish you are about hand-trawling through the bin to retrieve your precious worms – though squeamishness is unlikely to survive long after the Catastrophe.

b) Medical Maggots

Proper sterilized medical maggots in their nice little bags are available by doctor or veterinary prescription only in the US and UK, although the flies that produce them are free for the catching (assuming you are confident in your identification) and quite happy to carry out their life-cycles in a screened aquarium, raising their young on clean meat provided by humans in a regularly-sterilized environment. Or a survival-minded doctor or vet could simply order some and keep a generational maggot-farm going against times of need. Some people's spouses have been known to react adversely to this suggestion, however. The same spousal lack of enthusiasm has also been observed in regards to keeping a colony of medical leeches.

c) Hops Strains, Seeds, and Rhizomes

Many home-brewers and herbalists today grow their own hops. One or two plants will quite suffice for even a very industrious home-brewer; indeed, if left unattended for two or three years, they will quite suffice for covering most of a large garden. A hops plant can produce vigorously for twenty years or more. Hops come in a variety of strains, suitable to different climates and with different flavour profiles and (presumably) somewhat differing medical effects, although the latter have not been investigated much. "Noble hops" are a class of European strains that have a strong scent but less bitterness, and are characteristic of most German and Czech beers (particularly the "Pilsner" type...since it no longer contains actual Pilsenkraut unless you put it there yourself).

There are four main strains: Tettnanger (from southwestern Germany), mild, slightly spicy, and floral; Saaz (Bohemia, Czechoslovakia), mild, spicy, and earthy; Spalt (southern Germany), mild, slightly spicy, notably strong aroma, an old traditional hop that may be difficult to come by; and Hallertau (Bavaria; strongly floral, slightly earthy, used in Sam Adams Boston lager among many others). The two varieties of hops that are most popular in England and Ireland are English Fuggles and East Kent Golding. Many British and Irish brewers consider the latter to be the single finest hops variety in existence (it's the variety I grow, myself). Like the noble hops, these are strongly aromatic and relatively less bitter. The British Hops Association website offers a much longer, detailed list of the varieties usually grown and available in Britain: https://www.britishhops.org.uk/varieties/.

British hops varieties have been bred for resistance to the scourge of verticillium wilt (a soil-borne disease). There is at least one "dwarf hops" variety, Prima Donna. This is bred to grow to no more than 2-3 metres (6.5 – 9.8 ft.), and can be planted in hedgerows or grown on a trellis or over an arch as usual. It may be more suitable for the smaller garden unless you enjoy pruning a lot, and has the advantage of easier harvest with less training effort when grown in multiples. Seeds can be difficult to germinate. They require autumn planting or scarification (put them in a box with a piece of medium sandpaper and shake a bit) and 3-4 weeks in wet sand in the refrigerator followed by 1-2 months in soil at ca. 68 F/20C. Most growers start with rhizomes (live root sections).

Seeds of specific varieties are also difficult to find. Even notable sources of interesting seeds such as Seedman (not Seedsman, they're the cannabis place!) only offer a generic "hops seeds". The eBay store Exotic Garden (search "Exotic Garden eBay Store" to find a link) does have a wide selection of varietal seeds, but only seems to sell on eBay. Rhizomes (dormant bare-roots, sold between November and March; optimum if you must mail-order) are more generally available. A good selection of US varieties can be found at buyhoprhizomes.com; Burpee also carries a few US hops varieties as plants or bare roots (https://www.burpee.com/fruit/hops/). The Thyme Garden is mostly US varieties, but includes some English varieties and all four of the German noble hops (https://www.thymegarden.com/rhizomes).

How to Neuter a Male Animal

In real life, get the vet to do it – they can do it a lot more safely and with less pain. After the Catastrophe, for a cat or dog (at least 6 months old – only vets should neuter earlier): anesthetize – general if you have someone experienced, local otherwise. Lidocaine is used in cats and dogs. The maximum cat dose is 1-2.5 mg/kg or 0.5-1.25 mg/lb; for a dog, 1-5 mg/kg or .5-2.5 mg/lb. While putting the cat's front end into an old boot may be traditional, doing a purrito wrap with a heavy towel (looks like a kitty burrito, keeps the cat effectively immobilized) and getting someone else to hold him is greatly preferable.

With local anaesthetic, the animal is first injected in each testicle, then subcutaneously around the sac in three or four individual jabs (at least half the total dose goes into the testicles; the rest is divided evenly around the sac). When the anaesthetic has taken effect (give it ten minutes and flick the sac or prod gently with a sterile needletip), cut a short slit in the sac. Pop each testicle out; tie the blood vessels and spermatic duct to prevent bleeding; sever the vas deferens; suture the incision.

Rubber band castration (affixing a tight rubber band around the scrotal sac until the whole thing withers and falls off) does not work on cats or dogs, because they can chew their genital region, and their testicles don't hang down like larger livestock's do, which means banding wouldn't work anyway. It works a treat on goats, sheep, cattle, pigs, horses, etc., and is ideally done ca. 1-2 days old. If possible, use the ones made for the purpose (Elastrator), which are particularly heavy-duty, smaller than you'd expect, and come with an application tool to get them over the testicles.

Caponizing requires tying the young rooster's wings and legs to weights; pulling the skin back tightly across his ribcage; making a slit into the body cavity between the lowest two ribs on each side; spreading the ribs; and scooping out the organ (an elongated, pale yellow, bean-shaped item). The incision is not sutured; anaesthetics and antibiotics are not required. There will be losses: this is very invasive surgery and the testes are right next to major blood vessels. Practice on a few dead roosters first.

On the other side of the Atlantic, Willingham Nurseries has an excellent selection of rhizomes and plants including the noble hops and a wide range of English and North American varieties, and they will ship outside the UK (http://www.willingham-nurseries.co.uk/hop3.html), though they strongly recommend ordering rhizomes during the November-March period for longer-distance shipping. Essentially Hops also has a fine selection, and will ship rhizomes outside the UK or EU (https://www.essentiallyhops.co.uk/acatalog/Bare-Root-Hop-Plants.html).

D) CATS

If you live in the country, excellent hunting cats may be readily and freely obtained from your neighbours. Otherwise, your local rescue centres are the best bet. The ideal is to get a well-tempered, but experienced, pregnant female so that she can teach her kittens, while you raise them to be healthy and affectionate little personal heaters as well as rodent control experts.

Mama Cat should be spayed as soon as she has weaned her babies (earlier runs the risk of death by milk fever); if you can, keep her indoors until then to avoid further pregnancies. Should she get pregnant while nursing – and cats can get pregnant even in mid-birthing – an early spay/termination is no risk to her and the potential kittens are not developed enough to be guilty about.

The babies should be spayed/neutered as soon as they are old enough, generally around 4 or 5 months at the vet's office, or 6 months for males at home if you no longer have a vet after the Catastrophe. In those circumstances, you may well be kind of hosed on the spaying thing: to spay a cat or dog requires a vet or surgeon and feline-appropriate anaesthetics and someone who knows how to use them. But at least you can neuter the males without significant risk to their lives – and you want to. Only one tom is needed for a rotating supply of barn cats, even in a high-mortality area.

If you have no full tom on your farm, Freyja and Bast will reliably provide one or many when a queen comes into season (you may wish to keep a supply of old boots on hand at night). It is unknown whether human pregnancy-discouraging herbs such as wild carrot seeds will do anything for female cats, but it might be worth a try after the Catastrophe. Cats such as the Norwegian Forest Cat and Maine Coon are excellent survival breeds, but they do not come with more hunting skills built in than the average moggy, except for the Forest Cat's inclination to hunt cooperatively. They have to learn from other cats just as any feline does. A rescued barn cat who knows what she's doing already and can teach a few kittens is a better choice, particularly as her maternal instincts are likely to incline her to teach any other young cats that come her way. Further information on the cultivation of barn cats, as mentioned above, can be found in Melodi Grundy's book, The Happy Barn Cat (insert ordering link here when available if publishing schedule permits).

IV. References

Flythe MD, Kagan IA, Wang Y, Narvaez N. Hops (Humulus lupulus L.) Bitter Acids: Modulation of Rumen Fermentation and Potential As an Alternative Growth Promoter. Front Vet. Sci. 2017; 4:131.

Grundy, Melodi. The Happy Barn Cat. (The Three Little Sisters April 17, 2019). https://www.the3littlesisters.com/book/barncat/. ISBN-13: 978-1989033166

Le Conte, Joseph. "Instructions for the Manufacture of Saltpetre" (Columbia: Charles C. Pelham, 1862). https://docsouth.unc.edu/imls/lecontesalt/leconte.html

Rozalski M., Micota B, Sandowska B, Stochmal A, Jedrejek D, Wieckowska-Szakiel M, Rozalska B. Antiadherent and Antibiofilm Activity of Humulus lupulus L. Derived Products: New Pharmacological Properties. Biomed Research International. 2013, Article ID 101089, 7 pp. http://dx.doi.org/10.1155/2013/101089

An illustrated guide to caponizing can be found at http://www.afn.org/~poultry/capon.htm; actual photos and discussion at https://www.backyardchickens.com/threads/how-to-caponize-a-rooster-warning-graphic-pics.210041/. There are also many YouTube videos, including: https://www.youtube.com/watch?v=pSUx5d31BKk and https://www.youtube.com/watch?v=WOhfBWZtiuU. Caponizing makes roosters fatter, less gamy-tasting, and milder-tempered, all of which are generally desirable for any roosters who are not intended for breeding and hen-protection.

Appendix II: Weights and Measurements

Length:
1 cm = 0.394 inches
1 inch = 2.54 cm.
1 metre = 39.4 inches

Weight:
1 oz = 28.34 gr
1 lb = 454 gr
1 kilogram (1000 gr) = 2.2 pounds

Volume to weight (water; note that other liquids, and even more, dry substances, may vary considerably! An ounce of dried plant leaf will usually take up quite a bit more than ¼ cup volume; and its final volume can depend on whether it was powdered or used whole, how finely it was powdered, u.s.w.)

1 ml = 1 g
¼ tsp = 1.25 ml
1 tsp = 5 ml
1 TB = 15 ml
1 cup = 237 ml
1 litre = 1000 ml

Drops to millilitres: 20 drops is normally considered to = 1 millilitre.

Apothecary measurements: If using a calculation programme (if you have such a thing available after the Catastrophe), be aware that the apothecary measurements are different from standard measurements of the same name. 1 apothecary drachm, for instance, is 3.89 g; but one standard drachm is 1.77 g; and one apothecary ounce is nearly 3 g heavier than a standard ounce.

- 1 lb divided into 12 oz
- 1 apothecary oz = 8 drachms
- 1 drachm = 3 scruples
- 1 scruple = 20 grains.
- 1 apothecary oz = 31.1 g (vs the standard 28.34 g). Also called "fluid oz." Ca. 1/5 cup
- 1 apothecary drachm = 3.89 g. One fluid drachm = 3.89 ml or just over ¾ tsp.
- 1 scruple = 1.296 g. One fluid scruple = 1.296 ml or just over ¼ tsp (1.25 ml)
- 1 grain = 65 mg. Fluid equivalent = 1 minim/0.065 ml

These are the measurements Mrs. Grieves, and most other authors on herbalism (as well as many medical books) up to the middle of the 20th century, use. Learn them, because after the Catastrophe, you won't be able to get a handy conversion programme on the Internet! Apothecary Weight set at Health Care Logistics – ½ grain to 5 oz. weights. If using a professional weight set, weigh the weights to make sure that they correspond to the above values. http://shop.gohcl.com/default.aspx?page=item+detail&itemcode=4027

Appendix III: Herbal Fertility Reduction (and sexual health)

This is a matter which will be of considerable concern after the Catastrophe, and is of no little concern now, although there are many fairly good and some very effective methods currently available. Fortunately for the author, the element of chance is such that pregnancy can occur or be avoided as necessary for the plot-line. But that avoidance still has to be presented in a plausible manner, whether in a medical sense or whether (as in, for instance, most religious stories, including the Old and New Testaments), a narrative context is presented in which "miracles" may be considered believable.

The Internet is full of sites purporting to teach women how to perform their own contraception and/or abortions with herbs, not least as a response to the imminent or current suppression of women's right to control their own bodies and reproduction. Many of these sites present information that is inaccurate; would be ineffective; or is actively dangerous...and you, the author, can be sure that some of your readers will recognise these faults if they appear in your work. If you, for instance, have a character inducing an abortion by inserting sprigs of fresh parsley, or slugging down pennyroyal and tansy oil without untowards consequences, the suspension of disbelief will come crashing down, down, down! And your book may go crashing against the wall.

I use the term "fertility reduction" rather than "contraception", because there are no herbal treatments that have proven beyond very small studies indeed to be at least 90% reliable at preventing pregnancy (wild carrot seed is the closest to demonstrating efficacy comparable to most pharmaceutical methods). This is also true in practice for many modern "contraceptives": barrier control (condoms), for instance, are hypothetically 98% effective, but in practice, due to user error and other factors (age-related degradation, accidental damage), are no better than 82%. The only forms that are at least 99% effective are those which do not allow for user error: implants, intra-uterine systems, and intra-uterine devices.

Even injections, which have to be repeated every 8-12 weeks, do not approach better than 94% in practice (6 of 100 women using them will become pregnant in the course of a year); most hypothetically 99+% effective methods are no better than 91-92% effective in practice. "Natural family planning" (monitoring a woman's fertile periods via menstrual timing, temperature fluctuations, and cervical mucus secretions) is also 99% effective in theory, but no better than 76% effective in practice, comparable to diaphragms and caps (92-96% effective with perfect use, 71-88% effective in reality). In real life – don't try any of the no-other-alternative post-Catastrophe possibilities suggested here if you can possibly avoid it, except perhaps contraceptive wild carrot/carrot seed, which seems to have good efficacy and an excellent safety profile. Menstrual extraction is still practiced occasionally, but it is usually done by qualified medical personnel in a setting designed for relatively invasive but low-risk procedures, such as the GP office. Go where you can be taken care of by qualified medical personnel, if you have any option to do so. In fact, this advice applies to the majority of this book.

I. Basics of Fertility Reduction and Control

Fertility reduction and control has been a human concern since we realized that we (1) had the capability to control our reproduction to some degree, and (2) had a significant need to do so. Nursing reduces fertility, which is a major reason why many traditional hunter-gatherer societies nursed until the age of four, and there were often taboos or social restraints against having sex with a nursing woman. Among the Apache, for instance, it was noted that, "A man who is so importunate as to demand connection with his wife too soon is subject to sharp criticism and is said to have acted 'against' his growing child.

'There is a man whose child is not walking yet and his wife is pregnant. The Indians think he is no good. We are ashamed to have a second child on the way before the first is weaned." Nonetheless, I have personally seen a patient who was not only nursing after a recent birth, but on the micro-Pill...and still managed to conceive (and another who was using condoms, spermicidal cream, and then the morning-after pill; whose daughter, conceived at that time, is now a sturdy and healthy child). Nothing short of never having conception-type sex or an absence of the necessary organs is 100% effective.

In a post-Catastrophe world, a practice that is a good idea now (keeping track of the days of one's menstrual cycle), will become a great deal more important, both in regards to becoming pregnant when that is desired, and not becoming pregnant when it isn't. While the rhythm method alone is notoriously ineffective, as mentioned above, tracking one's cycle plus temperature and cervical mucus checks is moderately effective. Responsible parents or adult caregivers will teach this to their daughters and encourage them to get into the habit of tracking their cycles. Whether the object is to conceive, or not to conceive, this is something that a woman probably wants to know now, and will absolutely need to know after the Catastrophe.

It may only be 76% effective in practice (or lower if one is a bit lax about keeping track), and certainty will require additional methods of fertility reduction if you definitely don't want to become pregnant; but it will make a very significant difference, and does not require anything but a working thermometer. A woman's body temperature rises at the point of ovulation, and remains higher until just before the point of menstruation, when it drops. To use this as a guide, it is important to track the changes daily for several months in order to establish a reference. Temperature needs to be taken in the morning before getting out of bed; even getting up to urinate will affect it. Use the same thermometer and take your temperature at the same time every morning, after having had ca. 3-4 hours sleep (staying up all night will also interfere with accurate results).

Cervical mucus (found by inserting a well-washed finger as deeply into the vagina as possible; you may or may not be able to actually touch your cervix, but the closer to it you can get your sample, the better. Observe visually, then press finger and thumb together, roll slightly to judge consistency, and pull them slowly apart to check for the stretchiness of ovulation) alters noticeably during the various phases of the menstrual cycle. Dry, sticky mucus = not ovulating. The mucus becomes more creamy as ovulation approaches; wet and watery just before ovulation. At the time of ovulation, it is said to resemble a raw egg white, very wet, and stretchy; this is considered "fertile mucus".

After ovulation, it becomes sticky and thick, though some women experience the "fertile mucus" phase for a day or two before their periods, for reasons unknown; and multiple brief incidences of "fertile mucus" may suggest an issue such as polycystic ovarian syndrome and interfere with the use of cervical mucus quality as a guide to ovulation. The reason for the alterations in cervical mucus is that hormonal changes alter mucus composition either to keep sperm out of the uterus as best as possible (non-fertile times), or to help transport it up the uterus and towards the ovaries (fertile period). Mark your cervical mucus status on the chart with your body temperature readings. Remember that, although rare, it is quite possible to become pregnant while menstruating. Changes in circumstance can throw off the ovulation cycle even of a woman who is normally quite regular.

If you are not willing to become pregnant, or at least to take the chance and let your god, goddess, or fate and chance decide, always use the fertility-control means available to you, every time. Some women experience, or are conscious of, a phenomenon called Mittelschmertz ("middle-pain"): a single sharp pain at the time of ovulating. Women who reliably get this pang, and who have tracked it along with the rest of their menstrual chart, may well be able to exert an enhanced control over conception timing by means of chart and cervical mucus tracking. After the Catastrophe, as is usual among agricultural peoples, more children will be wanted than is the case now.

Children swiftly become useful in an agricultural setting, and without modern medicine, sadly, infant and child mortality rates tend to be significantly higher. Nonetheless, pregnancy and childbirth are very physically stressful – are, along with smoking, the greatest risk factor for almost every major health problem that exists. When I was in medical school, one of my fellow students was quite pregnant and another had a pregnant wife, and I remember everyone in the room cringing every time the pregnancy-increased risks and dangers of most conditions were brought up.

Avoiding pregnancy before the age of sixteen at the earliest to twenty (there is no hard and fast rule; some women mature earlier than others, but usually risks rise significantly below the age of sixteen, and eighteen to twenty is considered optimal for most women), and spacing pregnancies by at least two years between one birth and the next conception in fully mature women, is strongly to be recommended if at all possible. In harsher circumstances where the food supply is more irregular, four years is preferable, which is why it is the common nursing (and often hence taboo or at least socially-discouraged conceptive sex) period for many hunter-gatherer peoples. There are four points at which herbs, or any medications, can work to discourage conception.

1) Preventing ovulation
2) Preventing fertilization
3) Preventing implantation
4) Early termination

Medications discouraging or potentially discouraging ovulation include poppy (Papaver somniferum) latex, turmeric (Cucurma longa; may suppress GnRH, or gonadotrophin releasing hormone, which stimulates the hormones that cause ova to mature and be released), high levels of glucocorticoid drugs (or endogenous glucocorticoids, as seen in Cushing's syndrome), and hormonal birth control methods (some of which also thicken cervical mucus, which discourages fertilization by providing a partial barrier to sperm). The "morning-after pill" RU-486 (mifepristone) is an anti-progestogen and prevents ovulation, as well as other effects.

Herbs containing high amounts of phytoestrogens or oestrogenic precursors such as hops and black cohosh have not been fully studied in this regard. The phytoestrogen coumestrol has been observed to reduce fertility in ewes, and soy products in cheetahs. It is currently recommended not to use these herbs or plants (possibly including large amounts of soy products) while taking hormonal birth control medications, as they may interfere with the chemically-regulated anti-conception hormonal balance produced by these medications. They may also be dangerous in pregnancy, as there is also some evidence leading to a strong suspicion that they could cause foetal developmental abnormalities, particularly in regards to hormone balances and sex hormone-regulated development.

Methods discouraging fertilization include progesterone (thickens cervical mucus, helping to form a sort of barrier at the cervical opening) and herbs that reduce sperm production, density, and/or motility such as tulsi ("holy basil", Ocimum tenuiflorum); curcumin, from turmeric, also suppresses sperm motility. Barrier contraceptives, including everything from condoms to IUDs, also fall into this category. Medications discouraging implantation include onion (Allium cepa), COX inhibitors such as indomethacin and celecoxib, unripe papaya (blocks progesterone synthesis), and possibly levonorgestrel.

Medications causing early termination include, though are by no means limited to, RU-486 (the "morning-after" pill) plus a prostaglandin analogue, tansy, pennyroyal, and methotrexate (often used to terminate an ectopic pregnancy and/or eliminate remaining foetal cells before they can become metastatic or foci for infection). Often birth control herbs in this category work by inducing oxytocin, which causes uterine contractions and content expulsion. The effectiveness of herbal contraceptives of this type is hard to judge. Not only are attempts seldom reported unless something goes disastrously wrong, but unless a woman has actually had an early pregnancy test – assuming that the result was a true positive – it is impossible to be sure whether the herbal treatment caused termination, or whether her cycle was simply a little irregular. In addition, it is estimated that 50-75% of conceptions may end naturally before a pregnancy test is utilized to detect their presence (usually within the first two weeks; the menses occur on time, and the pregnancy was never known to have happened).

Pregnancy tests vary by sensitivity; some might be able to pick up the hormone tested for (hCG) as early as eight days after conception, when it first appears in the bloodstream; but women who test negative at that time may test positive later in their cycle. User error, misrecollection of date of last menses/misestimation of likely fertilization time, etc., all play a part in the variability of these tests. The percentage most usually quoted for loss after clinical diagnosis (most commonly done in the 4-6 week period...after a period is late enough for pregnancy to be suspected) is 10-15%. This is why herbs used for contraception via early termination are generally called "emmenagogues" (menstrual stimulants). Short of a very accurate, very early pregnancy test, which have only been available comparatively recently, there is no way to tell if a woman was pregnant at all, let alone whether she suffered a natural very early loss...or induced it. Historically, there have been no legal, social, or religious stigma attached to bringing down a period at the general time when it is due.

Sensitivity, Specificity, False and True Positives and Negatives

The sensitivity of a test describes its ability to pick up the presence of whatever is being tested for. The specificity of a test describes its ability to pick up only the presence of what is being tested for.

Thus, a test with a sensitivity of 90% and a specificity of 60% will produce:

90% of true positives, 10% false negatives. False negatives are the failure to pick up the presence of the tested subject when it is actually present.

60% of true negatives; 40% false positives. 40% of tests that score positive will declare the presence of the tested subject when it is actually absent.

If this were a pregnancy test, that would mean that 10% of women who received a negative were actually pregnant; 40% of women who received a positive were actually not pregnant.

Most pregnancy tests available today claim 99% accuracy, but that is in laboratory conditions with trained testers. Home tests may vary considerably.

II. The Rabbit Test

For pregnancy testing after the Catastrophe, almost anyone with a little basic knowledge and access to rabbits can perform the traditional "rabbit test". This may be diagnostic as early as four to six weeks after conception, though is probably more accurate from six weeks onwards (just about the end of the period when a herbal or medical termination is likely to be effective, and pushing the absolute outer limit for menstrual evacuation, as described below).

Mice can also be used, but rabbits were preferred because the ovarian changes are easily visible to the naked eye (mice often required microscopy); the test was a day quicker; and the rabbit can be anaesthetized and opened, and if the test is negative, it can be closed up and re-used for another test.

The woman's first morning urine, collected in the middle of the flow (0.2-0.4 cc/dose for mice, injected subcutaneously 6 times over 48 hours; 10 cc for rabbits, injected into the ear vein once) was injected into the immature female rodent. Mice were euthanized 96 hours after the first injection; rabbits were examined 48 hours after the single injection.

The ovaries were examined. A pregnant woman's urine would cause the rodent ovaries to enlarge and its follicles to mature. From a pale, firm, bean-shaped organ about 1 cm long, the pregnant rabbit ovary becomes pink, softly swollen with fluid, and lumpy with what may look like tiny cysts (the follicles), some dark with haemorrhage; and some tiny yellow spots (the corpus luteum enlargement typical of pregnancy).

"The bunny died" comes from the common belief that the rabbit died naturally if the woman was pregnant. Actually, the rabbit was usually killed by the testers if the test was positive, since it could not be re-used as it could if the test was negative (and if a supply of rabbits was readily available, it was considerably easier to just kill and dissect the rabbit in any case). If the rabbit is simply killed and dissected, the urine injection does not render it unfit to eat, an important thing to know after the Catastrophe if you're raising rabbits mainly for food. It is, of course, crucial to make sure that rabbits whose future lies in pregnancy testing are separated from their brothers before three months of age.

III. A Selection of Emmenagoguic and Abortifacient Herbs

Some of the herbs used for contraception, particularly those causing early termination, are significantly toxic: multiple deaths have been reported from several of them. Mrs. Grieve gives dosages according to the British pharmacopeia of her era; these should be considered with the usual warnings about variable strength of plants from place to place and year to year, and also the notation that the dosages and usage she knew were based on empirical evidence in an era with rather lower concerns about safety than ours, not on the exhaustive large-scale, double-blinded clinical studies and more rigorous safety protocols we use now. Some of the herbs and other things widely used, and promoted, for fertility control – or warned against using in pregnancy – are also what can most politely be described as myths. I mention a couple of the most widespread ones here, and the evidence, or lack thereof, as well. It should be noted that one of the largest difficulties in obtaining reliable information on herbal effects, outside of the current shortage of scientific evaluation, is the tendency for almost any published statement to spread by repetition.

One person prints a piece of information that is inaccurate; another references them; and in a short while, one will find a pile of sources appearing to support the assertion made by a single problematic original. When it comes to herbal information and seeking documentation, quantity does not "have a quality all its own"! Angelica root (Angelica archangelica) acts by inducing uterine contractions, which may cause the early expulsion of the uterine lining and developing foetus. It is most effective in the first four weeks of pregnancy. Oral use of angelica root is relatively safe in general, although it may increase the sensitivity of skin to sunlight, leading to burning and blistering. Photosensitivity is generally focused on as the primary danger of taking this herb, and direct sunlight or UV lamps should be avoided when one is using it, especially when the dilute essential oil is used topically.

Although some sources list fresh angelica root as a deadly poison, upon investigation, this was found to stem from a single historical report of Native American use repeated in more recent herbals, and the reporter may well have confused it with a deadly look-alike such as one of the water hemlocks (the Cicuta species), which closely resemble the angelicas and grow in the same habitat, often side-by-side with angelica – or the users themselves, from tragic experience, may not have been sure of the distinction. The aerial parts and root have been used in Europe for literally thousands of years, and there have been no recorded European instances of angelica poisoning, nor any folk knowledge or recent analyses of the plant suggesting that the fresh root might be unsafe, though it is most often used dried. There have been no poisoning cases reported from any of the American species, nor have any significant toxins been identified in them. In fact, it can be stated quite confidently that no one, anywhere, has ever been poisoned by an accurately-identified fresh angelica root, although people most certainly have been poisoned by mistaking a Cicuta or poison hemlock (Conium maculatum) for an Angelica.

Which is why one should not be casual about gathering wild angelica. Angelica may raise blood sugar levels, and is generally avoided in diabetes. It also contains coumarins, which inhibit clotting; it should not be used with warfarin or other anticoagulants without medical supervision. Angelica archangelica essential oil has been shown to have significant antimicrobial action against Clostridium difficile, E. faecalis, and Candida albicans, among others, although oral administration is unlikely to be effective in the former cases (as with most antibiotics, which are ineffective against C. difficile, the GI system would probably absorb the substance before it could reach the region where the bacteria live), and using it for vaginal yeast infections would require dilution, probably down at least as low as 3%, to prevent damage to the delicate mucosa.

For emmenagoguic purposes, Mrs Grieve recommends pouring a pint of boiling water on an ounce of the bruised (which would, in fact, be fresh) root, and administering 2 tablespoons three or four times a day, or else 10-30 grains (650-1950 mg) of the powdered (dry) root given with the same timing (p. 38). Kress suggests ¼ cup herb to 1 quart water, made into a tea. The dosage recommended by the American Botanical Council for general purposes is 4.5 g of cut dried root or up to 4 grams simmered in 150 ml boiling water, drunk warm several times a day before meals.

The acute oral LD50 of angelica root oil in rats is 1.116 g/kg; for angelica seed oil, it is >5 g/kg. 5-10 mg/kg may be a safe oral dose of the root oil, but no studies have been done in humans, and cases of poisoning have been reported from high doses. It is probably better to use decoctions of the whole herb, though, absent allergy, a normal oral dose of 1-3 drops (20 drops in 1 ml) is also probably safe. Topical applications of the essential oil are relatively safe; it should be diluted to ca. 5%, and the skin must not be exposed to sunlight afterwards. However, the efficacy of absorption and total dosage levels in topical use are not known.

Like many herbal treatments, topical angelica oil is in that gray area of, “probably best not used in a desired pregnancy at all, just to be sure; but no way to guarantee that using it will prevent or halt pregnancy”.

Angelica is difficult to start from storebought seed unless it is extremely fresh, but self-seeds readily: once you have obtained a plant and it has seeded, you will have all the angelica you want and then some. It is a biennial, sometimes a triennial; in the second year (usually) it very rapidly sends up a tall stalk with a large ball-like flower-head sometime between the end of April and mid-June, depending on your climate (in full flower in Ireland in mid-May). Roots are generally harvested in autumn of the first year, when they are at their strongest; after flowering, they are exhausted. Angelica prefers a rich, moist soil and a partially shaded situation. It grows wild throughout Northern Europe, and the young shoots were a staple spring vegetable in Iceland and Norway.

Angelica root, Chinese, best-known as Dong Quai (Angelica sinensis) is a close relative of the European angelica, and is more often used for treating menopausal symptoms and other difficulties related to female hormones, though no direct comparisons have been done; this may or may not simply be a matter of Chinese vs Western medical traditions. Dong quai has been alleged to be more likely to exacerbate bleeding than European angelica. I could find no direct experimental comparisons or comparisons of tested coumarin levels; even the EMEA (European Medicines Agency) analysis covering different angelica species did not give a quantitative report on many of the coumarins that were found present in Angelica archangelica, and other reports on the individual species' coumarin contents vary wildly, probably due to the normal active-constituent variation of any whole-herb medicine which has not been pharmacologically tested and standardized.

Dong Quai has been shown to contain coumarins on several tests, which means that it is potentially dangerous in combination with warfarin, and the increased bleeding risk presents the major possible hazard with any of the angelicas in the case of a difficult termination or if subsequent surgical intervention is required for success. Because of its significance in Chinese medicine, Dong Quai appears to have been more thoroughly studied in recent times than its European cousin, and compounds found in it potentially have a wide range of beneficial effects (anti-inflammatory; neuroprotective; anti-hepatotoxic; anti-cardiovascular disease; immunostimulatory; anti-cancer). Growing dong quai is very similar to growing Angelica archangelica, except that the roots take three years to reach maturity. It is tolerant of both full sun and woodland conditions, but partial shade is probably ideal.

Anise (Pimpinella anisum). The major constituent of anise essential oil is trans-anethole. In rats at high doses (50-80 mg/kg), trans-anethole has shown dose-dependent implantation prevention, abortifacient, and anti-fertility effects in rats. The maximum safe dosage for humans is noted to be 2 mg/kg. 1-5 ml aniseed oil has been observed to cause nausea, vomiting, seizures, and pulmonary oedema. 1 ml = 1 gram = 1000 mg/kg, or the rat-effective dose of 50 mg/kg for a 20-kg person, who is unlikely to be pregnant in the first place; and anise essential oil is not 100% composed of trans-anethole. The safe daily oral maximum cited by Tisserand and Young is 70 mg (0.07 ml)/day. The likely-effective dose, in short, would seem to be equal to or greater than the dosage causing significant toxicity.

Asafoetida (Ferula foetida) resin is best-known as one of those ethnic spices that you kind of have to grow up eating to appreciate. While it is popular in Indian food, Westerners often find the scent objectionable, maybe very objectionable, as suggested by the appetizing folk names such as "devil's dung". It is also one of the folk-medicine emmenagogues/abortifacients that modern research is proving to be effective for the traditional purposes. In rats, the ethanolic extract of asafoetida resin from days 1-7 of pregnancy (the equivalent of up to 84 days of human pregnancy – rat speed of gestation is 12x human speed), caused "pregnancy failure" in 65-85% of rats, apparently due to interference with the enzymes necessary to energy metabolism in the rat uterus.

Another rat study, using doses of 400 mg/kg for 10 days on post-coital rats, showed prevention of pregnancy in 80%; lower doses also reduced implantation significantly. Asafoetida also interferes with foetal haemoglobin, and should not be given to infants. While generally considered safe (except for pregnant women who want to stay pregnant, infants, and breast-feeding women, for whom it is strongly disrecommended), asafoetida has mild anti-coagulant activity (may increase bleeding or potentiate anticoagulant medication); in high doses, there is a risk of triggering seizures in vulnerable persons even at low dosage; and it can be irritating to the stomach lining. 300-1000 mg of resin/day is the general medicinal dosage, and considered sufficient to significantly increase the risk of miscarriage in a safe manner.

Asafoetida is a giant fennel, used by Romans back in the day as a substitute for the culinary/birth control giant fennel (probably) silphium, though it was considered inferior. It can grow in most temperate climates; the foliage is very like parsley, but the plant can get 6-10' (roughly 2-3 metres) tall. It prefers full sun, requires excellent drainage, and seeds may benefit from exposure to cold and dampness (an autumn sowing or a few weeks of stratification in the refrigerator, if you have a refrigerator). Like most of the Umbelliferae, asafoetida self-sows readily. The young shoots may be cooked and eaten as a vegetable; the resin is harvested in June by exposing and slashing the roots of plants ca. 4 years old and allowing it to leak out (Grieve, p. 64).

Black cohosh (Cimicifuga racemosa a.k.a. Actaea racemosa) is often used to relieve menopausal symptoms. It is, in fact, so effective at this that one of my colleagues (and his patient) got a nasty scare from what appeared to be a case of a solidly post-menopausal woman suddenly starting to bleed vaginally – not something one wants to see. Everyone was much relieved when the problem was finally traced to nothing more threatening than using black cohosh, which had actually given her internal apparatus enough of a boost to make and shed a bit of uterine lining. In short, while not containing actual oestrogens, black cohosh has significant oestrogen-like effects in humans. It also stimulates uterine contractions, which can cause miscarriage even at an extremely early stage, and can be used in childbirth to help "ripen" and open the cervix as well.

Kress lists the contraceptive dosage for this herb at 3 tsp (root)/cup, 4x/day. A recommendation for abortifacient purposes is 1-4 tablespoons, simmered in water for ten minutes, 3-4x/day, taken for no longer than 10 days. Be aware that black cohosh toxicity can cause dizziness, diarrhea, decreased heart rate, tremors, liver damage, and death. Because of its strong oestrogenic effects, it, like pharmaceutical oestrogens, can promote blood clotting, increasing the risk of deep vein thrombosis and subsequent pulmonary embolisms. For menopausal symptoms, the dosage is 20-80 mg once or twice daily; for female osteoporosis or osteopaenia (the milder form of osteoporosis), it is 40 mg daily.

Black cohosh is a woodland plant, requiring a shaded or partially shaded site and rich, moist, but well-drained soil. Seeds have to be stratified (warm-cold-warm cycle – 70 F for 2 weeks, followed by 40 F for three months), and thus are best sown directly in autumn for spring germination; roots are not ready for harvest until 4-6 years after germination. It is more commonly propagated by root division in spring or autumn, which yields harvest-ready roots much more swiftly.

Blue cohosh (Caulophylum thalictroides) is sometimes used for early termination or abortion as well. It is less well-studied, and appears to have a worse safety profile, than black cohosh. It contains oestrogen-like substances, and is an inducer of oxytocin (causes uterine contractions). Tripathi mentions that it should be continued for 1 day after bleeding starts to make sure that all material is expelled from the uterus, and observes that it is often used with black cohosh, which may moderate and coordinate the uterine contractions. Kress recommends 3 tsp herb per cup, taken 3x/day until bleeding starts or up to a maximum of six days. Grieve was not familiar with either black or blue cohosh.

While blue cohosh is also used as a labour inductor for desired children, there is some evidence that it may cause severe problems in the infant; infant heart attack, stroke, and severe hypoxemia leading to multiorgan damage have all been recorded. Blue cohosh has been found to disrupt cellular mitochondria, and in general does not seem to be a good choice for the delivery of a living baby. Maternal toxicity includes nausea/vomiting, headaches, seizures at high doses, and kidney and liver damage. If the patient experiences chest pain, pallor and blueness of finger- and toe-nails, extreme thirst/urination/dry mouth, headache, pounding or irregular heartbeat, or any other symptoms of either cardiovascular problems or diabetes, she should stop taking it at once and go to her primary care doctor. Despite the name, blue cohosh is not actually related to black cohosh.

Cannabis (Cannabis sativa) – as discussed in Section II, 3b and 3f, it has been suggested that there is a possibility that the endocannabinoid system is involved in embryonic transport, implantation, and development. However, the large study cited in 3f showed no difference in fertility or reported outcomes (such as, for instance, ectopic pregnancy rates).

While it might be more prudent to avoid hemp when trying to conceive and for the first few weeks after probable (or at least courted and hoped-for) conception, there is no reason at this time to think it might be relied on as a preventative; and if it does show efficacy for this purpose in future, the possibility of interfering with embryonic transport, which would lead to an increased likelihood of ectopic pregnancy if cannabis has this result, would still make it a bad choice for the purpose.

As per section 3f, while hemp does seem to lower sperm count, the impact has not been shown to be significant enough to affect male fertility except possibly in borderline cases.

Chamomiles (German – Matricaria recutica, Roman – Chamaemelum nobile). German chamomile essential oil: unknown; incredibly non-toxic, but it has been advised not to use it simultaneously with birth control pills as it may disrupt the medical hormonal regulation. Herbal sites often warn against the use of the chamomiles in pregnancy due to the risk of inducing a miscarriage; to the point where it has become virtually viral, and indeed has lead to some distress in women who had been drinking it for things like pregnancy-related stomach upset before hearing this particular rumour; the essential oil of German chamomile is listed as a treatment for "delayed menses". However, it proves nearly impossible to find any scientific information supporting any of these claims. References, when given, consistently trace back to nonsupported sources.

The presence of a minute amount of thujone has been mentioned. Thujone is a toxic compound found in wormwood, tansy, and pennyroyal, as well as, in smaller amounts, in more innocuous herbs such as rosemary and sage. The level of thujone in the chamomiles is so low that even their essential oils are among the very, very few considered safe to use on infants, who are generally extremely sensitive to essential oils due to both metabolic factors and bodyweight. A small study (37 women who used herbal teas during pregnancy) showed that ca. 78% consumed chamomile tea at some point during their pregnancies (p. 27); 27% drank it throughout pregnancy (p. 28); one took it daily throughout the first 12 weeks. The only indications of an adverse result were occasional allergic reactions, which is the primary concern with the chamomiles.

No adverse pregnancy-related outcomes were reported. On reviewing the scientific literature, it seems probable that the only benefit of the chamomiles to a woman who thinks she might be pregnant and needs not to be is to calm her anxiety until her menses occur on their own – which is not always the best solution for a woman who really needs not to be pregnant. Roman chamomile is a perennial herb, short and bushy, covered with daisy-like white flowers in the summer. German chamomile is a small annual, each plant producing only a few daisy-like white flowers. In both cases, the part generally used is the dried flower-head (the yellow bit in the middle).

German chamomile self-seeds widely and enthusiastically, growing well on disturbed ground, particularly sandy and well-drained soil, but not competing well with grass. It takes a great many chamomile plants to produce any reasonable amount of chamomile flowers, particularly German chamomile. Both prefer full sun. The essential oil of German chamomile is a deep rich blue; the essential oil of Roman chamomile is a pale gold. For practical purposes, they are essentially the same, although many essential oil therapists are of the opinion that German chamomile is the more effective of the two. Given a choice, German chamomile is the one that I would prefer for the uses for which it actually works (calmative, anti-inflammatory, digestive).

Fennel (Foeniculum vulgare) has oestrogen-like effects, and is used for both painful menstruation and easing menopausal symptoms. The seed extract causes shrinkage of the chorion (outer membrane of the embryonic sac). Toxicity is low: the whole herb is edible as a vegetable raw or cooked, and stuffed fennel is quite popular in several parts of Europe. Like the angelicas, however, it has a certain degree of anti-coagulant effect, making bleeding more of a concern if difficulties arise; and also causes or exacerbates photosensitivity. Its oestrogen-like effects may interfere with hormonal birth control. Fennel seed is most commonly used medicinally for relieving digestive problems, for which Mrs. Grieve recommends half a pint of boiling water to a teaspoonful of bruised fennel seed (p. 196). As much as 4 tsp seed in one cup of water, 3x/day is considered quite safe.

There is some doubt as to the actual effects of fennel in terms of effective birth control or abortifacient potential. It is often cited as an inducer of uterine contractions. However, sweet fennel oil has been demonstrated to reduce oxytocin- and prostaglandin-stimulated contractions,, which would be desirable in preventing early labour, but is the opposite of what would be wanted in terminations. It is used effectively for diminishing menstrual cramps for this reason.

Fennel is a perennial that grows easily from seed. It requires a sunny situation, can tolerate a wide range of soils, and self-seeds readily. It is one of the more common plants to be found in herb gardens, for its culinary uses and because its delicate plumes of bright green foliage are extremely attractive; and even garden centres with meagre herb sections usually carry it.

The near-legendary Roman plant silphium, used for birth control by Roman women and presumed for nearly two thousand years to have been driven to extinction by Roman medicinal and culinary demand (the last stalk found is said to have been sent to the Emperor Nero for the price of its weight in gold), is believed to have been a species of giant fennel, of which asafoetida, another contraceptive herb, is a living relative.

Holy basil (tulsi, Thai basil; Ocimum tenuiflorum): has been shown to significantly decrease sperm count in animal models (rabbits) by raising testosterone while decreasing follicular hormone (FH) and lutenizing hormone (LH), probably as a feedback response to the testosterone increase. It is under consideration as a potential source of male medical contraception. Suppression of FH and LH would also decrease female fertility, but the effects in women, particularly regarding sex steroid hormones, have not been tested.

It is suspected that this herb may contain an androgenic analogue, which, with daily usage, could have possibly undesirable side effects in women (virilisation – facial hair, vocal changes, alteration in body-fat/muscle ratio, and possibly longer-term compromises of fertility). Human dosage for sperm reduction also has not been tested, but the equivalents by weight to animal dosage would be: 5.5 grams (fresh leaves) for a 150 lb man; 7.3 grams for a 200 lb. man. This plant would also be a good choice for men who require exogenous testosterone supplementation, being quite safe to eat and easy to grow in a wide range of situations.

Animal models are reported as showing that holy basil inhibits implantation, so it is considered contraindicated in pregnancy or when attempting to conceive. It is unlikely that female use for no more than ca. 3-5 days a month would cause any significant androgenic side effects; but if the beginnings of these are noticed, it would be wisest to discontinue at once if the effects are unwanted (gender identity and the individual expressions of same being the wide and variable spectrum that they are, this would have to be up to the individual. Some women, or people who are biologically female, may not be bothered in the slightest; others may find androgenic effects extremely distressing).

Holy basil, otherwise, has anti-inflammatory, adaptogenic, and anxiolytic uses. It is a major herb in Ayurvedic medicine and Indian religious practice.

Holy basil is closely related to common basil (an oxymoron, to be sure!), and is grown in the same way: easy to start from seed; site in full sun and good warmth, likes plenty of water but not being waterlogged, does well in northerly climates over the summer if it doesn't damp off from cold and wet in the spring, though cooler summers may require a greenhouse. It can be grown outdoors or in a sunny window and takes well to containers. And even if you put up barrier defences, slugs will actually paratroop off your garden walls to get at it.

In temperate climates, holy basil is an annual; but it can also be grown as a perennial in warmer areas. Tulsi loves being harvested; and once it is established, the more leaves you pick, the more leaves will grow. And it is a very pleasant culinary herb as well, spicier than regular basil, with elements of pepper and clove to the flavour, and particularly popular for cooking Siamese – no, I mean Thai! For culinary purposes, it is best used fresh. The red strain (dark tulsi, Shyama tulsi) is somewhat hotter-flavoured than the white strain (light tulsi, Rama tulsi).

Juniper (Juniperus communis) causes decreased uterine blood flow via high levels of isocupressic acid. It may also have anti-implantation effects. Taking juniper in pregnancy is strongly disrecommended if one wants to continue the pregnancy. It is generally believed that the abortifacient properties of juniper were the reason why gin (in effect a weak tincture of juniper) was commonly used in large doses in hopes of causing abortion when medical recourse was legally unavailable. Juniper is excreted through the kidneys, making juniper tea a good prophylactic and anti-microbial for urinary infections, but also meaning that it should be avoided by those with kidney disease. It is diuretic and may decrease blood sugar; if under treatment for hyperglycaemic conditions (specifically diabetes), medical supervision is recommended when using this herb to avoid unintentional hypoglycaemia. Large doses may cause digestive problems. Ripe berries – 500 ml. water over 30 g berries (ca. one pint to one ounce), steep for 10-20 minutes; 60-80 ml (ca. 4-5.25 tablespoons) 2-3x day. Leaves – same proportions; 1-3 tablespoons 2-3x day. Mrs. Grieve recommends the same dose of 1 pint to 1 ounce, but for more general purposes, the pint is to be taken over the course of 24 hours.

The bark of Utah juniper (Juniperus osteosperma) has been shown to cause abortions in late-term cattle. Effects and safety in humans are not known. Juniper is common as a decorative tree/shrub, growing in a wide variety of conditions and climates – from the Mediterranean up through Sweden, Norway, and Finland - though a sunny site is best for maximum medicinal production. Juniperus communis is dioecious, pollinated by wind; so if procuring plants for medicinal use, make sure you get berry-bearing females and one male to fertilize the flowers! Berries take 2-3 years to ripen, at which time they turn from green to blue.

Juniper berries are often used for culinary purposes, particularly to season game. In Scandinavia, they are still used instead of hops as a very pleasant beer additive and preservative; and traditionally in Norway, juniper water was used for mopping and washing the house, fronds were used as strewing herbs, and juniper fumigation was practiced (particularly after someone had died of illness), all of which which probably had good disinfectant effects as well as producing a pleasant scent. The anti-microbial characteristics of juniper indicate that a strong decoction of water boiled for 20 minutes with juniper berries then steeped in it for another 10-20 minutes (the essential oils are highly volatile, making this an excellent inhalant for lung infections; but 20 minutes boiling would probably release them all into the air) would make a pretty fair antiseptic wash.

Parsley (Petroselinum crispum) contains a substance called apiole, which has been used on its own as an abortifacient. While apiole and parsley (whole or as an essential oil or extract) are considered some of the most effective herbal abortifacients, they are also among the more dangerous, at least for later terminations; Tisserand and Young note that both have been repeatedly documented as leading to extreme post-termination bleeding, massive organ failure, and death. The safety and efficacy profiles for early (post-intercourse contraceptive) use are unknown, as the use of "emmenagogues" is almost never recorded unless there are significant negative consequences.

The lowest dose of apiole which appears effective for later abortions (likely to be significantly higher than for contraception by early termination) is 900 mg/8 days; the lowest fatal daily dose recorded was 770 mg/14 days, suggesting that the therapeutic index (between "successful abortion" and "death") is both extremely low and varies by individual to a degree that makes judging it virtually impossible. Fresh parsley, fortunately, is sufficiently low in apiole that normal culinary uses seldom present a threat even during a wanted pregnancy.

Some sources recommend the insertion of raw parsley into the vagina, either as an early inducer in itself, or to "ripen" the cervix in the manner of mifepristone. There is absolutely no data that can be evaluated on whether or not this actually works to any degree. Very few women seem to use, or at least report having used, the insertion method alone – normally it is combined with oral herbs of some sort – and if it had even the most marginal chance of being effective by itself, that would probably be in the early period before diagnosis, making it impossible to determine whether (1) the woman was pregnant at all, (2) the termination occurred naturally regardless of the parsley, or (3) the parsley caused the termination.

Herbalist Henrietta Kress observes that she has never personally even heard of anyone bringing on a delayed period by this means, let alone successfully terminating a pregnancy. Given the low level of apiole in fresh parsley, it seems awesomely unlikely to work. This is another of those, "one person said it and a few others picked it up, and now a lot of sources will support each other on it; but it's still complete hooey" things.

Pennyroyal (Mentha pulegium) is one of the best-known herbs used to terminate pregnancies. It is also highly dangerous. Deaths have occurred from both the essential oil (single uses, taken orally) and the regular use of an alcoholic tincture over two weeks. No safety profile is known on tea. Grieve recommends 1 oz herb/1 pint of boiling water, taken at ca. 4 oz doses, "frequently repeated"; she also mentions an essential oil oral dosage of ½-3 drops (p. 626). Kress suggests ¼ cup herb to 1 quart of water, once a day, for no more than six days.

In small doses, pennyroyal is used for digestive problems. Otherwise, it is probably best left to the use from which it got its name, "fleamint"; that is to say, using dried pennyroyal in clothes and bedding to discourage fleas (be careful that cats don't get the opportunity to nibble on it).

Like most of the mint family, pennyroyal is a perennial that prefers plenty of sun and water. It can be grown from seed, and once well-established, can easily be propagated by division.

Red raspberry leaf (Rubus idaeus) is a uterine stimulant, often used to speed labour. However, a small study (51 participants) indicated that it might actually also decrease the likelihood of premature labour. It is not recommended in pregnancy, particularly early pregnancy, because of the uterine stimulant effects; but anecdotal reports are all over the place, some suggesting that it may actually aid in becoming and/or remaining pregnant. It may also interfere with hormonal birth control.

It should probably not be considered a reliable choice as a contraceptive until we know more about how it works and why. After birthing, red raspberry leaf tea is well-known and well-documented in regards to increasing milk production in the nursing mother. Raspberry plants grow almost as easily and enthusiastically in a wide range of climates and situations as their cousin the blackberry or bramble; once established, a fair amount of energetic pruning is often required to keep them under control.

Rue (ruda, Rutens graveolens) induces contractions and decreases the blood flow to the endometrium; the uterine lining is thus unable to provide enough nourishment to the foetus for it to survive, even as the uterus attempts to expel its contents. However, the use of rue as an abortifacient has been demonstrated, albeit in a very small study, to cause multiple organ failure and deaths very significantly more often than any of the other 29 plant species mentioned by women in that study. It should not be used unless all other alternatives, such as continued maternal life, are even worse.

Rue prefers full sun, and can grow in a variety of well-drained soils, even very rocky, sandy soil. One should be careful handling it, as it can cause burns and rashes to sensitive skin. Like pennyroyal, dried rue makes an excellent insect repellent in the household, something that will be of no little concern after the Catastrophe when you can't get flea powders and mothballs; but do not use it directly on animals for flea control. For both convenience and safety, it is best to sew the dried leaves up in cloth packets for household insect repulsion.

Smartweed (Polygonum hydropiper a.k.a. Persicaria hydropiper; also called marsh pepper). The root extract demonstrates substantial oestrogenic effects, comparable to estradiol 17; it causes follicular recruitment and endometrial hyperplasia initially; but were shown to reduce protein expression 5-6 days after implantation, to which the plant's antifertility action, traditional in several parts of the world, is attributed. Other herbs in the polygonum family, such as bistort, have not yet been scientifically evaluated for possible antifertility activity. However, the root of bistort (Bistorta officinalis a.k.a. Persicaria bistorta, Polygonum bistorta, snakeweed, twice-writhen) has traditionally been used as a mild contraceptive occasionally (and is definitely a very powerful astringent, effective against diarrhoea and useful in tanning leather; dried and powdered, it is a good styptic or blood-stopper).

Saltpetre

Saltpetre can be readily produced on the farm, assuming a good supply of amnure-producing animals. Joseph LeConte's "Instructions for the manufacture of saltpetre" (1862) advises beginning with "a good quantity" of well-rotted manure on a bed of well-rammed clay (limited or no drainage – don't want the stuff leaching out into the ground). Wood ash, unleached or leached, leaves, straw, twigs, and a "considerable quantity" of ordinary dirt are mixed in; the lot is covered with a rough roof to protect from rain, which may or may not have side protection. It is watered weekly with urine, liquefied manure, or similar, the object being to keep it moist but not wet.

The materials are turned weekly to ca. 5-6" (12.5-15 cm) deep, and the whole heap turned over monthly. During the last few months, it is moistened with water alone. The saltpetre appears on the top as a whitish bloom or crust; the top 2-3" (5-7.5 cm) are removed, put aside under shelter, and kept moist. When enough has been collected for leaching, usually by autumn or early winter, the small heap left becomes the nucleus of the next one. Soak the earth for leaching in water for 12 hours and drain; repeat. Each 12-hour soaking leaches ca. ½ the nitrates present into the water.

The water (ley) is then run through fresh batches of nitrate/earth until the solution is strong enough to float an egg. Wood ashes are then mixed in, or the ley can be filtered through them. Then it is poured off whatever has precipitated out, and crystallized by boiling (periodically removing other salts from the bottom and organic scuzz from the top) until a drop on a cold metallic surface quickly crystallizes. It is now left to cool. The saltpetre precipitates as crystals.

The crystals are boiled in water again (added gradually up to 40 lbs/1 gallon, which is saturation point). Again, organic scuzz from the top and crystals of common salt precipitating to the bottom are removed. .6 gallons of cold water is added slowly. 1-1.5 lbs of dissolved hoof/skin glue or blood/100 gallons are added to finish purifying; this binds to any remaining organic matter, which rises to the top and can be skimmed off. The liquid is cooled with constant stirring; the saltpetre crystallizes as very fine needlelike crystals ("flour"). This is put into a drainage box (perforated tray above the bottom) and moistened with a saturated solution of pure nitrate, then left for 3-4 hours and drained off. A small quantity of pure water (1 pint/454 ml to 53 lbs (24 kg) of saltpetre is added and drained off after 2 hours. The nitre is dried by low heat and constant stirring; congratulations, you now have refined saltpetre.

Tansy (Tanacetum vulgare): 1 oz leaves and tops, harvested in August at first flowering, to 1 pint boiling water; 4 oz. twice a day on an empty stomach (Grieve, p. 790). More recent herbalists such as Henrietta Kress suggest lower doses to be used if at all: e.g., 4-8 tsp dried herb/quart of boiling water, sipped throughout the day. Both the essential oil and other extracts, as well as the raw herb have been recorded to cause death. The fatal dose of the essential oil has been noted to be ca. 10-12 drops.

John Ringo's novella, "In the Time of Darkness" (included as a bonus at the end of The Emerald Sea) presented a character refining tansy essential oil for contraceptive purposes when she is in a fairly dire situation (captive in a powerful lunatic's breeding harem). However, quite appropriately, the character is shown to be extremely well aware of the toxic and potentially fatal nature of the substance she is using, and titrates her doses very slowly and with the greatest caution. And, needless to say, since she is a major heroine in the next couple of books, her author really needed her not to kill herself with the stuff. Your author may not be so kindly. Tansy is an extremely hardy perennial (can take winter temperatures down to -40 C/-40 F), preferring full sun or light shade and well-drained, fertile soil. It grows well from seed.

Turmeric (Curcuma longa). A minimum dose of 1000 mg of curcumin daily, found at ca. 3% in turmeric, disrupts sperm production and motility. Either stockpile a stabilized extract, or learn to love fresh turmeric. The dosage required with the whole herb, assuming that it is <6 months from harvest, is probably lower than the 30 grams (a bit over 1 oz) per day indicated by the supplement dosing and plant percentage: curcumin alone has very low bioavailability, but it is more effectively absorbed when the whole herb is taken.

Turmeric is traditionally used in the Barghar District of India as a female contraceptive, a piece of rhizome being ground and taken on an empty stomach once daily for two weeks from day 5 of the menstrual cycle (the fifth day after menstruation begins), in order to prevent pregnancy for a year. How effective this actually is, at what point the regimen becomes effective, and how much rhizome is actually eaten, remains unknown; although if suppression of GnRH (gonadotropin-releasing hormone) is indeed the mechanism of action, it could be expected to be effective each month that it is taken at the appropriate time in the cycle; and the traditional timing is consistent with the proposed mechanism.

This plant, or more specifically its constituent curcumin, has a great many proven health benefits, as an anti-oxidant, anti-inflammatory (particularly useful in chronic inflammatory conditions such as both osteoarthritis and rheumatoid arthritis, and auto-immune conditions characterized by chronic inflammation), and counteractor of atherosclerosis. The poor bioavailability of isolated curcumin is improved by adding piperine (a component of black pepper) and much improved when ingesting the whole herb. Unfortunately, once turmeric is dried and ground, the curcumin degrades within a few months, so it cannot be relied on from the shop, or stockpiled except as live rhizomes.

Turmeric, like ginger, is a hot-weather plant that can be grown quite easily in greenhouses or even warm rooms with good window lighting. The rhizomes (roots) can be kept dormant in cool sandy soil indoors overwinter, and will come back nicely in spring if not allowed to freeze. Most Indian food shops and many cosmopolitan supermarkets sell the fresh rhizomes, which – again, like ginger – are happy to sprout and grow if put in damp soil in a comfortably warm place. Turmeric (and ginger) can be propagated indefinitely by root division.

Vitamin C: high doses of vitamin C are reputed to have abortifacient effects, but the evidence is extremely sketchy and unreliable at best. Even in the anecdotal reports, the women who successfully aborted seldom used vitamin C alone. It seems to be in the same category as the recommendation of the chamomiles as a means of early termination: something that got into the water and has been repeated often enough that an uncritical general search makes it look as if it were a proven fact. Vitamin C should not be considered a remotely plausible means even of implantation prevention or initial-termination birth control, let alone termination within the first 4-6 weeks or later.

Wild yam (Dioscorea villosa) appears to have some oestrogenic effects, but is not a plant source of oestrogen itself unless you have access to a laboratory to process it. The human body cannot change the wild yam-produced steroid-precursor diosgenin into oestrogens, and the oestrogen-like effects of wild yam are quite mild, making it possibly well-suited towards gently easing a woman into menopause, but not at all suited to contraception. Kress states straight-out that, "Wild yam (Dioscorea villosa) does not work as a herbal birth control. People who try it invariably end up being called "Mom", unless they're naturally infertile." Mexican yam is a closely related species, Dioscorea mexicana, and similar to wild yam in active constituents and effects.

Wild carrot seed (Dauca carota, a.k.a. Queen Anne's Lace) is probably, both in terms of efficacy and in terms of safety, the best choice of all the herbal contraceptives known. Wild carrot is the most commonly used contraceptive herb in Western folk medicine; it is also the safest by a long way. Although reports of its efficacy are largely anecdotal or individual-retrospective, they are widespread, consistent, and have received at least a little attention in terms of evaluating efficacy and safety in multiple women over a period of time. If my wife or daughter were in the position of needing something of this sort after the Catastrophe, wild carrot seeds would certainly be my first-line recommendation for her.

Wild carrot seed is a progesterone-blocker with anti-oestrogenic effects (discouraging ovulation), anti-implantation effects, and may also contribute to early termination. The alcoholic extract totally inhibited implantation in mice at 4-6 days post-coitally, and had no effect at 8-10 days post-coitally; petroleum ether extract (subcutaneous) caused abortion in rats and inhibited implantation in rabbits except when supplementary progesterone was administered simultaneously; both intramuscular alcoholic extracts and oral extracts in water showed significant disruption to the oestrous cycles of rats and rabbits.

So far, in the admittedly uncontrolled human studies done by Robin Bennett, there have been no indications of harm done to either the women using the herb, or the children that they conceived when they discontinued/forgot to use it. One teaspoon to one tablespoon a day, chewed or taken with water (the former said to be more effective) is anecdotally reported to be an effective dose. Opinions vary as to whether the dose should be taken every day; only during and for seven days following the fertile period; or as three doses at eight-hour intervals following potentially-fertilizing intercourse. There was at least one case of a woman who took it daily for ten years, and conceived a healthy child with no difficulty, on the single occasion of going on vacation with her husband and forgetting to bring her carrot seeds with her.

Herbalist Robin Bennett has worked and experimented with this plant for many years, and found it to be efficacious with intermittent use as a post-intercourse contraceptive, as long as three doses are taken at 8-hour intervals, with the first dose no more than 8 hours after intercourse. The dosage she used was 15 drops of flower tincture and 15 drops of seed tincture, or an unstated amount of seeds (elsewhere she recommends 1 tsp seeds as an alternative, with the same timing for taking the 3 post-intercourse doses). She did also note that failures which occurred due to causes other than specific and documented user error were matched to strong and long-term systemic responses to the dosing: sensitive breasts and increasingly shortened menstrual cycles; spotting before and increasingly after menstruation; which suggests that a woman whose body responds to wild carrot seed with altered hormonal production (perhaps compensating for the hormonal effects of progesterone blockage?) is unlikely to find it an effective contraceptive.

Cultivated carrot seeds and foliage are similar to those of wild carrot; the breeding which gave us our garden carrots was deliberately directed only towards qualities of the root (larger, less woody, introducing orange, purple, red, and yellow strains as well as the original white). However, food carrots are generally harvested before they have a chance to flower and go to seed, as the root becomes very woody and far less pleasant to eat.

It is occasionally stated that cultivated carrots are weaker medicinally than wild carrots. This does not seem to have been tested experimentally. Jansen and Wolmuth comment that, "Most of the literature does not clearly identify the taxonomic status of the plant material used, and it has therefore not been possible to discriminate between results obtained with "wild carrot" and cultivated forms of the plant. Most chemical and pharmacological work on carrot seed has undoubtedly been conducted using cultivated material, but information is not available to establish the degree to which this may differ from "wild carrot" seed in terms of chemistry and pharmacological activity" (p. 11).

However, an analysis of the essential oil content of wild carrot seeds vs. cultivated carrot seeds showed that wild carrot seeds (from northern Serbia) contained 1.67% essential oil, whereas cultivated carrot seeds from the same region contained 0.55%. The constituents of the essential oils were largely similar, but the proportions were different, wild carrot being higher in sabinene and -pinene, and cultivated carrot being much higher in carotol. The difference in essential oil content is usually a good guide to the overall strength of a herbal medication, so this can be taken as reasonable verification of the idea that wild carrots are medicinally stronger.

Wild and cultivated carrots, both Dauca carota, are, in any case, similar in kind if not in degree. Wild carrot would be the preferable choice for contraception, since it is the one that we know the most about for this purpose and has the higher proportion of active constituents. But if you didn't manage to plant wild carrot before the Catastrophe and can't find any growing that you can identify with absolute certainty as not being any of the fatally poisonous look-alikes where you live, it is safe enough to triple the amount of cultivated carrot seed, using a tablespoon rather than a teaspoon; this dosage has been used for wild carrot seeds.

If you (or your patient) start showing signs of overall hormonal disruption, cut back until you have gotten down to a teaspoon per dose; either the particular seeds are stronger than estimated, or your body is counter-reacting more strongly than usual and the medication may not work for you (if the 1 teaspoon dose continues to affect your system, you know the latter is the case).

Note: if the Catastrophe caught you without a back stock of birth control, and all you have is the carrot seeds you picked up at that abandoned garden centre... commercial seeds are often treated in various manners, which frequently include poisonous substances, to protect them from insects, various pathogens, etc. Unless the packet says specifically that the seeds are either untreated or organic, don't eat them! In the vast majority of circumstances, pregnancy is a better outcome than death (if you're in a situation where it's not, and such things have happened in real life and definitely do happen in fiction, you are in a bad situation indeed).

In addition to its contraceptive qualities, wild carrot (decoction of the whole herb, 1 oz to 1 pint boiling water) is an effective diuretic, which was often used to relieve the symptoms of congestive heart failure, some kidney and bladder problems, and aid in passing urinary microstones ("gravel"). The seeds relieve gas and flatulence, and aid digestion (Grieve, p. 163). The root of both the wild and the cultivated carrot is helpful in speeding wound healing and may have anti-diabetic, cholesterol-lowering, and hepatoprotective functions, among other things; the seeds appear to have both anti-inflammatory and analgesic effects.

Wild carrot grows wild in many places in Europe and North America. Like the cultivated strains, it can be grown just about anywhere short of the most extreme climactic regions. Unfortunately, if looking for it in the wild, it is one of those hemlock look-alikes that I warned you about in Section III, but the stem is hairy (hemlock has a smooth stem; a mnemonic often used by wildcrafters is, "The Queen has hairy legs") and wild carrot has a sweet carrot-like scent instead of the unpleasant scent produced by hemlock (though if you suspect a plant of being hemlock, you probably oughtn't be sniffing it at all, let alone crushing the leaves for a good whiff).

It prefers a light sandy or chalk soil, but can grow very well in richer soils; it requires full sun. Wild carrot grows well from seed and self-seeds regularly and enthusiastically; in some places, it is considered an invasive weed. Seeds can be sown in autumn to overwinter, or in spring after the last frost. If you grow it within 1 km (0.6 miles) of your cultivated carrots and let both flower and seed, they will pollinate each other. This will not improve the culinary character of your cultivated carrots, nor the medicinal character of your wild ones. Carrots are insect-pollinated, so, if planting your own wild carrots, it would probably be best to cover the umbels of those cultivated carrots which you are letting run to provide next year's seed with mesh bags and do hand-pollination, as described for preserving distinct poppy varieties.

The root resembles a small cultivated carrot, but is white and very woody, without the typical cultivated carrot sweetness, though it is quite edible and rich in vitamin A. Wild carrot, like cultivated carrot, is a tall, lacy-leaved plant, with tiny white flowers produced in large flat umbels. The name Queen Anne's Lace refers to the dainty "lace-like" look of the flower heads. Most wild carrot flower clusters have a single deep red or black flower in the centre, which is striking of appearance and bears the legend that it comes from Queen Anne pricking her finger on a needle. Some have also associated it with menstrual blood, making the obvious connection with the plant's use. If you see this flower, then you can be confident that you have identified the plant correctly.

Mark the plant and return in autumn to collect the seeds. As the seed forms, the umbel head curls up into a very distinctive cupped shape (as contrasted to hemlock, which retains the splayed positioning of the original umbel stalks); the seeds of wild carrot are covered with tiny spikelets (if you get them from a garden centre, the spikelets have usually gone, but they should definitely be there when you first collect them in the wild – the same is true for cultivated carrot seeds. If in doubt, let a cultivated carrot run to seed and observe the seeds for yourself so you can recognise them in the wild in future), whereas hemlock seeds are always smoothly fluted.

Wild carrot is a biennial (flowers in second year and dies) or short-lived perennial. Like most wild plants, and indeed like other carrots, wild carrot is hardy and requires little maintenance. The seeds are quite small, but prolifically produced. One umbel may produce a thousand seeds – but that is only a gram in weight. To be sure of a year's supply for one woman if using the daily dose method, you will want to grow a number of plants. If you're short on plants, Robin Bennett's post-intercourse method may be your only option.

Of the herbal fertility reducers, Dauca carota has one of the best safety profiles and seems to be the best-defined in terms of dosage and efficacy in humans. And if carrots aren't part of your diet now, you certainly will want them to be after the Catastrophe, given their range of benefits and the ease with which they grow.

IV. Contraception and Supernatural Persons

It is generally accepted that vampire women (assuming that vampirism is the result of supernatural forces or a supernatural-acting virus, rather than vampires being a fully separate species of their own) cannot give birth, so no contraception is needed there. Whether a vampire man can father children on a non-vampire woman or not depends on the world and sometimes special circumstances; if it's possible, barrier devices (for the man) or female contraception of some sort (for his partner) are probably the best options. Oral sperm-reducers are unlikely to affect vampires unless taken secondhand (through the blood of someone who has taken the medication), though this is likely to be quite effective, given that the sperm count of undead vampires can hardly be particularly high if it exists at all.

In those instances where vampires are a separate, true-breeding species, it is commonly observed that they breed less frequently and often less successfully than humans. Contraceptives working by any mechanism are likely to require lower doses than is the case in humans, unless the vampiric physiology includes a powerful breeding cycle (as in J.R. Ward's Black Dagger Brotherhood novels). Lycanthrope men can usually reproduce, either with women of their own kind or of others. Barrier contraception and female contraception are the best options. However efficacious holy basil and turmeric might be (if they are) on human men, the lycanthrope sperm is likely to be more resistant and the lycanthrope metabolism less affected and more quickly cleared. Significantly higher doses would be required for sperm suppression, and might well not work at all.

Whether lycanthrope women can bear children depends on the world and sometimes special circumstances. Some authors claim the trauma of shapeshifting invariably dislodges embryos; others have female lycanthropes producing children by ones, twos, or litters; and whether the children can change shape from birth or not is also variable. Assuming a dominant hereditary lycanthropy or two lycanthrope parents (if lycanthrope women can carry to term), it can probably be assumed that post-implantation termination will be significantly more difficult to achieve than with a human child, given the usual increased vigour and healing ability of lycanthropes (especially if the mother is one). Implantation may also be more difficult to block. The focus for contraception in lycanthrope women with the capability for successful pregnancy should be on discouraging ovulation and fertilization.

Other biological and social elements may also present a challenge in regards to lycanthrope contraception, if lycanthrope women of your world have reproductive cycles with the intensity and pheromonal inducement characteristic of their animal form. Such potentially troublesome situations are often socially and/or ritually circumscribed, and there may be a conflict between a social expectation and the woman's own desires. Both an expectation of mating/reproduction, and a denial of the right of women to choose to procreate based on social position within the group, are possible. In such cases, the caregiver's first responsibility is to respect the autonomy of the individual patient in making her decision and either provide her with the assistance she has chosen, or refuse to force contraception/termination on her if she is unwilling to accept it.

By all accounts, both in folklore and in the fiction based on it, the main fey fertility problem is not avoiding conception, but achieving it, towards which end they make considerable efforts. It is quite possible, however, for a human to end up with an unwanted half-fey pregnancy. In this case, the safest first line would be a combination of prophylactic wild carrot with substances toxic to the fey but not, except in excessive doses, to humans: iron, rowan, St. John's wort. All mechanisms of contraception are likely to be significantly more effective with the fey, including and perhaps especially those which diminish sperm motility (fey men are likely to have low sperm counts in any case, given the constantly-documented reproductive issues).

V. Other Post-Catastrophe Fertility Reduction Possibilities

a) The IUD

After the Catastrophe, the copper IUD will probably be the one continuous contraception method that can be made even in very primitive circumstances. Copper is strongly spermicidal, and also provokes a mild inflammatory reaction in the uterus by which the woman's own immune system attacks the sperm. The fundamental principle of all non-hormonal IUDs is to maintain the presence of copper in the uterus in a manner which neither risks damage nor is likely to suffer spontaneous expulsion. The efficacy of the copper IUD is 99%+, and user error is not a factor, as once it is in it generally stays in and continues to work until the copper has fully dissolved (a minimum of three years; most current copper IUDs last for five, and some can last up to fifteen years; but for any homemade version, three years should be considered the upper limit).

Because it prevents implantation as well as conception, the copper IUD can also be used for emergency contraception within five days of the concern-raising sex. Although copper poisoning is sometimes a concern when, for example, cooking primarily in copper utensils, there has never yet been a recorded case of a woman getting copper poisoning from an IUD. The copper-based IUD raises plasma copper concentrations slightly, but not to toxic levels; and IUDs of this type have been used long-term by a large population over a period of decades. It is safe to say that this is not a concern for either the real-life user or the Catastrophe survivor.

The Graefenburg ring, invented by a German physician in the early 20th century, is considered the original form of the modern IUD. Graefenburg's version was a ring of high-copper-content (27%) silver wire coiled around a silk thread. The most common version of the non-hormonal IUD today is a soft plastic T-frame with the long arm of the T covered in copper (coating, wire-wrap, or cylindrical hollow beads. The cross-arms of the T hold the device in place within the uterus; two small strings depend from the end of the long arm and pass out through the cervix so that the IUD may be readily removed when the woman wishes to have it out. The main problem is that not all uteri are the same size or shape. The adolescent woman and the nullipara (woman who has never given birth) generally have smaller uterine cavities; some women have cylindrical cavities instead of the typical one that is wider at the top.

Therefore, in some women, the T-frame can be too large or just shaped wrong, causing pain, cramping, bleeding, and general unhappiness and a need to have it out. The horror stories of embedded IUDs which require general anaesthesia for removal are almost inevitably about T-frames, and the cause is inevitably that the crossbars were too wide for the specific uterus. The "frameless" IUD is a more recent and far superior invention, which works on the same general principle as the T-frame (plastic with a form of copper sheathing), but instead of cross-arms to keep it in, the top terminates in an anchor knot which is implanted into the myometrium (muscular wall of the uterus). This is proving preferable in real life for several reasons: far less bleeding, cramping, and pain; no issues selecting the correct size or just even finding one small enough to fit a young nullipara; the shaft is extremely flexible, moving easily with the normal uterine movements; and the anchoring knot, in practice, is secure enough to prevent migration or evacuation, but not so secure that the device cannot readily be removed when a woman wants it out. Sadly, there will be issues post-Catastrophe.

To wit: it must be established that the myometrium is thick enough to take a knot (we generally use ultrasound; there's not a way to detect it unaided); and the device requires a specialized implanter to set the knot, so unless you had a way to stock up on the actual devices and implanters beforehand, it's pretty much not going to work. The essence of a copper based IUD is: the copper has to get into the uterus and fairly reliably stay there, without risking perforation (ca. 1:1000 during implantation with T-frame or frameless modern IUDs) or excessive irritation; and it has to be easily removable when the woman using it wants it out, which means soft, but durable (i.e., silk) threads hanging down through the cervical opening and into the vagina, long enough that they are unlikely to be rolled back up into the uterine cavity with device movement (because you don't want your midwife, doctor, or best buddy to have to dilate your cervix and go fishing in there when you've decided it's time to have it out).

Under no circumstances can there be sharp or rough edges anywhere on the item. If wire is used, the ends must be soldered down and smoothed, or heated until they bead and smoothed; tucking them under the coils is not good enough for parts of something that will be moved about a bit when, if they got loose, they could go right through the uterine wall. Do not use any lead-containing solder on any form of IUD! Being able to prevent pregnancy when you don't want to get pregnant is excellent. Getting lead poisoning is not excellent. If using pewter as an improvised solder, you have to be sure that it is lead-free – a lot of older pieces do contain lead, and again, you absolutely do not want lead in your uterus. Plumber's solder also needs to be verified: some of it contains lead and some is lead-free, although if it was manufactured any time in the last few years, it should be clearly labelled. Solder used on fittings through which drinking water may pass is legally required to be lead-free; because leaded solder is often easier to use, it is frequently utilized in heating and gas systems. If you're in Britain or Ireland and the original label on a roll you found is missing, look for the stamp YP (Yorkshire Potable), which is lead-free and designed for drinking-water fittings.

A COUPLE OF POSSIBLE POST-CATASTROPHE IMPROVISATIONS MIGHT BE:

» Copper beads sewn into a coil or a ring on silk thread (cotton is more absorbent, faster to disintegrate, and has a worse record with nurturing bacteria). Flexible enough; but you still have to get it in through the uterine opening in as sterile a fashion as possible (see below on menstrual evacuation). This is not a do-it-yourself procedure; you at least need a friend who is capable of using a speculum (and a speculum or reasonable equivalent). A copper version of the Graefenburg ring will also be an option, but be aware that the risk of bleeding, infection, etc., and especially pain and cramping, will be higher, as the item is not as flexible as the beads-on-a-coil. If you have soldering capacities, stringing a number of small copper rings together on a silk thread might also be preferable to the Graefenburg single wire coiled around and around the thread.

» Probably the easiest version to make and insert – take a large spherical or ovoid copper bead (ovoid goes in more easily and will probably be more comfortable for the young and/or nulliparous with that narrow little uterine cavity and small cervical os; spherical will probably stay in more reliably).

» The size will depend on the woman: about a third of nulliparous women have uterine cavities as narrow as 2 cm (4/5 inch), and some are smaller than that – which is why the T-frames are not reliably user-friendly. Run silk thread up through it, through a smaller copper bead (just needs to be bigger than the hole in the large one; it's a stopper), and back down; then tie both around a second copper bead (the stopper to keep the removal threads from rolling back into the primary bead), and leave enough length that, if the bead goes all the way up to the top of the uterus, it will still be possible to grab them and remove the device when required. The main potential fault with this is that accidental evacuation will be easier than with other shapes such as the coil or ring, especially for a woman who has already borne children. But replacement will also be easier. Repeated or excessively easy evacuations (as in, if the thing pops out every few times its user has menstrual cramps or successful sex) probably indicate that a larger primary bead is needed.

» Silver might gainfully be mixed with the copper, either as the secondary beads in the three-bead version, intermittent silver beads around the sewn/beaded coil version, or bits of wire added to the copper Graefenburg ring. This will not increase efficacy, but is unlikely to decrease it, and the anti-microbial properties of the silver may prove beneficial in regards to lowering the risk of infection.

» Uterine cavity sizes vary widely. The common ranges, though individual women may differ more widely on either end of the curve, are:

  » Anterior-posterior: 6.29-38.2 mm. (0.27 to 1.5 inches).

  » Cavity width: ca. 32% of nulliparous women have a cavity width < 20 mm (4/5"), but a multiparous woman (several births) might have a cavity of 38 mm or greater - say, effectively twice that of her thirteen year-old daughter. Some very small uterine cavities can be as narrow as 7 mm (0.28 inches).

» Length: ranges from ca. 25 to 40 mm. (1 to 1.6").

Inserting the IUD safely does not require medically-trained personnel; just someone who has a clue about womb anatomy and can learn to keep sterile protocol and use a speculum. The procedure is, ideally, the same as that detailed below for inserting the cannula to perform a menstrual evacuation. The same anesthetics and relaxants are appropriate, although a higher dose of opiate might be required without implying that something is actually going wrong with the procedure, especially in the nullipara, since the cervix has to be dilated a lot wider with the IUD than with a cannula – and many women have reported that cervical dilation, as, for instance, when having a T-frame IUD placed, can be very bloody painful.

The cleansing procedure and the effort to maintain sterility are also the same as with the menstrual evacuation cannula. It's not a DIY procedure unless you absolutely have no choice; in which case, the three-bead method is definitely your best bet. That version may pop out more easily, especially in women who have had babies and therefore have larger and differently shaped (a vertical slit instead of a small round opening in the middle) cervical openings, but it also goes in more easily than the other options).

B) The Sponge

If you live near a coast, or have trade routes with people on the coast, the sea sponge is a fair option as a one-use contraceptive (or, if you can sterilize it between uses, a resuable one). You could also use a salvaged synthetic sponge for the purpose, as long as it has never been used for any other purpose; those, too, can be sterilized and re-used if needed. Efficacy for the modern contraceptive sponge (synthetic, containing spermicide) is variable. Planned Parenthood estimates that theoretically, assuming perfect placement every time, it would be 91% effective for women who have never given birth; in practice, it runs around ca. 88% for nulliparous women. For women who have given birth, the theoretical perfect use would give 80% and the practical runs around 76%. The sponge is inserted all the way into the vagina to form a cup over the cervix (a natural sea-sponge can easily be trimmed suitably to the individual cervical size), providing a physical barrier as well as a source of spermicide.

c. Spermicides

Post-Catastrophe options for spermicidal creams, douches, sponge soaks, etc., will largely be herbal. It appears, so far, that combinations of herbs are more effective than single-plant mixtures. Some of those you might wish to use in compounding your own include:

» Bergamot mint/pineapple mint (Mentha citrata, also known by several other common names: lemon mint, orange mint, water/wild water mint, and others). A component in the herbal spermicidal pessary compound Praneem (the other two elements are soapberry and neem seed extracts); the efficacy gained by combining the three was estimated at an 8-fold improvement, and, although the rabbit study was quite small, 13 out of 15 controls got pregnant, while 15 out of 15 of the Praneem test group did not.

» Clove pink (Dianthus caryophyllus – carnation, but note that "carnation" also describes other dianthus varieties; and garden carnations are often crosses between the original clove pink and other dianthus. The caryophyllus is the only one that has been tested in this regard. Still, if standard garden carnations are all you've got, it can't hurt to add some to your spermicidal mix) – a gel made with an extract from dried stems and leaves was shown to have spermicidal activity (affecting both motility and viability), with relatively minimal cytotoxicity in regards to vaginal/uterine cells.

» Fat hen (Chenopodium album; also called lamb's quarters, white goosefoot, pigweed) seeds, even prepared as a simple water-based decoction, showed marked spermicidal effect; its constituent desgalactotigogen appears to be an extremely effective spermicide, which, unlike nonoxynol-9, does not affect the endogenous lactobacilli (maintain a more acid environment, protective against diseases). Fat hen is a common "weed" throughout most of the world, formerly used frequently in European, British, and Irish folk cooking (and, as the name suggests, as poultry food); and is a popular food crop in Northern India, closely related to quinoa. The seeds contain protein, potassium, vitamin A, B-complex vitamins, calcium, and phosphorus, and can be ground into porridge, sprouted like alfalfa or mung beans, and generally treated like most grains. The leaves and young shoots are used in a manner similar to spinach, and serve as a fair spinach substitute. The green parts do contain a high amount of oxalic acid, so should be eaten in moderation (steamed is preferable to fresh for this reason, as well); however, beekeepers should know that oxalic acid can be used as a miticide against varroa. Fat hen is an annual that can get very large (up to 3 metres, or ca. 10 feet, tall) in good soil and good sunlight. It grows enthusiastically from seed, germinating only a few days from sowing, and is a hardy and vigorous plant, one might even say rather invasive (hence its frequent definition as a "weed").

Once you have started some, it is hardly necessary even to bother replanting the next year unless you managed to harvest every seed the previous late autumn/early winter. Fat hen is native to Europe, but quickly escaped early European gardens in North America (or came over accidentally in animal fodder and bedding), and now grows throughout the continent, as well as in South America, Africa, Australia, and Russia up through Siberia. It should be discouraged from growing among your other grains and various food crops due to its invasive and vigorous character. Still, it will thrive in conditions that are hard on more usual crops, and that could save your life in a bad year.

» Lemon juice: undiluted lemon juice kills sperm instantly, but is pretty rough on the vaginal mucosa as well. Diluted 1:1 with water, it was generally comparable to apple juice, both killing sperm steadily over a longer period (up to 60 minutes), although the pineapple was the most effective of the five juices tested (lemon, diluted lemon, pineapple, apple, aloe vera). The aloe vera was the least effective, but more effective than the control. The conclusion is that the acidity of the various juices was the primary cause of their effectiveness as spermicides (suggesting that vinegar would also do the job - Wolfe); high alkalinity may have a similar effect, but the juices tested in the study were all acid, with pH levels ranging from 2-3 (undiluted lemon juice) to 6 (aloe vera juice).

» Neem (Azadirachta indica) has been proven to be an effective spermicide, both in the form of the oil (from the seeds) and the form of extracts made from the leaves with water. Neem is also excellent for treating skin conditions and infections; the twigs make effective anti-microbial toothbrushes when chewed; the flowers are used for treating digestive disturbances; it lowers blood sugar well enough to be a concern regarding hypoglycaemia in people already on medication for that purpose; and it is a substantial enough booster of the immune system that it is not recommended for people with auto-immune diseases. Note that the seeds and oil can also be dangerous to children, though toxicity in adults is low! Neem grows readily from seed, and tolerates heat well (up to 50 C/122 F), but drops its leaves with any extended period below 5 C/41 F and tends to die when the temperatures get below freezing. While its soil should be moistened regularly, neem does not tolerate wet feet or poor draining; let the soil dry out between waterings. Growing it in pots that can be brought indoors during the winter (I recommend a pot on wheels, since neem is a tree that naturally has a very large root system; the bigger the pot, the happier the tree will be) is probably the best choice in most of Europe and North America. A healthy neem tree takes pruning, even fairly extensive pruning, quite in its stride; and you will need to do this for growing it in a pot.

» Soapberry, Chinese (Sapindus mukorossi) cream. The current product Consap, which is a cream made from the saponins in this tree's berries (which are also called "soap nuts", has been demonstrated to be efficacious, safe, and less irritating than common pharmaceutical spermicides such as nonoxynol-9.

» Chinese soapberry is native to the foothills of the Himalayas. It can be grown from seed, but the seeds are quite hard-shelled. They must be rubbed lightly with fine sandpaper (scarification), then soaked for 24 hours in warm water (a thermos and occasional replacement to keep the water warm are recommended; ½ tsp (2.5 gr) saltpetre to 1 pint of warm water may be helpful in softening the coat as well. It prefers warmth, full sunshine, and a well-drained clay-loam soil (as with most plants, drainage failure may lead to root rot), but is not particular about pH. Soapberry can tolerate poor and rocky soil quite well, but is not cold-tolerant and cannot take frosty winters; like neem, it may have to be pot-grown and pruned to keep it to a plausible height (outdoors it reaches 30-40 ft, or ca. 9-12 metres), and brought indoors in the wintertime. A soapberry tree takes ca. 10 years to start producing fruit. As well as its contraceptive uses, the hulls of the seeds can also be added, for instance, to one's laundry; they make an excellent gentle detergent that is currently gaining popularity in real life.

> » Extracts of the Southern Asian soapnut (Sapindus emarginatus) kill larvae and pupae of the Aedes aegypti mosquito, one of the main vectors of viral diseases such as dengue, yellow fever, and Zika, among others; this trait is likely to be shared among the other soapberries, but S. emarginatus was the one tested in the particular study. Likewise, Chinese soapberry (S. mukorossi) is the only tree in this family to have been specifically tested for spermicidal properties, but it is probable that the other soapberries (Western soapberry, Sapindus saponaria var. drummondi – Mexico and the southern United States; Florida, Sapindus marginatus – South Carolina to Florida; wingleaf, Sapindus saponaria var. saponaria – Florida Keys, Central America, Caribbean islands), which also contain high amounts of saponins and are used in the same manner as Chinese soapberry, would be efficacious for the purpose as well.

» Soapwort (Saponaria officinalis – also known as wild Sweet William, Bouncing Bet, and a number of other folk names). Thus far, all plant saponins tested (which include soapwort) have shown significant spermicidal activity. Saponins are the source of the mildly frothing "soap" that some plants produce naturally. In fact, you will want to grow soapwort for its hygienic purposes alone; it is an excellent source of soap which can be used straight from the plant (leaves and roots can both be used). Many European museums use soapwort for cleaning delicate old fabrics, as it is effective, but gentler and less likely to cause untowards effects than commercial soaps! It is also highly suited for sensitive skin, especially for infants. Soapwort is also a first-rate and attractive garden ground cover, hardy and spreading quickly by underground rhizome runners, with pretty small pale pink flowers and lush green foliage.

It grows very well in most temperate climates; it likes full sun to partial shade and moist, well-drained soil, but can tolerate a fair range of other conditions. Soapwort sprouts easily by seed, and can be propagated even more easily by rhizome division. In fact, if it likes its garden situation, it is inclined to become quite invasive; gardeners who are not depending on it to provide most of their hygienic needs (or as a spermicide) generally plant it in pots or other circumstances where it can be restrained from taking over the garden.

» Castile soap: the saponins in castile soap come from the plant oil, and are released by the reaction of the oil with the potassium hydroxide (lye). It is also a "gentler" soap than either most commercial soaps or soaps made from animal fat; less drying and less potentially irritating. If making a spermicidal cream, castile soap is really your only choice, since not only is it easier on the delicate internal membranes, but its plant saponins, though not yet studied regarding this purpose, are likely to contribute to the overall spermicidal effect. Directions for making castile soap are given in the sidebar to section II, 6f ("Ointments and Creams").

» Ionic (or colloidal) copper: unlike silver or gold, copper naturally dissolves slowly into ionic form in a liquid medium (this is why it is so effective for IUD use). Keep a piece of copper soaking in water constantly, boiling the two together to sterilize the water before use; or pressure-can a bunch of small jars of water with some copper in each. This is, in principle a short-term version of the copper IUD's constant slow ionic dissolution, although probably should be a supplementary spermicide, not the only substance relied on at any given time, since it has never been experimentally tested. Unlike ionic (or colloidal) silver, transmucosal absorption of ionic copper is considered quite safe.

d) Condoms

Before the prevention of HIV transmission became one of the main reasons for condom use – and even more, before rubber condoms became commonly available – condoms were made out of animal intestines (commonly lamb) or bladders, and soaked in brine to keep them flexible until needed. Bladders need only to be thoroughly washed and sterilized. Intestine condoms need rather more work to make them safe from use. The part of the intestine used is the caecum (a pouch found in sheep between the joining of upper and lower intestine), because sewing would be rather counter-productive, putting holes in something that is meant to contain small and very active cells. A nineteenth-century American receipt for home condom production goes as follows:

--Take the caecum of the sheep; soak it first in water, turn it on both sides, then repeat the operation in a weak ley of soda (potassium hydroxide lye – directions for making it are in a sidebar to section II, 6f – Wolfe), which must be changed every four or five hours for five or six successive times; then remove the mucus membrane with the nail; sulphur, wash in clean water, and then in soap and water; rinse, inflate, and dry.

--Next cut it to the required length and attach a piece of ribbon to the open end. Used to prevent infection or pregnancy. The different qualities consist of extra pains being taken in the above process, and in polishing, scenting, &c.

"Sulfuring" means fumigating with sulphur. The book from which this comes, The United States Practical Receipts Book (1849), may also be useful to you in a number of other regards, because it really does cover just about everything imaginable; though care must be taken to evaluate its recommendations in terms of modern knowledge. I am indebted to Esther Inglis-Arkell for printing the condom recipe and for the book recommendation and link (see above end-note for details on her article).

Another recipe, from ca. 1824, describes the manufacturing process as follows:

--Ordinary Condoms (Armour, Baudruches, Redingotes Anglaises) (Used to prevent venereal disease or pregnancy) are made from sheeps' intestina caeca soaked in water for some hours, turned inside out, macerated again in weak alkaline changed every 12 hours, scraped carefully to remove the mucous membrane, leaving the peritoneal and muscular coats; exposed to the vapour of burning brimstone (sulphur – Wolfe), washed with soap and water; blown up, dried, cut to length of 7-8 inches, bordered at the open end with a riband.

--Baudruches fines: soaked in weak ley (water drained from wood-ash – the lye-water from which soap is made, but diluted to avoid destroying the condom – Wolfe), turned inside out, dressed as before. Soaked in ley again, brimstoned, drawn smooth upon oiled moulds of a proper size, with the external coat of the gut next to the mould.

--Baudruches superfines: washed in 2 soapy waters after soaking in them for 24 hrs and very carefully dressed with the knife. Soaked in hard water for 3 days, the water being often changed; dried with a clean cloth, scented with essences, and being stretched on a glass mould, rubbed with a glass to polish them.

--Baudruches superfine doubles: in their moist state being on the mould, another is drawn over also moist, the 2 insides adhere together.

--Condoms should be soaked in water before use to make them supple.

If, for whatever reason, you have to sew the intestine's end, a French seam enclosing a regular seam, sewn with cotton thread if possible (absorbent, swells a little) and the tiniest needle you can find, is probably the best way to do this. The integrity of the condom is tested by the traditional method of, "fill it with water and see if it leaks anywhere"...because, as everyone knows, one little pinhole leak in a condom is quite enough to invalidate it! Even if no leaks can be found with the water test – well, a spermicide together with a condom is always a good idea, but I'd consider it absolutely necessary if the condom had to be sewn, and would maybe also use a sponge as well.

At least a sewn condom will contain the majority of the sperm; but there's too much risk that a few will escape and start their trek up into the uterus to rely on that method alone. Condoms that do not come with a handy rubber ring at the bottom to help them stay on need something else to secure them. Falloppio (yes, the guy who identified Fallopian tubes) used a ribbon about the bottom of his linen sheaths (soaked and lubricated with a herbal solution...a spermicidal combination with castile soap might be a really good idea if you have to try this) in the 16th century.

Interestingly, Falloppio performed one of the West's first large-scale trials - on the efficacy of his linen condoms as a prevention against syphilis, noting in De Morbo Gallico ("The French Disease") that he had provided these items to > 1000 soldiers, and not one of those men had contracted the disease. This can't really be called a proper clinical trial – no control group, no evaluation of their activities with the condoms or the disease-status of their partners, no information about how, or for how long, he followed his test subjects up. But then, considering the undeveloped state of medical ethics at the time, and the atrocities perpetuated by twentieth-century American medical researchers in the interest of establishing "control groups" for studying this disease in Tuskegee and Guatemala, it may be just as well that Falloppio didn't think about the issue.

Still, even given the uncontrolled state of his proto-trial, when we remember that syphilis was a great deal more virulent in his era than it is today, and had become a major scourge in Europe, his results says quite a lot about how well the Falloppio condom worked against very small and mobile organisms (yes, spirochaetes can swim, especially in viscous fluids that stop most other bacteria. So what blocks them from passing, also has a pretty good chance of blocking sperm). As well as sheep intestines, various animal bladders (including fish bladders), and linen, silk was also used, particularly in the Orient.

Very tight-woven silk such as parachute silk (or the more currently available nylon equivalent) would be particularly well-suited for this process: that which is airtight is definitely going to be semen-tight! Unlike the convenient rubber condom, condoms made of intestines, bladder, or cloth all can be sterilized and re-used – a good thing, since one sheep can only provide two condoms (caecum and bladder) unless you want to take the extra risk of sewing the business end!

E) Other Barrier Methods

i. The Cervical Cap

The cervical cap is a deep silicone or latex cup which fits over the external opening of the cervix to physically block sperm from entering. The edge is folded back to create a groove between the rim and the dome, into which, along with the bowl (the part in direct contact with the cervix) and the brim (the cervical-side edge), spermicidal gel is placed before the cap is inserted. It is held on by suction, and there is a small silicone or latex strap across the outer part of the dome so that it can easily be removed. While it may not be possible to make these after the Catastrophe, they are reusable (after cleaning), portable, and suitable for stockpiling. Advantages include: easily inserted and removed by oneself; low (though still always present) risk of pain, bleeding, or infection; no interference with the enjoyment of either partner; and no longer-term fertility restrictions. You can decide to use it, or not to use it, on the spot at any time, so if you have been using it regularly, but your heart suddenly tells you one evening that it's time for you to make a baby, all you have to do is not put it in that night.

The main disadvantage of the cervical cap is relatively lower effectiveness, especially for women who have already given birth. Efficacy is estimated at 84% for nulliparous women, but only 68-71% after having given birth. And that is with spermicidal gel. Also, you have to use it every single time you have sex, and keep adding spermicide before each go if you have multiple rounds in that 6-48 hour period that you're wearing it. The cervical cap does not work for emergency contraception. Once the sperm has reached the uterus, the cap is useless.

The cap can be inserted without assistance. It should be cleaned and sterilized if possible before each use, but the insertion process itself does not have to be sterile, as the vagina is not a sterile environment to begin with, and the cap never enters the womb. Just be careful that your hands have been well-washed first, and that you have no ragged edges on your nails or any other opportunity to scratch yourself, both in regards to insertion and in regards to position checks and removal later. Reach in with a finger until you feel your cervix (it is sometimes described as feeling "like the tip of a nose).

Once you have identified the position of your cervix – it may vary depending on stage of cycle and body position – put your spermicide in the bowl and grove and on the brim and the rim. Slide it into your vagina along the rear wall, keeping the tip of one finger on your cervix so that you can position the cup correctly, and slip the bowl over your cervix. Press the rim around your cervix until you are sure it is completely covered. The cervical cap should stay in place for at least six hours, and ideally up to two days (but no more than two days at one time, after sex. If you are going for seconds or thirds in a session, check the positioning between rounds to make sure it is still where it needs to be; if you are having sex multiple times in those two days, check the positioning shortly before each occasion and put more spermicide into your vagina. Since it is made of a very soft and flexible material, it should not cause any discomfort to you or your partner, however energetic you get.

To remove, squat, reach in and catch the strap, bear down, and gently rotate the cap to break the suction. Pull out by the strap. Wash with a mild soap and water (castile soap, soapwort, and soapberry are all very well suited to the purpose), and allow to air-dry for reuse. Do not powder it with anything. Between uses, check to confirm that no holes, cracks, or severely worn spots have developed. Mild changes in colour may occur, but do not mean anything. The cervical cap's integrity can be tested in the same way as a condom's: fill it with water and see if it leaks. Do not use the cervical cap while menstruating, or leave it on more than six hours as you approach the time of month when menstruation is expected, as it would significantly increase your risk of toxic shock syndrome.

Your chances of becoming pregnant at this time are very low in any case. Not non-existent – depending on length and regularity of your cycle, which can vary quite substantially both according to the individual and according to her circumstances, it is entirely possible to become pregnant while menstruating (lowest risk is in the first two days of menstruation) – but quite low. As mentioned above, if you are quite committed to not becoming pregnant under your current circumstances, it is important to use some method or combination of methods of birth control even during menstruation. Just not the cervical cap.

Using the cap should also be avoided if you are allergic or highly sensitive to silicone/latex; within six weeks of the end of a pregnancy (regardless of outcome, timing, etc.); if you have ever had toxic shock syndrome or a cervical condition (such as a diagnosis of dysplasia); or if you or your partner is HIV-positive. Do not use a spermicide to which you are sensitive or allergic; many people find nonoxynol-9 intolerable, and anyone can find themselves allergic to any plant. Cervical caps in regular use generally stay good for about a year.

The only warning is: cervical size may increase following pregnancy (regardless of the outcome or its cause), and a refitting is usually required at that time. Significant weight loss (> 15 lbs/7 kg or so) may also change the size required, which is important to consider, as the odds are that you will lose weight after the Catastrophe – maybe a lot of weight, depending on your body-fat and activity levels (and food storage/access) when the Catastrophe hit. The FemCap brand, according to the company's safety guidelines, comes in three sizes, measured at the inner rim diameter. 22 mm – nullipara. 28 mm – woman who has been pregnant, but not had a vaginal delivery of a full or close to full-term-sized (> roughly 2 kg/4.5 lb birthweight) baby. 30 mm – vaginal delivery of full or close to full-term-sized baby. If you don't get the chance to visit a health-care practitioner for a personal fitting, these are not bad guidelines to go by.

Surgically scrubbing your hands requires antiseptic soap, a small sterilized sponge and nail pick, and running water. If you don't have a pump, you may need an assistant with a bucket and a large quantity of clean water.

Your hands must stay above your elbows at all times, so that runoff (and accompanying bacteria drip off your elbows, not back onto your hands. Wet your hands and forearms and scrub with the soap. Wash from palm to elbows in a series of straight downwards motions. Soap again and rub palms and finger undersides together, interlacing extended and slightly spread fingers and rubbing vigorously to get the spaces between them. More soap, and proceed to the sides and backs; again, rubbing between the fingers, this time with the palm-side of each hand against the back of the other. Grasp each thumb in the palm of the other hand and rotate several times. Scrub fingernail beds and fingertips in a circular motion on the palm of the opposite hand. Rinse soap off, being very sure that all water drips down towards your elbows, and repeat.

Clean under your nails with the sterilized nail pick. Soap and wash as before using the sterilized sponge. Rinse and repeat the first sequence again. If you do not have a sterilized towel, allow your hands to air-dry before gloving. Do not touch anything with them! Unless your hands are actually doing something, they should stay ca. 6-8" from your body, in the area between your shoulders and waist (commonly known as the T-rex position).

Shelf life (again, according to FemCap safety guidelines) has been tested at ca. 3 years. This, unfortunately, means that you can't just stock up enough cervical caps to get you through your fertile years. This means you may have to improvise a mold and make your own after three years. When scavenging or stockpiling, keep an eye out for silicone that is food-safe (intended for making molds for candy, etc). Aquarium silicone is also a good choice, because, by its nature, it is specifically designed not to contain any toxic chemicals (given that it is constantly in contact with water in which creatures live). Unless you or one of your survival group is particularly good at fine crafts, a homemade cap (or diaphragm) is unlikely to be even as effective as a commercial one, which is not exactly the most effective method to begin with even when spermicide is added, so don't depend on it alone to do the job!

II. The Diaphragm

The diaphragm is similar to the cervical cap: a small, flexible blocking device that fits over the end of your cervix to physically block sperm from entering your womb. It resembles a tiny bowler hat with a rolled rim. It is usually larger than the cervical cap, and may not be quite as comfortable.Like the cervical cap, it is filled and coated with spermicide; it is inserted and placed over the cervix in much the same way.

Leaving it in for 6-24 hours after sex (and adding vaginal spermicide each time if having more sex while it is still in) is recommended; leaving it longer, or using it during menstruation, presents a risk of toxic shock syndrome. Also like the cervical cap, the diaphragm usually requires an initial fitting, and a different size may be required after any pregnancy (again, regardless of outcome). Storage, use life, and shelf life are similar to those of the cervical cap.

!

Sterile gloving (if you have stocked up on packs of sterile gloves):

Either pull the pack open by the corner, touching only the outside of the pack, before you scrub, or get an assistant to do it for you.

Slide one hand into the appropriate glove. You will see that the cuffs are folded over. With your bare hand, touching only the part of the cuff that will be on the inside (in contact with you), pull the glove down into place, but do not turn the cuff back yet.

Put on the other glove. Since your gloved hand is sterile, you may touch the second glove anywhere. Flip down the cuff (if you have a sterile gown, it goes over the cuff of the gown). Insert a couple of fingers of the fully gloved hand inside the cuff of the first one (touching only the part that will be on the outside, because the gloved hand is now sterile) and flip it down in the same manner.

Return hands to the T-Rex position. You will hold them in this position whenever they are not doing anything, until you are ready to take them off.

If you touch anything non-sterile with them (such as, if you have to connect up the Del-Em cannula yourself), you must put on a new pair of gloves. Have one ready just in case (not on the sterile field, the wrappers are not sterile!).

III. Menstrual Extraction

If herbal methods fail or if the toxicity of available herbs is a problem, perhaps the best post-Catastrophe option when lacking the ability to perform surgical abortions is a recent technique known as "menstrual extraction". While no invasive procedure can be called perfectly safe, menstrual extraction is considerably safer than a D&C, as no rigid or edged items are introduced into the uterus. The technique was designed, at least in part, as a way to avoid restrictive abortion laws in a manner which women without specific medical training could apply themselves and which was safer than most herbal remedies, restoring women's personal bodily autonomy where it had been denied.

It has also been used in the medical profession, in many cases by general practitioners who wished to offer this service to their patient (because of the relative ease and low risk, it is a suitable procedure for a GP office). In legal terms, if the woman has not had a positive, recorded pregnancy diagnosis, menstrual evacuation is not considered to be "abortion"; merely a safety procedure to avoid toxicity from retained menstrual substances.

This procedure is meant to be performed no later than 7 weeks from the end of the last menstrual period, and, assuming that to be the case, is 99% successful and notable for its safety profile, ease of performance, and cheapness. The apparatus, known as a Del-Em after its creators, is easily constructed. It requires a Mason jar or something similar (tight-fitting lid in which two holes can be made), flexible tubing small enough that the end of a 4-5 mm cannula can fit tightly into it at one end and the syringe tip at the other, caulking, a one-way valve, a soft flexible 4 or 5 mm cannula, a large syringe (without a needle!), and a speculum.

If you cannot get a cannula, two sections of tubing, each 2-3" long, are inserted through the holes in the jar lid, with caulking put around them to ensure that the jar stays airtight. One end of the tube is connected to the one-way valve in such a manner that the air will not flow up to the cannula. A short piece of tubing is connected to the syringe on the other side of the valve. It should not be possible to fully empty the air in the syringe if this has been done correctly (valve pointing the right direction, connection secure. The end of the other tube will be connected to the cannula.

Place that end into a cup of antiseptic/antibacterial liquid (e.g. Betadine, or ethanol if you cannot get Betadine) and pull the syringe; if all connections are secure, liquid will flow into the tube. Expel the liquid and wrap the apparatus in a sterilized cloth. To perform the procedure, sterilize all items that are not already in sterile packaging (these items are opened without touching the inside of the packaging and dropped from the package directly onto the sterilized tray), and use sterilized tongs to place them on a sterilized tray where they can easily be reached. This is your sterile field! Do not allow anything non-sterilized to touch it!

If you have not stockpiled Betadine or similar, or have run out, high-percentage (ideally 90% plus – what you get out of a still before diluting it for human consumption) ethanol may be used for sterilization, or metal tools may be boiled at a rolling boil for 20 minutes. Allow the sterilizing solution to air-dry. You will need: sterile gloves if available or a complete surgical scrub-in of your hands and forearms if there are no rubber gloves any more (if there are, still do the scrub-in before you put the gloves on); sterilizable tray or tabletop (smooth copper, smooth silver, or sheathing of either metal is a good choice, given that both have antimicrobial functions even before being wiped down with alcohol or another sterilizing solution) your Del-Em apparatus; a 4-5 mm sterilized cannula or equivalent (thin flexible plastic tube with a smooth pointed, perforated tip); sterilized and, if there is any way for you to manage it, warmed speculum (cold specula are.

I am firmly informed, particularly not nice in one's tender areas); at least two sets of sterilized tongs; cotton swabs; Betadine or sterilized water, which may also be copper-infused (boil at least 20 minutes and allow to cool; adding ionic copper, putting a piece of copper into the water at the start of the boiling process, or leaving copper to steep in the water for several days beforehand and then boiling, may provide some extra antimicrobial protection. Do not do this with silver, which is considerably less safe in regards to absorption through mucosa); flashlight (if possible – otherwise you may have to resort to a candle and an extra mirror to reflect the light where you want it); possibly a mirror; and ideally at least one assistant to hold the latter items for you and connect up the cannula to the tube when the time comes. Half an hour to an hour before the procedure, depending on the medication used, the woman should be given moderate relaxant/analgesic drugs to limit uterine cramping and discomfort.

Valerian (or Valium, if you've still got any) is often recommended for its relaxant effects; hemp flowers (ingestion method of the patient's choice, but if a lipid extract is being used, administer ca. 2 hours before the procedure) or a small amount of poppy extract (equivalent to no more than 25 mg codeine/2.5 mg morphine – you do not want to hurt the patient, but if something starts to go very wrong, she needs to be able to tell you right away) may also be used. Inhaled cannabis, being quick to take effect, may be administered by an assistant as requested during the procedure. This is preferable to inhaled opium, as cannabis has direct muscle-relaxant and antispasmodic effects, and if the patient is in enough pain to need more opium than the minimum initial amount, something may be going wrong and you seriously need to back off and reconsider.

The woman is placed in "lithotomy position", on her back with her legs spread, knees bent, and feet up (a position familiar to anyone who has ever experienced or performed a vaginal examination). OB/GYN stirrups are ideal, but assistants to support her legs may be required if you don't have stirrups, as the position is very uncomfortable to maintain without support. The speculum is lubricated by your assistant (you're still keeping your hands sterile, but the vagina is not a sterile environment, so at this point it is a "clean" procedure, not a "sterile" one), gently inserted, and the vagina opened. Be as gentle as possible, especially if you are a man and have never experienced it for yourself; this is not a pleasant experience for the patient!

Take one of your sets of sterilized tongs and dip a cotton ball in Betadine or sterilized water/water-copper solution (do not use alcohol, it is far too harsh for the delicate mucosa. Sterilized water proved as effective for the purpose as chlorhexidine, the other surgical antiseptic cleaner). Clean the vaginal walls and the cervix. Your assistant is shining the flashlight (or your best approximation) in so that you can see what you are doing. The external os (mouth) of the cervix looks like a raised ring around a round perforation (woman who has never delivered) or vertical slit (woman who has delivered).

The cannula should only be touched by hand at the last 2" of the end furthest from entry. Use sterilized tongs to guide it more closely. Do not let it touch the non-sterile vaginal walls. Insert the cannula slowly into the opening. After ca. ¾"(roughly 2 cm), you should feel resistance; this is the internal os. Cramping may begin at this point. Continue, gently but firmly, to push until you are past the resistance. The cannula is now inside the uterus. Your assistant will now remove all the air from the Del-Em jar with the syringe, putting one finger over the end of the open tube to create a vacuum; attach the far end of the cannula; and slowly remove any remaining air. Begin to move the cannula in a slow sideways back-and-forth manner, rotating it as you go. Remain in each area until you feel it go from soft to ribbed and hard.

There will be some blood and white material (the foetal tissue) coming through the cannula. When the whole uterus is hard, and no more blood or white material is coming out, the uterus may be considered clean. Remove the cannula and cover the patient. If she wishes to be alone, check in on her every 15 minutes or so to make sure she is doing all right, and check her vital signs (pulse, breathing, blood pressure if you can) at least hourly or if she starts showing any indications of distress. Keep someone with her overnight unless she requests otherwise; if she seems well, check vital signs ca. every 2 hours after the first four have passed without incident, and make sure that someone at least stays within earshot so that she can call if she experiences anything untowards. The complex aftercare is not considered necessary in a GP setting or the like in real life – the procedure actually is very simple and low-risk, as it was designed to be carried out by people with minimal training in order to avoid having to go into a hostile medical/legal system - but the improvisations that the Catastrophe may require in terms of sterilization and apparatus construction make it a good idea to be even excessively careful; no harm can be done by excess caution in this instance.

Finding a sterile lubricant will probably be your biggest challenge, once you have run out of all those nice plastic packages of the stuff that health-care professionals use in real life now. Your best option will probably be pressure-canning a number of tiny jars of oil or a herbal ointment formulated for anti-microbial action (no need to worry about volatile components escaping when you pressure-can!). While it is reportedly tricky to maintain the heat precisely enough to reliably sterilize the jars' contents on a wood-fired stove or the like, requiring constant monitoring of fire and temperature - this is a skill which all survivors, or at least someone in every family or group, had better have in any case in order to keep their people fed and not dying of botulism.

IV. Later Herbal Terminations

The further along a pregnancy is, the more significant any attempt to terminate it has to be, and the more dangerous and more often unsuccessful the process is (even leaving out the increased risk of herbal toxicity with higher dosages and/or more prolonged use). The herbs classed as "emmenagogues" (menstruation inducers – usually a term meaning, "terminates a pregnancy before it could have been ascertained by anything but a missed period in the past, thereby avoiding legal and social difficulties") are most effective and safest in the first four to six weeks, and ideally administered shortly after the intercourse of concern, or at least as soon as the first menstrual period fails to occur on time (assuming that the woman in question is normally reasonably regular).

As well as being notoriously unsafe, herbal abortions after a maximum time of six weeks from conception are notoriously inefficient. In real life, it appears to be quite common for a herbal abortion attempt to require a follow-up clinical abortion - although considerable question remains as to how many successful herbal abortions are never reported at all/are passed off as natural miscarriages, especially in areas where social stigmata or legal penalties are a concern. Among reported herbal abortion attempts, ratios vary but are invariably <50% successful, including the cases where additional methods are used (for instance, herbs plus instrumental manipulation or self-trauma).

However, many herbal abortions are only reported because of adverse effects requiring medical intervention or because the woman has sought out clinical assistance after failure of self-treatment, which makes it probable that an accurate evaluation of the success rate of all herbal abortions cannot be obtained...especially since the most common use is in situations where a woman cannot procure a safer medical or surgical abortion for legal or sometimes financial reasons, and will therefore not report an herbal attempt unless she is in danger of death (and sometimes, sadly, not even then). A recent scientific article stated, "The purpose of this report is to describe the herbal products used to induce abortions, and to enhance awareness and understanding of their toxic effects." They achieved this by basing their study entirely on calls received by the Montevideo Poison Center regarding herbs taken with the intention of causing abortion: that is, selecting only instances that either had failed and caused poisoning or had succeeded but also caused very significant poisoning.

Only 23 out of 86 cases (in which 8 of the 23 had also used other methods) actually aborted; and five of those (one with instrumental manipulation, the other four with herbs alone) died. These figures appear terrifying, and do present some real and serious warnings. For instance, "ruda" (the Spanish name for rue; Ruta graveolens), was used in four of the deaths and the traditional mixed herbal remedy Carachipita (pennyroyal, oregano, pearlfruit [Margyricarpus pennatus], and marsh rosemary [Limonium brasiliensis aka Statice brasiliensis]) in one; multiple organ failure occurred with rue, Carachipita, arnica (Arnica montana - excellent topical for bruises, and every herbalist in the world will start out by warning you that arnica-containing products should never be taken internally or even used on broken skin), and greater burdock (Arctium lappa).

Clearly, these are not good herbs to try ingesting. However, what we do not have is any data on the overall number of herbal abortions attempted in the place and time period of the study, or on how many of them were successful without major incident (or, contrariwise, how many attempts resulted in trips directly to the hospital or morgue rather than calls to the Poison Center). There was also no indication regarding how far along any of the pregnancies in the study were at the time when the attempts were made. Tisserand and Young observe, regarding the toxicity and abortifacient qualities of parsley essential oil, that "The cases recorded tend to be the worst ones, in which medical attention has been urgently sought".

In hospital, severe bleeding following any delivery (regardless of the age or vitality status of the deliveree) is treated with:

IV fluid resuscitation (normal saline or Ringer's lactate).

Blood transfusions if more than 2 liters (roughly 4 pints) is lost. Bimanual compression/massage: the person present with the best combination of small hands and experience puts one hand into the woman's vagina to press on the uterus from inside its anterior fornix (the little cavity at the front, on top of the exterior cervical opening), and presses on the abdomen from the outside with the other hand set on the fundus (top) of the womb.

This is as close to direct pressure as possible, and the massage also helps stimulate the uterus to regain its muscle tone and activity. Manual examination and cleaning may be necessary if there is a suspicion of retained placenta or other materials. This generally requires some degree of anaesthesia, the degree depending on the patient, the situation, and the urgency.

Injection of oxytocin (a bolus of 5 IU, or 20 IU in a litre of normal saline run as fast as possible, intravenously) promotes uterine contraction, which puts pressure on the blood vessels. Note that in a post-Catastrophe emergency, if herbs are being used for this purpose, they need to not be ones with a high toxicity; it would be far too easy to fatally poison the mother while trying to save her life. Consider other relevant factors as well; for instance, if an angelica must be used (not the best idea in an haemorrhagic emergency) Angelica archangelica might be a better choice than dong quai, if it is true that its effects in suppressing clotting are lesser; but this is not certain. A strong raspberry leaf tea may be the best choice, as it stimulates the uterus and has few side effects.

Uterine packing (preferably including a liberal addition of astyptic such as bistort), ligation of uterine blood supply, arterial embolization, and even hysterectomy if necessary, are all options if the bleeding persists.

This may be a situation like the "high Swedish suicide rates" of the 1960s – where it was eventually established, not that Swedes were more likely to kill themselves than people from other countries (they weren't), but that they were markedly more willing to acknowledge and record death by suicide than other Westerners in general; the trend evened out sharply as international means of reporting and recording suicide standardized.

Or it may not. We have no way of telling. In terms of efficiency, however, we do know that medical abortions (by means of ingesting pharmaceutical drugs, as opposed to surgical abortions) have a high success rate in the first eight weeks, ca. 97-98%.

This drops significantly after eight weeks. It can, therefore, be said with considerable confidence that the efficiency of herbal abortions - which function by similar mechanisms - whatever the initial success rate, will follow a similar pattern: the earlier measures are taken, the more successful (and safer) they will be. Timing is, in short, crucial.

After six to eight weeks from conception, the success rates even of modern pharmaceutical abortions plummet rapidly; surgery may be the only reliably effective and reasonably safe recourse thereafter.

A trained person with the right tools can undoubtedly perform a D&C without much risk even in a post-Catastrophe environment...or one of the other, more gruesome, extractions that necessity sometimes requires to save the mother's life (intrauterine death, if spontaneous stillbirth does not occur quickly, may require transvaginal intrauterine dismemberment, up to and including, at a late stage, syringe extraction of the deceased baby's brain/collapse of the skull to allow extraction with minimal physical trauma – an extremely horrible thing to perform or contemplate, but still far less horrible than a woman dying of sepsis from the dead child in her womb); or even the final and most dangerous resort, breaching the body cavity to perform a premature Caesarian.

But if your survival group does not include a health-care professional with the appropriate experience to perform whatever procedure is needed, then even a fairly simple procedure such as a D&C becomes vastly more dangerous both in terms of bleeding and in terms of infection. This was the cause of many terrible and unnecessary deaths among young women before abortion became legal in most Western countries, and still casts its nightmarish shadow today.

Ultimately, there is no one with the moral right to make the final risk-benefit judgement and decision in such cases but the woman herself; however, making good judgements requires good information. The author may, of course, have deliberately put you in a situation where a high-risk abortion is your only alternative.

The favourite version is the repressive theocracy of one kind or another; but one can equally envision, say, a situation such as the Chinese, except with a demand for population growth rather than the enforced abortions which were one means of upholding the one-child-per-family law. If that is the case...well, as an author of fiction myself, I can only say that I am very grateful that there is no way for a character to effectively sue (or beat up or execute) their author, but I can certainly see why some characters would want to.

The major risks are:

Herbal poisoning. Many of the best-known herbal abortifacients can be fatal in larger doses, especially if an essential oil or strong extract is used. These include tansy, pennyroyal, rue, black cohosh, and parsley, among many others. It is an unfortunate fact that, generally, if an herb is strong enough to kill the more developed foetus and/or force the mother's uterus to expel its contents prematurely, it is strong enough to present a danger to the mother.

The pharmaceuticals used for medical abortions are safer because they more accurately mimic the body's endogenous molecules (mifepristone, misoprostol), or else, like chemotherapy, target a difference between the activity of the developing foetal cells and the maternal cells (methotrexate); and again, they are limited in the time range of their efficacy.

Bleeding. This is a significant risk and one of the most common causes of death in any delivery of foetus from uterus, no matter how premature or timely, natural or induced. The highest risk is when an untrained person attempts a surgical abortion; but many women have bled to death following apparently trouble-free natural births, even in hospital with all possible care to hand.

Infection. As with bleeding, infection is a huge risk at and shortly following the conclusion of any pregnancy, regardless of timing or outcome, or whether natural or induced. It was one of the major causes, probably the major cause, of maternal and infant death in the era before sterilization was understood and instituted.

In current practice, a significant rise in maternal temperature during delivery is grounds to switch a natural delivery to an emergency Caesarian and dose both mother and baby with empirical antibiotics until the lab results come back. The highest infection risk is in surgical abortions, particularly in circumstances where these cannot be performed in a proper hospital or clinic; the lowest risk by far is in very early miscarriage (whether natural or induced); but the possibility must be considered in all cases. Proper medical hygiene is the best defence, but often insufficient.

If antibiotics are still available, the caregiver or individual should be alert for symptoms such as a significant rise or drop in temperature (38 C/100-100.4 F or above, or 36 C/96.8 F or below, are usually considered the points at which significant concern starts) and be ready to administer them.

If not, Appendix IV lists a number of possible antibacterial herbs which have proven to be potentially effective in the lab, though in most cases have not yet been examined in live animals or humans. Since E. coli contamination from either the anal region or a urinary tract infection is very much a concern in this case, as are Gram-positives such as Streptococcus and Staphylococcus species, keeping both Gram-negative and Gram-positive, and/or general broad-spectrum coverage in mind when preparing aftercare for a birth, natural miscarriage, or abortion is of significant importance.

Undiagnosed ectopic pregnancy. Inducing an abortion in what turns out to have been an ectopic pregnancy (embryo implanted somewhere that is not the uterus) is the same as suffering a natural rupture of an ectopic pregnancy, which carries a risk of death now and will carry a far greater one after the Catastrophe. Whether you triggered the rupture or it happened because the surrounding structures could not support the embryo (which probably was going to occur in the relatively short term anyway, regardless of anything you did or didn't do) does not matter – the results will be the same - but at least in real life, in the Western world, most women do get ultrasounds to guard against this possibility (as well as many other things that can go wrong).

Of course, in real life, if the pregnancy is ectopic, you no longer have to be concerned about an herbal abortion. Even in a country such as Ireland, the medical system will provide a medical and/or surgical one in order to save your life from an embryo that never had a chance of survival – a truly heartbreaking situation when the child is wanted, but quite possibly a relief when an abortion is needed for other reasons. The characteristic symptoms of ectopic pregnancy are pain, amenorrhea, and bleeding – but only 50% of patients present with all three, and many patients present with one or all three for other reasons. Sometimes a mass can be felt in the area surrounding the uterus (suggesting Fallopian tube implantation, which is a particularly bad thing due to the likelihood of tubal rupture); the abdomen is tender in most.

But unless the embryo can be physically felt where it shouldn't be, it is virtually impossible to diagnose an ectopic pregnancy with true certainty by clinical examination; an ultrasound is required. Caught early, the treatment is usually a medical abortion via methotrexate which causes the death and allows the reabsorption of the misplaced foetus. If this is ineffective or other problems such as local rupture, etc., present, laparoscopic surgery may be needed to remove the foetus and/or deal with any damage that has occurred.

Failure of complete expulsion of all uterine contents. As after delivering a live child, any portion of the uterine contents remaining inside after either a natural or an induced foetal death provides a quick road to infection, sepsis, and maternal death. The risk is present even in otherwise apparently uncomplicated normal deliveries, very serious in deliveries where the placenta has broken up; and intermediate (depending on stage of pregnancy and circumstances) in both natural and induced miscarriages, more so as the pregnancy advances.

!

Normal saline contains salt and water in roughly the same proportions as most human body fluids. It is water with 0.9% regular salt (as in, table salt) added. The proportions are measured as 9 grams to a litre, or 1.5 teaspoons to roughly a quart (salt is heavier than water, weighing 6 gr/teaspoon).

Warning: the first site that came up in a Google search on this subject was prepared by someone clueless about measurements, and recommended 9 grams per litre or one teaspoon per cup – a smidgen over 24 grams per litre. Several other sites on the same first search page repeated the error.

If the Imperial proportions, instead of the metric proportions, of this recommendation were used on a patient who needed fluid replacement, they would shortly be in far worse need of fluid replacement (and if it was used IV, quite possibly in danger of brain damage and death).

As for the Falloppio condom – a higher percentage of salt could be used without risking severe damage, but it depends on how tolerant the user and his partner are regarding, "how it feels to have seawater dry on your privates without getting a chance to shower it off".

Treatment may involve induction of further uterine contractions in hopes of clearing the remnants, or physical cleaning of the uterus by means of suction (see below, "Menstrual Evacuation"), dilation and curettage (D&C), or sometimes manually where the internal space has been sufficiently enlarged. Non-fatal but severe damage to the foetus. If other methods of removal are not available following a failed attempt at herbal termination, toxicity can cause an increased risk of delivering a child that is not only already unwanted and possibly disastrous to the mother's life/health/well-being, but damaged physically and/or mentally, compounding the fundamental problem.

Medical abortions are currently performed by administering mifepristone (an anti-progesterone drug which causes endometrial breakdown and encourages detachment of the embryo, softens and dilates the cervix, stimulates prostaglandin release, and makes the uterus more prone to prostaglandin-induced contraction), usually followed by misoprostol (a prostaglandin analogue). Misoprostol is also used with methotrexate (blocks folic acid, preventing DNA synthesis and hence cellular reproduction), particularly in regards to terminating ectopic pregnancies.

Therefore, if absolutely necessary after the Catastrophe, when the safer and more effective drugs are no longer available and if there is no one around who can perform a surgical abortion in a reasonably safe manner, a combination of juniper berry decoction, wild carrot seeds, and asafoetida if available, taken for up to five days, followed by one of the herbs that stimulate uterine contractions if needed, might be attempted. Success is possible, especially in the first four to six weeks after conception (or if the plot needs you to succeed at it), but – at least as far as the limited and problematical data we have tends to show – failure might be more likely.

V. Bacterial Venereal Disease and Yeast

In real life, Westerners often tend to underestimate the dangers prevented by the bacterial venereal diseases (syphilis, gonorrhoea, chlamydia), because these are usually easily and effectively treated by antibiotics. Although resistance has slowly been developing, notably in some strains of gonorrhoea, syphilis and gonorrhoea are generally still quite vulnerable to a penicillin injection (or azithromycin, doxycycline, or ceftriaxone for those allergic to penicillin; although drug resistance has led to recent guidelines recommending two antibiotics: a cephalosporin such as ceftriaxone or cefuroxime plus either azithromycin or doxycycline). A single dose of azithromycin or doxycycline usually suffices for chlamydia, and is commonly given on principle along with treatment for either of the other two, given how common and easily spread chlamydia is.

These drugs may not be available even shortly after the Catastrophe, depending on circumstances; and definitely won't be available forever, unless you learn how to recognise the penicillin mould under a microscope and refine your own. If you do (or if you have a stash of pre-Catastrophe pharmaceuticals), know that the teas of rosehips and pomegranate blossoms have been shown to have a synergistic anti-microbial effect when used with ampicillin (a penicillin-drug), although they are antagonistic to ceftriaxone and erythromycin (in the same antibiotic family as azithromycin) and should not be used with those drugs.

Since homemade penicillin is not exactly going to be of the most reliable concentration, the concurrent use of rosehips, which grow in almost any climate imaginable, would probably be an extremely good idea. For the author, in the interest of realism, the spread and damage of venereal diseases after the Catastrophe (or in a pre-penicillin era) is something that cannot be readily ignored or discounted. Diana Gabaldon emphasises this point very well, although her heroine is able to deal with the problem via syringes of home-cultured penicillin; and as mentioned before, the eighteenth century may have had many health problems – but antibiotic-resistant bacterial strains were not among them.

S.M. Stirling brings venereal diseases up as a plot point in the Emberverse series, but fails to follow through: a remarkably promiscuous early warlord catches gonorrhoea (probably, from the description) from one of his "numberless concubines", and passes it on to his wife, who is only able, with great difficulty, to bear one child (required by the entire plot arc of the series. With a 50% male-female transmission rate, and given the nightly activity and varied companionship of the warlord in question, it is safe to assume that quite a lot of young women left his bed with a dose before he got treated himself; and half of those would not have shown any symptoms.

Given described behaviours of the male portion of that society at that time (and for generations to come), Patient Zero (the unidentified woman from whom the warlord caught it) could well have ended up infecting a significant proportion of the society; while other groups in the same world were notably free about sleeping around and reproducing as the spirit moved them – even with an interesting stranger who just rode into town - when not committed to a relationship, if equally reliable about keeping oaths of marriage once made.

It seems likely that venereal disease would swiftly have become a major problem in the world of the Emberverse – as it would in any circumstances with dwindling supplies of antibiotics and rubber condoms, and no health departments to trace, inform, and offer treatment to contacts of identified cases. But then, that world differs slightly from our own in many ways prior to the Change, so maybe these diseases just weren't as prevalent or easily transmitted? Only the author knows – and a lot of faults can be glossed over with the "It's my world and it's not quite the same as our world" line.

The Falloppio linen condom, as mentioned above, proved to be a remarkably effective protector against syphilis, and given the mobility of spirochaetes, would very likely work as well against gonorrhoea and chlamydia, or better. Unfortunately, we do not know exactly what Dr. Falloppio was soaking his prophylactics in; only that it was a solution of salts and/or herbs. Bismuth subsalicylate (the active ingredient of Pepto-Bismol and several other digestive remedies) or another soluble bismuth salt would probably be the best option if you have no other choice, along with several of the herbs with Gram-negative antimicrobial effects listed at the end of this section.

The water-soluble copper salts, unfortunately, tend to burn or severely irritate skin on contact (and are quite toxic via inhalation or oral ingestion); but there might be something to be gained by storing the Falloppio condom in water or a normal saline mixture, perhaps laid between a couple of sheets of copper in hopes of absorbing enough ions to make a difference (not to mention discouraging other bacteria from invading during storage). Other antibacterials such as honey could present certain issues of practicality and comfort, though an oil soak (essential oils suitably diluted in a carrier oil for mucous membranes, ca. 3-5% total) might actually aid in sealing and lubricating a cloth condom.

A) Syphilis (Treponema pallidum pallidum)

Although it is not the extremely virulent, literally face-eating and often fairly swiftly fatal, disease it was when it first hit Europe, untreated syphilis still presents a number of major dangers. Long-term syphilis can cause severe neurological damage, as well as potentially damage to the aorta (the major blood vessel leaving the heart). Syphilis in a pregnant woman can also cross the placental barrier, resulting in deformity and neurological damage to the child. The estimated prevalence of syphilis worldwide is 0.5% in men, 0.2-1.3% in women worldwide.

The first symptom of syphilis is a firm, usually (but not always) painless and non-itchy genital chancre or set of chancres, appearing 3-90 days (average 21 days) after the initial infection. The chancre may occur externally or, for the receptive party, internally (e.g., cervix, anus, mouth/throat). First-stage syphilitic chancres are very contagious; most transmission occurs via these sores. The chancre may be as small as 3 mm or as large as slightly over an inch (30 mm), and characteristically starts as a spot which raises into a lump and then ulcerates, usually with clean, sharp, borders. Lymph nodes in the area may become enlarged ca. 7-10 days after the chancre first appears.

A fairly high proportion of people either do not show, or (particularly women, where the manifestation is often internal and would not be noticed unless she is regularly, for instance, inserting and removing a cervical cap or diaphragm and feels a lump or rough spot) do not notice the first-stage chancre. Second-stage syphilis normally appears ca. 4-10 weeks after the primary infection, though it may take longer if the first stage has a more delayed appearance. It is characterized by a symmetrical, reddish-pink rash on the body and extremities (including palms and soles), which does not itch and may become bumpy (papular) or form pustules.

Flat or warty white patches (condyloma latum) may appear on the genitals and other mucous membranes (rectum, mouth, throat, inside of the nose). Vaguer systemic symptoms are common, including malaise, fever, sore throat, headaches, hair loss, and headaches; rarely, there is inflammation of the joints, liver, kidneys, or individual nerves. These symptoms usually resolve within three to six weeks, but may reoccur. Third-stage syphilis can be gummous (largely benign, but may be disfiguring and distressing; characterized by soft inflammatory lumps that resemble tumours; these appear 1-46 years after the initial infection); neurological (syphilitic meningitis; general or partial paralysis; tabes dorsalis, which is a degeneration of spinal tracts causing loss of balance, loss of sensation, and often shooting pains in the legs, and is frequently associated with syphilitic dementia.

The pupils may constrict when focusing on close objects, but not in response to bright light); or cardiovascular (syphilitic aortitis; may lead to aortic aneurysms, which, if they burst, are often fatal even with immediate response and full modern hospital resources). Late stage neurosyphilis is likely to require hospitalization and IV penicillin (or alternate antibiotic for the allergic). Congenital syphilis is the form passed down to infants in the womb. If the child survives to birth, characteristics include the "saddle-nose" deformity (the bridge of the nose is sunken); unilateral enlargement of the sternal end of the collarbone; "saber shins" (shins are bowed sharply forwards); liver and spleen enlargement; lung inflammation; and fevers, among other maladies.

These may only become apparent in the first two years (early congenital) or even later (late congenital), rather than being obvious at birth. Poor feeding and (very contagious) runny nose are common early signs; deafness, anaemia, and jaundice also occurs. Death is usually by bleeding into the lungs. Prior to the development of penicillin, there were many quack remedies for syphilis, mercury (both oral and via genital irrigation) being both the most common and the most dangerous in and of itself. There was one that actually worked, although it sounds more bizarre than the quack cures. Namely: an Austrian physician by the name of Julius Wagner-Jauregg discovered that the repeated high fevers caused by malaria (he used Plasmodium vivax, the least aggressive form of malarial parasite) actually could cure syphilis; the malaria itself could then be cured by the application of quinine. Dr. Wagner-Jauregg received the Nobel Prize for this in 1927.

The treatment itself was still dangerous (ca. 15% mortality rate), and was gratefully abandoned as soon as penicillin showed itself effective against syphilis; but it is worth knowing about. Other means of raising body temperature were also used; syphilis has been demonstrated to be susceptible to high body temperatures. The chief problem with fever therapy for syphilis is that the therapeutic index is quite low: the body temperature needs to be raised as high as possible for as long as possible (Wagner-Jauregg allowed 12-15 febrile episodes before initiating treatment for the malaria). Spirochaetes and syphilitic cankers disappeared in rabbits whose body temperatures were kept at 42-44 C/107.6-111.2 F for thirty minutes; but maximum temperatures in adult humans are limited to no more than five hours of 41.5-41.7 C/106.7-107 F, and a temperature of 42 C/107.6 F becomes dangerous after a much shorter period.

Rabbits given syphilis inoculations did resist infection if placed in a hot bath (45 C/113 F) for fifteen minutes daily on eleven consecutive days. Injecting the blood of a malarial patient directly is also a bad idea in general for all sorts of reasons (when were they last tested for HIV and hepatitis? I bet it was before the Catastrophe). The sauna (at proper heats, ca. 80 C/176 F) generally does not raise the body temperature to over 39 C/102.2 F in any given 20-minute session, which might not suffice – it has not been tested – but, on the other hand, is a good deal safer in every regard than injecting blood from a malarial patient (when were they last tested for HIV or hepatitis? I bet it was before the Catastrophe). The hot bath rabbit experiment suggests that repeated sessions of Finnish-style sauna might have the potential to be effective between infection and first-stage symptoms, though less likely to be curative for established disease.

The temperature of the sauna itself is ca. 80 degrees (some like it hotter, especially if about to jump through a hole in thick ice and into a freezing lake); the maximum internal human temperature achieved after a standard twenty-minute session is only 39 C/102.2 F., but successive repeated sessions might do the job of prophylaxis (the moral of which is: if you're going to sleep with people who might have contracted syphilis after the Catastrophe, limit yourself to traditional Finns). Happily, a Finnish-style sauna can easily be constructed with hand tools as long as you have trees and a minimal concept of carpentry; many Finns pride themselves on being able to go from trees to sauna in the traditional manner without needing electrical tools.

Be careful to maintain constant hydration and electrolyte balance - water, fruit juice, and a little bit of salt should be taken constantly throughout the process; to monitor the patient temperature; and, if the patient is not used to intense sauna, to make sure that they are monitored to guard against loss of consciousness, etc., and to ensure that there are no signs of carbon monoxide poisoning (always a slight potential risk with home-constructed saunas). A slow cooling between sessions, rather than the traditional cold lake or snow, may be preferable in terms of syphilis prophylaxis, as the elevated temperature will be retained longer. Slow-releasing bismuth (as from a "plug" or implant") was shown to have significant prophylactic effects, and was also used in treatment, while bismuth salts were injected.

Bismuth is the material of choice for non-lead-containing shotgun pellets (the use of lead pellets is no longer allowed in some countries, and bismuth pellets are available everywhere); the object is that, should the animal escape with a few embedded pellets, it will not die of lead poisoning or, if it dies of its wounds, poison any scavenger that feeds on it. This is important to know if you are short on other options and need to find out whether an implanted plug of bismuth protects you as well as it protects a rabbit: at least the treatment won't harm you, although it may or may not do you any good.

As mentioned above, the soluble bismuth salt bismuth subsalicylate is readily available over the counter in Pepto-Bismol and in various other digestive medications, making it something easy to stockpile (or reasonably likely that a character might be able to scavenge after the Catastrophe). The syphilis bacterium is very, very weakly Gram-negative. The most effective stain is the Dieterle stain, of which silver nitrate is the main component. Syphilis bacteria (Treponema pallidum pallidum) appear as spiral-shaped rods, grey or black against a yellow background. Dark-field microscopy is usually recommended; smears must be checked within 10 minutes of taking the sample.

B) Gonorrhea (Neisseria gonorrheae)

Gonorrhea is a remarkably common disease; in 2012, it was estimated as affecting 0.3-1.2% of women and 0.6% of men worldwide. It is the second most common venereal disease, outstripped only by chlamydia. The characteristic symptoms are: discharge (vaginal or penile), inflammation (cervix, penile urethra); burning urination, chiefly in men; lower abdominal pain, chiefly in women. Oral gonorrhoea may cause a sore throat. Skin lesions and joint inflammation (usually single-joint, unilateral; knees are probably the most common site) are rare, but are seen: a single inflamed joint, particularly in a younger patient with no history of trauma or autoimmune disease, should always put gonorrhoea on the list of possible diagnoses. However, ca, 50% of women are asymptomatic, and many more have only slight generalized symptoms which may not readily be clinically identified as gonorrhoea.

One Canadian study also identified as many as 42% of men with gonorrhoea as asymptomatic, excluding patients with even slight generalized symptoms; another study indicated that 2.2% of 2628 sexually active US Army enlisted men had gonorrhoea, and 68% were asymptomatic. A man has a minimum 20% chance of contracting gonorrhoea from an infected woman; a woman has a 60-80% chance of contracting gonorrhoea from an infected man. Gonorrhoea may be passed to an infant from the mother (approximately 28%). It is not possible to evolve immunity to gonorrhoea; one may catch it many times. The prevalence of asymptomatic carriage has contributed very considerably to the difficulty of eradicating gonorrhoea.

Many cases are only discovered by means of tracking contacts of people known to be infected, which is not going to happen with much efficiency after the Catastrophe outside of small and close-knit groups or villages. Together with the increasing lack of access to reliable disease-preventing prophylactics (specifically rubber condoms), and, unfortunately, the high likelihood of a significant increase in rape (physically traumatic sex vastly increases the likelihood of disease transmission) means that the prevalence is likely to increase very significantly. If symptoms appear, they normally begin 4-6 days from the initial infection (the incubation period can be as short as 2 days, or as long as 14).

Complications of gonorrhoea include: systemic inflammation (pustular rash, septic arthritis, meningitis, endocarditis, conjunctivitis). In women, pelvic inflammatory disease and possible infertility due to scarring is a major complication; men may suffer inflammation of the epididymis, urethra, and prostate, and have a higher risk for prostate cancer. Prophylactic drops of 1% silver nitrate are put in the eyes of all babies whose mothers are suspected to suffer from gonorrhoea, to prevent blindness. N. gonorrheae is a Gram-negative diplococcus; it appears as two pink (as opposed to the deep purple of Gram-positive) comma-shaped bacteria facing each other. After the Catastrophe (absent various pre-made culture dishes and carefully temperature-controlled incubators), direct microscopy of smears will still be possible – assuming that you have and, eventually, can make stains, and are able to make and fix slides. Otherwise, a high level of clinical suspicion and getting accurate sexual histories from your patients will have to suffice.

c) Chlamydia (Chlamydia trachomatis)

Chlamydia is an intracellular bacterium, and will be difficult to diagnose after the Catastrophe. It is not even particularly easy to diagnose now; patients treated for gonorrhoea are usually also just treated for chlamydia on general principles, as the two are often found together, and the signs and symptoms (when present) are virtually identical upon clinical examination. It is the most common venereal disease in the world, with a pooled prevalence: est. 2.7% of men, 2.4-6.9% of women worldwide. The common symptoms of chlamydia, when symptomatic (70-80% of infected women and ca. 50% of affected men are asymptomatic), are male urethritis with white pre-urination discharge, and female endocervicitis with odourless mucoid vaginal discharge, =/- painful urination. In men, chlamydia can lead to inflammation of the epididymis and prostate.

In women, though less commonly than gonorrhoea, it can cause pelvic inflammatory disease (PID), salpingitis, endometritis, tubal infertility, and ectopic pregnancies. Both genders are vulnerable to reactive arthritis (affects eyes, external urination, joints). Chlamydia also increases the risk of contracting or transmitting HIV; in pregnant women, it can cause premature membrane rupture/delivery, chorioammonitis, and puerpual and neonatal infections (conjunctivitis leading to blindness, pneumonia possibly leading to death). Even with modern treatment, it is a leading cause of PID and infertility throughout the world. Treatment is normally an injection of azithromycin + doxycycline (also treats gonorrhoea).

The herbal constituent berberine, found in European barberry (Berberis vulgaris), goldenseal (Hydrastis canadensis), and Oregon grape (Mahonia aquifolium, a.k.a. Berberis aquifolium), among others, seems to have strong anti-trachomal effects (both genitally and used for trachoma eye infections, which are still a leading cause of blindness in many countries). The herbal anti-conception compound remedies neem/soapnut saponins/quinine hydrochloride and aloe vera/Indian gooseberry (Phyllanthus emblica; also called amla)/curcumin/soapnut saponins have both shown efficacy against C. trachomatis. The former also showed activity against Gardnerella vaginalis and Candida albicans; The latter showed activity against gonorrhoea, HIV-1, HPV-16, and Candida spp.

d) Yeast infections (Candida albicans)

While the vast majority of yeast infections are not transmitted person-to-person, via sex or otherwise (though it can happen through sex), nor life-threatening in and of themselves, they are exceedingly miserable, and undoubtedly contributed to the earlier beliefs that women, or most women, found sexual intercourse intrinsically painful and unpleasant. If you have a vaginal yeast infection of any real severity, it probably is. Yeast infections also increase the risk of contracting any disease that can be contracted in the relevant location, however it may be transmitted. Yeast is a fungus, and often not subject to antibiotics; sometimes it is even exacerbated by antibiotic use. However, some herbal antimicrobials are also effective against Candida.

Herbs: Lemon juice and lemongrass (Cymbopogon citratus) infusion showed efficacy against oral thrush (C. albicans) in a small trial on HIV patients. Berberine (mentioned above: European barberry, goldenseal, Oregon grape) also showed anti-candidal action. Oregano (Origanum vulgaris) essential oil demonstrated a broad-spectrum antifungal effect, increasing with higher carvacrol content in the oil; it is potentially well-suited for treating both cutaneous and mucosal candida. Garlic, milk thistle extract, thyme, rosemary, dill seed, palmarosa and rose essential oils (high geraniol oil content), and peppermint, among others, have also shown significant anti-candidal action by a variety of mechanisms in vitro, and are considered suitable for further in vivo and clinical investigations.

Coconut oil has been shown to have significant anti-candidal effects, and is mentioned as a strongly possible treatment in real life for Candida, especially given the rise in resistance to current pharmaceutical fungicides. Its mechanism of action is probably based on a high content of capric acid a.k.a. decanoic acid (ca. 10% in coconut oil, vs palm kernel oil at ca. 4%), a fast and effective killer of C. albicans (lauric acid has a longer incubation time, but is more active at low levels). Lauric acid is also present in high amounts in coconut oil, palm kernel oil, and the essential oil of bay laurel (Laurus nobilis). Coconut oil appears to equal the usual pharmaceutical treatment, clotrimazole, in terms of efficacy, and to be superior in terms of side effect profile, cost, ease of use, and patient acceptability.

If available, it is probably the best choice as a carrier oil and a significant functional component of anti-candidal pessaries; as it is a non-toxic food oil, it can also be used safely for oral thrush. Dried coconut meat has lower amounts of capric and lauric acid than the oil, but still probably contains enough to be useful.

Goat milk fat contains ca. 9-14% capric acid; and ca. 3% lauric acid. Yoghurt made from goat cream or at least full-fat goat milk would probably prove a good choice for treating vaginal (or oral) candida as well.

Live yoghurt itself is often touted as a topical treatment for vaginal candidiasis. For once, common Internet lore is right. A small study done in pregnant women in 2012 compared local-topical live yoghurt and honey to pharmaceutical anti-fungal itraconazole. The clinical cure rate was higher in the yoghurt/honey group (87.8% vs. 72.3%), although the mycological cure rate (no yeast detectable microscopically) was higher in the pharmaceutical group (91.5% vs. 76.9%). suggesting that the woman who uses yoghurt and honey is likelier to obtain relief, but also has a higher chance of recurrence.

On the other hand, yoghurt and honey will be much easier to find years after the Catastrophe. A similar study was performed in 2015, comparing live yoghurt/honey to clotrimazole ("Canesten" – the most popular anti-candidal prescribed in real life). Again, the yoghurt/honey group had superior symptom relief ("clinical cure"), whereas the clotrimazole group had superior mycological cure rates.

These results suggest that the woman who uses yoghurt and honey is likelier to obtain relief, but also has a higher chance of recurrence. On the other hand, yoghurt and honey will be much easier to find years after the Catastrophe. Yoghurt is thought to work against candidiasis by means of providing lactobacilli to the vaginal environment, which means that it does have to be live yoghurt.

Honey itself, as well as being known for its antibacterial properties, has shown direct anti-candidal activity in human studies in which honey gel or ointment was used by one group and clotrimazole by the other. The results were largely similar between the two groups in both studies. One study found that itching was relieved to a greater degree by the honey gel and urinary problems (excluding painful urination) were relieved to a greater degree by clotrimazole. The other observed better recovery from inflammation and vaginal discharge in the clotrimazole groups, but no significant difference regarding irritation severity or patient satisfaction with the treatment results. Both recommended that honey be used either as a substitute for, or an adjuvant to, the usual pharmaceutical anti-fungals.

Anecdotally, lemongrass and oregano essential oils are often mentioned as functional treatments for C. albicans, with the usual cautions about dose and dilution. Bay laurel essential oil, due to its lauric acid content, might also be useful, particularly where coconut and palm kernel oils are not available. An in-vitro study investigating ca. 30 essential oils against C. albicans (agar disc diffusion) demonstrated that - as well as oregano - mint, basil, lavender, tea tree oil, and winter savory all performed better in inhibiting candida growth and activity, and inflicted more damage to yeast cell walls and membrane, than did clotrimazole. Fortunately, most of these are easy to grow and to distill the essential oils from (same type of still as you're using to distill your ethanol, although I wouldn't recommend using the same specific still, given the toxicity of some essentials). Pessaries should contain no more than 2 drops of each oil chosen, at a dilution no stronger than 5% maximum total essential oils.

APPENDIX IV:

SOME POSSIBLE ANTI-MICROBIAL HERBS

"First-pass metabolism" is based on the circulation of the human digestive system. Blood passing from anywhere in the GI tract, as well as the spleen and pancreas, drains into the portal vein and passes through the liver before returning to the heart.

At that time, any substances absorbed into the blood from the stomach and intestines are processed through the liver. They may be changed into a form with a different level of activity (inactivated or diminished, activated or enhanced) before reaching general circulation and beginning to take effect.

All ingested oral medications go through first-pass metabolism (if not destroyed by gastric acids first). Topical, inhaled, IM, IV, and mucosal applications avoid first-pass metabolism, and are thus considerably swifter to take effect (especially since the digestive process is not helping to slow absorption) and initially slower to be altered in character or concentration by the metabolic process, though that evens out after a period of time depending on that drug's metabolism in the individual body.

It should be noted that all the studies cited here are in vitro – that is, done with laboratory treatment of bacterial cultures – rather than in vivo – done in real living creatures. The first only shows the potential effectiveness of a substance against specific bacteria; the second is required for such crucial pieces of information as bioavailability (how much is actually absorbed by which routes of administration); concentrations needed to be effective; and, for oral medications, the degree of inactivation either by the digestive system or by first-pass metabolism (processing in the liver). This means, for instance, that even though ordinary black or green tea (Camellia sinensis) has considerable anti-bacterial potential, drinking a few cups of it every day is not guaranteed to dispose of any pathogenic bacteria that have invaded your body; otherwise there would be no bacterial illnesses in Ireland and Britain.

Modern medicine is only now, with the worrying increase in antibiotic-resistant strains of bacteria, beginning to explore the anti-bacterial properties of herbs and their constituents; probably a great deal more will be known about the clinical use of, at least, the effective herbal components in ten years, but we don't know it now. Therefore, if the Catastrophe doesn't hold off until we do know more, these herbs should not be relied upon to cure any serious infection; but when there are no other treatment options available, there is at least a chance that they may improve your odds – and give your author an opportunity to make your survival or recovery, if the plot demands it, at least theoretically plausible.

Be aware that we don't even have established dosages that are both reasonably safe and reasonably efficacious for anti-mycobacterial use for the vast majority of these plants – general safe doses can be checked, but that doesn't prove they're strong enough to work against TB or other mycobacteria - and many of them have the possibility to be very seriously toxic in overdose. Something crucial to keep in mind when administering any drug, whether it came directly from the hospital pharmacy or directly from your garden, is what we call the "Five Rights". Right patient (mainly a concern in the busy clinical setting, where, without proper identification precautions, patients have gotten treatment – sometimes major treatment – intended for someone else); right drug (meaning the correct treatment for the condition; an appropriate treatment for the individual; and making sure that the actual dose used is still within its date and has been stored properly, although more leeway will probably need to be taken with the latter in some cases after the Catastrophe than best practice really allows); right route of administration (people have died as a result of, for instance, receiving a drug that should have been given IV as a spinal injection; on the other side, a patient with a severe acute infection that requires the total absorption and swift action provided by IV antibiotic injection may well not receive sufficient benefit from oral administration to save their life); right dosage (that crucial therapeutic window in which safety and efficacy overlap); right timing (maintaining plasma concentration at the desired level, accounting for absorption and metabolism times).

Where there are only in vitro studies available, the last three rights are impossible to achieve with any kind of certainty. Except in cases where the alternative is certain death (situations that justify, for instance, the inclusion of part III in this book), one of the main goals of the caretaker is not to accidentally kill the patient with the wrong drug, too much of the right one or the right amount of the right one given by the wrong route – all of which can and do happen in real life; many medical protocols have been implemented specifically to prevent the recurrence of such tragedies. As the man said, "First, do no harm." With only a few exceptions (such as cannabis), the active principles of most herbs are extractable by water and ethanol; methanol is often used in laboratory tests, but is not recommended for human use due to being poisonous. Essential oils, as noted previously, are extremely potent concentrates. Some are safe to give orally in minute doses (1-3 drops/day), but topical administration, from which systemic absorption is fairly swift (though less efficient in terms of uptake), is widely considered to be a great deal safer, and also avoids the above-mentioned issue of first-pass metabolism.

I. Gram-positive bacteria and antibacterial herbs

Gram-positive bacteria include: Staphylococcus spp. (including MRSA); Streptococcus spp., Clostridium spp (including C. perfringens – gas gangrene; C tetani – tetanus; C botulinum – botulism; and C. difficile – cause of sometimes-fatal severe post-antibiotic diarrhoea); Listeria; Bacillus anthracis (anthrax); Corynebacterium diptheriae (diphtheria – now almost never seen due to the success of vaccination; but I have spoken to older Irish people who remember their siblings dying of it when they were children); and others. Even modern antibiotics do not always suffice to treat these bacteria – cutaneous anthrax, for instance, responds to antibiotic treatment; but maximal IV antibiotics and intensive care in hospital are by no means guaranteed to save the life of someone with inhalation anthrax (rare in normal life – cutaneous anthrax contracted by working with herbivores or their hides is far more common – but the distribution method of choice in biological warfare/ terrorism.

If that's part of your Catastrophe, be advised that herbal treatments are extremely unlikely to be very helpful). Gram-positive antibacterial herbs: plantain leaves (both Plantago major and Plantago lanceolata – this is the low-growing ground herb common on disturbed and grassy ground throughout Europe and North America, not the small bananas used in various types of ethnic cooking!) are one of the better-studied antibacterials. One component of the plantain has shown efficacy against Gram-positive bacteria in general; and since Staphylococcus and Streptococcus are the two most common causes of infections that start with damaged skin, this is very important to know.

Bay leaf (Laurus nobilis), as well as its potential anti-candidal effects, has also shown in vitro activity against Clostridium botulinum (botulism toxin). Adding bay leaves or a small quantity of bay essential oil (1 drop/3-4 estimated servings) to canned goods of the sort that will not be spoiled by the flavour of bay is likely to have some efficacy against botulism growth in those foods, since that basically is an in-vitro use (no human metabolism or bioavailability issues).

Gram-negative vs. Gram-positive

This distinction tells you what sort of outer coating protection a bacterium has. The Gram-part refers to a stain which soaks into the outer coat of the Gram +, but does not touch the outer coat of the Gram -.

This is important because some bacteria-killing substances can make it through the outer membrane of Gram +, but not Gram – bacteria, or vice versa. A broad-spectrum antibiotic is usually active against both.

After the Catastrophe, this will be very important indeed. Most herbs with anti-bacterial action (plantain, cannabis) only work on Gram + bacteria. Since the Gram + staphylococcus, streptococcus, and worse bacteria such as Clostridia spp (tetanus, gangrene, botulism) are significant threats, these herbs are important.

Verbena officinalis and a few other herbs (see Appendix IV) have been shown, at least in laboratory studies, to be effective against Gram – bacteria such as E. coli (also frequently the offender in urinary infections), S. typhi (typhoid fever), and many other bacterial terrors.

Cannabis (C. sativa) has also shown promising anti-Gram-positive effects (see part II, section I, 4k), as has its close relative hops (Humulus lupulus). Neither has any noticeable effect on Gram-negative bacteria; but both cannabinoids (part II, I, 4k) and hops have shown anti-protozoal capabities (malaria, the African sleeping sicknesses, Chagas disease in the Americas). A recipe from the Anglo-Saxon Bald's Leechbook caused considerable surprise in the medical community, when tested.

Equal parts of garlic and leeks were pounded together, mixed with wine and "bullock's gall" (the experimenters used the bovine bile salts used as supplements for people who have had their gall bladders removed), and left to stand for nine days in glass bottles with sheets of brass (the original called for performing the whole procedure in a brass pot, but there were sterilization issues. The brass of the period was primarily copper which had undergone an alloying reaction with zinc). Their product proved more effective against a multiply-resistant strain of MRSA than did vancomycin (the usual first-line alternative when MRSA has been diagnosed).

II. Gram-negative bacteria; Gram-negative and broad-spectrum antibacterial herbs

Gram-negative bacteria: E. coli; cholera (Vibrio cholerae) and other Vibrio species; the three major venereal diseases (S. pallidum, N. gonorrheae; C. trachomatis); bubonic plague (Yersinia pestis); various gastrointestinal infections (Salmonella, Shigella, Campylobacter, etc.), Helicobacter pylori (cause of stomach ulcers), glanders (Burkholderia mallei), and many, many others.

Gram-negative and broad-spectrum antibacterial herbs: Heal-all (Prunella vulgaris); greater burdock (Arctium lappa – not to be taken internally!); creeping saxifrage (Saxifraga stolonifera - also called Wandering Jew, and other folk names); barberry (Burberis vulgaris); spike lavender (Lavandula latifolia; also called Portugese lavender); corn mint or wild mint (Mentha arvensis); tea (Camellia sinensis – black and green tea both come from this plant; the difference is in preparation) ; Northern white cedar (Thuja occidentalis); white mulberry (Morus alba); thyme (Thymus vulgaris - enables better antibiotic penetration of bacteria), etc.

An ethanol extract of yarrow (Achilleum millefolium) demonstrated a range and efficacy comparable to most penicillin derivatives, though less than that of ampicillin. Water or ethanol extracts and essential oils of clove, cinnamon, oregano, thyme, rosemary, ginger, fennel, coriander, black pepper (particularly ethanol extract), Carum copticum (ajowan), sage (Salvia officialinis), and garlic (fresh being the most effective) all demonstrated antimicrobial effects on multiple Gram + and Gram – bacteria.

Holy basil (Ocimum tulsi), discussed as a contraceptive in the previous appendix, has shown efficacy against V. cholerae (cholera), Staphylococcus aureus, E. coli, Salmonella typhimurium (typhoid fever), Proteus mirabilis (often causes urinary infections esp. in women), Pseudomonas aerugosina (a generally hospital-acquired respiratory infection), and others. Extracted by water or ethanol. Also has immunomodulatory and antiviral properties.

Vervain (Verbena officinalis) demonstrated (ethanolic stem extract) particularly impressive broad-spectrum antibiotic effects in vitro; and as well as its anti-Gram- bacterial effects, was actually more effective against the Gram+ Staphylococcus aureus (the most common cause of staphylococcal infections) than amoxicillin. The stems were consistently the most potent part of this plant, and it produces quite a bit of stem.

Vervain seed has a fairly low germination rate. It needs either to be planted in late summer/early autumn for spring sprouting, or to be cold-stratified for two weeks in the refrigerator; seeds can take 2-3 months to germination. Once established, however, vervain is an extremely hardy plant which naturally self-seeds readily (and is very difficult to pull up when it grows where you don't want it). It can also be propagated by cuttings, usually taken in springtime. It likes full sun, but can tolerate partial shade. Vervain is a perennial.

Rosehip tea and pomegranate blossom tea were effective individually against a range of both Gram + and Gram - bacteria, including Staphlyococcus aureus (Gram +), E. coli (Gram -), E faecalis (Gram -), Klebsiella pneumoniae Gram -, and even Pseudomonas aerugosina (Gram -, and noted as one of the more challenging bacteria to treat with antibiotic therapy. They also had synergistic effects when used with ampicillin, but antagonistic effects towards ciprofloxacin, cefuroxime, erythromycin, and several other antibiotics; the recommendation of the study's authors was that these teas should be used with ampicillin and either avoided with the other antibiotics named, or used alone.

Honey is very well-known as an antimicrobial substance. It works through a combination of mechanisms: acid pH, slow hydrogen peroxide release (enough to damage bacteria, but not human cells), the bee immune system protein defensin-1 (produced by bees and added to honey), and bee lactobacteria (lactobacilli and bifidobacteria, found in bee stomachs and unprocessed honey), various of which have shown both very significant microbial and synergistic effects.

Honey's viscous nature and ability to keep the wound environment moist make it particularly suitable for treating burns, ulcers, deep and superficial infections, and conditions that involve skin damage.

Honey's hygroscopic (absorbs water) character makes it able to soak up fluids such as ulcer exudate, promoting the separation of slough and necrotic tissue from healing flesh; and it may also stimulate immune cells locally. There are some possible indications that certain types of honey (e.g., manuka, although it could probably be overpriced in specialty shops in comparison to the quality of the current evidence) might be more effective than the average; but all types of honey are effective for the purpose.

Two of the researchers on the effects of bee lactobacteria (Tobias Olafsson and Alejandra Vasquez, Lund University) are now studying the efficacy of mead brewed with unprocessed honey as a potential counter to antibiotic resistance. Commercial processing involves heating and sterilizing the honey, which also disposes of beneficial (and honey-tolerant) bee bacteria, and may, for instance, have other effects such as denaturing the defensin-1 protein. Their theory regarding the need to use unprocessed honey is supported by a second study considering the effects of various herbs and honeys against Yersinia enterocolitica (close relative of Y. pestis, or plague; but lacking the slight changes that made plague something more than a moderately annoying infection of the digestive system), unprocessed honey and the herbal extracts showed in vitro efficacy comparable to that of most antibiotics, whereas the effect of processed honey was essentially nil.

The Lund researchers' Honey Hunter's Elixir, developed with biotech company ConCellae AB, is now commercially available – and aside from its potential role in combating antibiotic resistance, is also very nice mead. The effect of fermentation on honey's antimicrobial capabilities is not fully determined yet, however. It should be noted that a certain amount of morphine may be found in honey produced near opium poppy fields, and rhododendron honey (contains grayanotoxin, which is found in many of the plants from the Ericaceae family) is not only a known somewhat-toxic hallucinogen, but used deliberately as an entheogen by the Nepalese Gurung tribe. This may or may not explain the reputation of the legendary Pictish drink "heather ale", which may well have contained heather honey as well as flowers (brewing with the flowers, pleasant as the flavour is, will not cause psychoactivity beyond the alcoholic in the drinker. I know this from experience. The grayanotoxin is concentrated in the honey).

Vinegar (ca. 6% acetic acid used, only marginally stronger than supermarket vinegar) demonstrated great effectiveness in killing TB bacteria (mycobacteria, below) on surfaces, and has been proposed as a possible anti-TB disinfectant which might prove to be extremely useful in low-resource countries/areas ...or after the Catastrophe. It is also effective against a wide range of bacterial pathogens; easy to make; and even in real life, is considered an optimum kitchen disinfectant even on wooden items into which meat, eggs, or fish might have soaked!

III. Mycobacteria and anti-mycobacterial herbs

The mycobacteria include two great cultural scourges: tuberculosis (Mycobacterium tuberculae) and leprosy (Mycobacterium leprae), as well as the more common atypical (sometimes "walking") pneumonia. Mycobacteria are intracellular, taking up residence inside the host cells, and therefore are difficult to eradicate with antibiotics. Usually at least a 6-12 month period of simultaneous treatment with multiple drugs, both for immediate effect and to diminish the evolution of resistance, is required for tuberculosis and leprosy.

Possible anti-mycobacterial herbs include (but are not limited to): Aloe vera (gel used directly); Andrographis panniculata; ashwaganda (Withania somnifera); black pepper (Piper nigrum); chaste tree (Vitex trifolium); cutch tree (Acacia catechu, a.k.a. black cutch) garlic (Allium sativum – 80 mg/ml of garlic essential oil was found comparable to anti-mycobacterial drug rifampicin); nettle (Urtica dioica), red onion (Allium cepa); St. John's wort (Hypericum perforatum) and other Hypericum species.

Many of these herbs are tropical by origin. Andrographis panniculata is an annual, growing well from seed and preferring full sun and humidity; it can be grown anywhere that has a warm summer, and if left to run to seed, self-seeds readily. Ashwaganda prefers temperatures between 70-90 F; likes being dry and tolerates drought; and is usually either harvested (roots) before first frost, or brought indoors over the winter.

Black pepper vines can be grown in a greenhouse or indoors with good light in temperate climates (most of Europe and North America), but start to die when temperatures get down to 60 F/16 C. They do not tolerate dry soil. Fresh peppercorns must be bought for viable seed; those found in grocery shops have been dried and probably given germination-discouraging treatment.

Chaste tree is hardier; it may suffer some frost-kill in winter, and should probably be grown in a pot and brought indoors for its first few winters, but generally revives as long as the winter is not too long or too harsh (not below -10 F/-23 C, which covers most of Western Europe and the US south of Idaho (moving upwards along the Pacific and Atlantic coasts). Garlic, stinging nettle, red onion, and St. John's wort are all easily grown throughout Europe and North America.

Sweet wormwood (Artemisa annua, a.k.a. Sweet Annie). Artemisinin, the compound derived from this plant from which artemether (now a first-line treatment for malaria as part of combination therapy) is made, does not directly kill mycobacteria, but prevents tuberculosis bacteria from becoming dormant and increases their susceptibility to antibiotics.

Other artemisias also contain artemisinin, but at lower concentrations. Artemisia absinthium, the common wormwood, had significantly higher concentrations in the flowers than in the leaves; root concentrations were very low for all tested species, and stem concentrations were consistently lower than flowers or leaves.

Artemisinin derivatives have been observed to kill other parasites such as Schistosoma spp (blood flukes); Toxoplasma gondii, Babesia, and trypanosomes (sleeping sickness – Africa; Chagas disease – Americas). They have also shown anti-viral activity (notably against hepatitis B and C, various herpesviruses, HIV-1, influenza A) and anti-cancer activity.

Be aware that the artemisias all contain fairly high percentages of thujone, which is quite toxic; the essential oils of any of these plants (mugwort, rue, various wormwoods) should be avoided in general; definitely not used orally; and totally avoided in anyone with a history of seizures, convulsions, or other neurological disorders. Sweet wormwood is a hardy perennial that, like the other wormwoods and artemisias in general, prefers full sun and a well-drained, somewhat dryish location. It can be grown from seed.

Ethanol extracts of hops (Humulus lupulus) are being very seriously considered in the management of rifampin-resistant tuberculosis, since, at least in vitro, this seems to work as effectively as rifampin – one of the standard elements of the anti-mycobacterial regimen! The concentrations used were 4 mg/ml and 8 mg/ml. Of course, we do not yet know the best way to deliver this to a real patient – it could be inactivated in the gut or liver with oral absorption. Inhalation by means of steam might be a therapeutic option for tuberculosis of the lungs; IV injection of homemade anything is generally not a good option, but dying of tuberculosis is a rather worse one.

IV. Antiviral Herbs

Basil (Ocimum basilicum; sweet or common basil) contains compounds effective against various DNA-viruses, in particular ursolic acid, apigenin, and linalool. Extracts showed activity against herpesviruses, adenoviruses (one of the types that cause cold), and hepatitis B, as well as the RNA-viruses coxsackie virus B1 and enterovirus 71.

Echinacea (Echinacea purpura). In vitro studies demonstrated that the A. Vogel preparation Echinaforce (1 dose = 20 drops = 614 mg fresh aerial parts + 32 mg roots, extracted into 65% ethanol) inactivated the influenza viruses H1N1 type 4, swine origin influenza virus, and highly pathogenic avian influenza viruses (HPAIV) H5 and H7 – that is, the strains of influenza currently considered to be among the most likely to mutate into pandemic-level outbreaks.

Effective concentrations in the culture dishes ranged from the recommended oral dose to several orders of magnitude lower, though of course there are always the issues of gastric inactivation and first-pass metabolism to be considered where efficacy for human use is concerned. Of some importance also is the fact that resistant strains did not appear to emerge from the echinacea tests, as they do with Tamiflu (oseltamivir – itself synthesized from shikimic acid, originally derived from Chinese star anise, Illicium verum).

Echinacea appears to inhibit haemoagglutinase, an enzyme which contributes to the virus' entry into cells; direct contact was required, suggesting that treatment early in infection is necessary for efficacy. The authors conclude that the potential efficacy, lack of resistance development, ready availability, and lack of toxicity in human use make echinacea extract a good possible option for controlling and treating influenza viruses. Echinacea has also been evaluated for possible interactions with pharmaceutical drugs metabolized by the liver's cytochrome P450 system, and there do not appear to be any such interactions. Echinacea is best known as an immunostimulant/immunomodulator, and pre-clinical studies have indeed demonstrated activation of various immune system cells.

There is little evidence for its effect in preventing, in particular, upper respiratory infections; rather more substantial evidence for its effect in treating those (and perhaps other viral infections). The antiviral effect may prove to be more significant in terms of clinical use of this herb than the general prophylactic use. Echinacea, a.k.a. "purple coneflower", is a hardy perennial that grows easily from seed and can flower from its first year, though may not flower consistently until its second. Native to prairies and open woodland, echinacea will grow in full sun or partial shade, and tolerates a wide range of soil conditions, although it does best in rich, well-drained soil with good sunlight. It likes a bit of moisture, but can tolerate long droughts very well; it is also quite able to withstand very hot summers and very cold winters, as one might expect of a plant that thrives on the North American plains.

Seeds germinate most easily with stratification; sow in the autumn for spring sprouting, and space at ca. 1' (roughly 32 cm.) apart. Echinacea will spread out on its own to form clumps and self-seed, and can also be propagated by root division in the autumn. In addition to its medicinal value, echinacea is also noted for its large purple, pink, or sometimes white daisy-like flowers with their golden-orange "cone" in the center, and its hardy perennial nature and reliable blooms make it a great favourite for the cottage or country garden. It stands 3-4' tall (or 1 metre, give or take a few centimetres either way) and will bloom throughout the summer, especially if deadheaded regularly and given the odd bit of extra nitrogen in the spring and potassium in the summer. Stems can be cut back in late autumn after the plant has gone to seed; it will renew itself quite vigorously in the spring.

Seeds of this plant are often available at garden centres, and are more likely to be classed as "ornamental flowers" than as herbs, often going by the alternate name of "purple coneflower". Look for the Linnean name Echinacea purpurea. E. angustifolia ("narrow-leaved purple coneflower") is also grown as a garden plant; it is not as well-studied as E. purpurea, but appears to be generally comparable, as does E. pallida. However, E. purpurea is generally the standard variety used by both pharmacological researchers and most herbal practitioners.

Elder (Sambuca nigra). The flowers, which usually appear in June, cover the tree with a great number of white umbels. The berries usually ripen between early September and the end of October. Flowers and berries are both used. An diluted elderberry liquid extract (standardized at 18:1 elderberry:extract ratio; dilutions showed significant efficacy at 5%, with maximum effect by 15%) demonstrated, in vitro, strong activity against both influenza B and the most common Gram-positive and Gram-negative bacteria which cause bacterial superinfections in patients with viral influenza (Streptococcus groups C, G, and pyogenes; Branhamella catarrhalis, Haemophilus influenzae).

Elderberry syrup (38% standardized extract; 15 ml 4x/day for 5 days) was shown in a clinical study to reduce influenza symptom duration by 4 days, with no reported adverse side effects.

Both flowers and berries are usually made into cordials, syrups, or wines/meads, although they can also be infused in hot water. They are used both dry and fresh. If brewing, the berries are acrid enough that some people find them unpleasant in conjunction with honey (as a mead), but the flowers are excellent in mead, brewed at a proportion of 3 lbs (approx. 1.5 kg, if you like) honey to 240 gr (roughly 8 oz) dried flowers to 1 gallon of water (if using berries, it's 3 lbs berries/3 lbs honey or sugar/1 gallon water).

Elder trees grow to ca. 30-40' tall, and are very quick to grow and produce flowers and fruit. They thrive in every climate from Texas to Scandinavia – in fact, I bought a small treelet in my first undergraduate year in Dallas, and when I moved out to graduate school, it took my mother about five seconds to execute it for the crime of having eaten half her backyard. I have seen elder trees thriving equally well halfway between the south of Sweden and the Arctic Circle.

Hops (Humulus lupulus) – In addition to their anti-bacterial and anti-plasmodial capabilities, hops – specifically the hops component xanthohumol – have been shown to have activity against cytomegalovirus, herpes simplex viruses 1 and 2, and HIV-1.

Lemon Balm (Melissa officinalis) has been shown to be active in vitro (water-based extract) against the herpes simplex virus; the main active component seems to be rosmarinic acid, also present in rosemary, basil, holy basil, thyme, marjoram, and self-heal (Prunella vulgaris). It is considered virucidal, and prevents the attachment of HSV to human cells. Lemon balm essential oil also showed antiviral effects at multiple stages of H292 influenza viral replication, and a synergistic effect when combined with oseltamivir.

Lemon balm should be used with caution in people with low thyroid function, as it can affect thyroid function and production, as well as interfering with thyroid hormone replacement.

KIOM-C consists of Scutellariae Radix, Glycyrrhizae Radix, Paeoniae Radix Alba, Platycodongrandiflorum, and Zingiberofficinaletc [7]. Fifty grams (g) of KIOM-C formula was placed in 1 liter of distilled water and extracted by heating for 3 hours (h) at 115°C using a medical heating plate (Gyeongseo Extractor Cosmos-600, Incheon, Korea). After extraction, KIOM-C was filtered out using testing sieves (150 μm) (Millex, Darmstadt, Germany), lyophilized, and stored in desiccators at 4°C. The extract was prepared by combining 10 g KIOM-C with 100 ml phosphate-buffered saline (PBS), vortexing for 30 min, and centrifuging the mixture at 2000 X g for 15 min. The supernatant was collected, and the pH was adjusted to 7.0.

The total aqueous extract was then subjected to membrane syringe filtration (0.45 and 0.22 μm) (Millex, Darmstadt, Germany) and stored at 4°C until administration. This combination demonstrated significant anti-viral effects in vitro, and significant protection of mice against fatal influenza infection (80-100% survival of various influenza subtypes, after inoculation with 5x the concentration of viruses required for lethality.

MECHANISM	INTERFERE WITH CELL WALL SYNTHESIS	Inhibit protein synthesis, preventing translation.	INHIBIT NUCLEIC ACID SYNTHESIS
BACTERIA	Gram-positives: streptococcus, staphylococcus, and others Gram-positives: streptococcus, staphylococcus, and others	BROAD SPECTRUM	Fluoroquinolones are usually broad spectrum; rifampicin is used for TB.
ANTIBIOTIC TYPES	BETA-LACTAM ANTIBIOTICS: PENICILLINS, CARBAPENEMS, CEPHALOSPORINS	Tetracyclines, macrolides,	Quinolones/ fluoroquinolones; metranidozole; rifampicin
SAMPLE ANTIBIOTICS	Penicillin, ampicillin meropenem; cephalexin (Keflex), ceftriaxone	Tetracycline, doxycycline; azithromycin, erythromycin, clarithromycin	Ciprofloxacin, ofloxacin, and others
HERBS	Self-heal (Prunella vulgaris) Vervain (Verbena officinalis)	Clustered gentian (Gentiana triflora), creeping saxifrage creeping saxifrage (Saxifraga stolonifera, self-heal	Berberine, found in European barberry (B. vulgaris), Oregon grape (Berberis aquifolium), goldenseal (Hydrastis canadensis)

V. Herbal antimicrobial action

BY MECHANISM: WHICH ANTIBIOTICS DO WHICH HERBS WORK LIKE? CCLXVIII

Appendix V: A Few Useful General Survival/Pre-20th Century Living Texts

A Practical Chemist. United States Practical Receipt Book, or, Complete Book of Reference for the Manufacturer, Tradesman, Agriculturalist, or Housewife, Containing Many Thousand Valuable Receipts in all the Useful and Domestic Arts (Philadelphia: Lindsay & Blakiston, 1849). And the author isn't overstating things in that description, either.

Cement-making, home-brewing, various home remedies (of, all right, possibly dubious character), varnish-making, and just about everything else you can imagine. Full text can be read on-line at https://babel.hathitrust.org/cgi/pt?id=mdp.39015093180779;view=1up;seq=9

Carla Emery. An Encyclopedia of Country Living, 10th edn (Seattle: Sasquatch Books, 2008). This book has just about everything you'd need to know; it is reliable, practical, and based on Carla Emery's own extensive experience. No survivalist or smallholder should be without it.

Mrs. M. Grieve. A Modern Herbal (London: Jonathan Cape, 1931; various reprints available). I've referenced and recommended this before in this book, but if you're planning to survive and stay well after the Catastrophe, you really can't do without it. Can be read online or ordered as a hardcopy at: https://botanical.com/botanical/mgmh/mgmh.html

John Seymour. The New Complete Guide to Self-Sufficiency, rev. edn. (Dorling Kimbersley, 2003). This book was the Bible of the self-sufficiency/smallholding movement that was particularly popular in Britain and Ireland in the nineties and the first decade of 2000. The one caveat: Seymour was born in 1914 and grew up as a smallholder, doing things in the old ways. His instructions do not always suffice completely for the newbie.

Things like making sausage casings out of intestines are not as easy for someone who didn't grow up doing it as he makes them sound (we gave up after our first go and just bought our sheep-gut sausage casings from a local company. Of course, after the Catastrophe, you'll have to stick with that kind of thing until you actually do get it right). A wide range of specialty books are readily available on every topic from slaughtering, butchering, and smoking your own meat, to various weapons and improvised devices for home/settlement defense. And, of course, there is a vast amount of material on the Internet, some of which is good.

One thing that the prepper character needs to remember when collecting sources for electronic reading: if you think you'll need it after the Catastrophe, print it out! You can't depend on the power being on when you need to check something crucial. There is an excellent list of recommendations on James Wesley Rowles' website. As an author of fiction, the guy is complete crap; and his personal focus is not on basic functional things like feeding and clothing the survivors, but on the other basic and necessary functional survivor thing that is "not getting killed by raiders or warlords", in regards to which he's pretty good. Apparently his wife did all the food/clothing stuff, so he thinks it's easy. Well, it is, if you can just say, "I need a warm jumper" and have it magically appear from your partner's skilled hands. I can vouch for that, because I do it all the time.

My wife, who can turn a sheep into a jumper in a couple of days (another two or three if colouring is requested), was not as impressed by his casual attitude. His recommendation list, however, is first-rate: https://survivalblog.com/bookshelf/. And I am amused to note that we have some rather similar tastes in survivalist fiction – he even gets in at least one rather good, but dead obscure novel (Vandenberg, by Oliver Lange), which I thought I was the only human being on earth that had read it outside of the author and his mother.

Also, his first novel (originally titled Triple-Ought) sucked the Mazola by all literary standards, but it had one thing going for it: the realistic portrayal of how, when the world falls apart, religion (he's apparently a fundie Christianoid fanatic himself; not an actual Christian in the sense of following Christ's teachings, but Christianoid, which shows up in his book – along with simple stupids such as thinking that major pain control is not necessary for major injuries, at least in the original Triple-Ought ms.; but he at least had the decency to recognise Judaism as a real religion) is one of the most important aspects in keeping people sane and functional through the worst times. Any religion in which people believe will do that crucial job. That makes slogging through his horrible prose worthwhile in itself, at least for one book.

Appendix VI: Some Fictional Works of Interest

Here I list some fictional works – several of which I have referenced in the text – which show a variety of approaches and possibilities for post-apocalyptic fiction, on the grounds that it is generally useful to know what other authors writing in your general category have done. Also, if you're interested enough in the genre to consider writing in it, you may just enjoy a lot of these.

Gordon Dickson
Wolf and Iron. The survivalist side is largely plausible (although the small nuclear family probably has roughly a monkey's chance of living long enough to see their kids grow up if they don't have any other support), and I can speak from experience when I say that the author has either raised a wolf, or did a lot of first-rate research. Actually, I found this work very useful when the time came that we had a wolf-cross (not even a full-blooded wolf, a medium-percentage cross) to care for, which inclines me to think highly about the realism-factor of the rest of it.

Pat Frank
Alas, Babylon (J.B. Lippincott, 1959). A classic post-nuke novel from the late '50s. Generally, together with Stewart's Earth Abides, regarded as one of the seminal novels of the post-apocalyptic genre.

Diana Gabaldon – Outlander series. In which a 20th century woman (a nurse in the first book; becomes a doctor in preparation for her return later in the series) is cast back into the 18th century. Particularly notable for its examination of medical possibilities for someone with 20th century knowledge in an 18th century situation – not a bad analogue for post-apocalyptic life – and for the extensive research done on real herbalism (and many other cultural, historical, and practical matters) by the author. The high degree of realism and exactitude of historical detail has undoubtedly contributed considerably to the great success of this series (although the whole big hairy manly kilted-Scot romance thing probably did too. One could, if one wished, describe these books as "the thinking person's romance novels", but there is a good bit more to them than that).

Outlander (UK title Cross-Stitch; Dell, 1990); Dragonfly in Amber (1992); Voyager (1994); Drums of Autumn (1997); The Fiery Cross (2001); A Breath of Snow and Ashes (2005); An Echo in the Bone (2009); Written in My Own Heart's Blood (2014).

Robert A. Heinlein
Expanded Universe (Ace, 1980). A selection of short stories and essays by The Master Himself, several of which deal with disaster/survival situations (focusing particularly on the US after losing a war to – specifically or implied – Russia).

Farnham's Freehold (Putnam, 1964). Another classic, pointing out the benefits (and some possible mistakes) in disaster preparation, and the kind of personal problems that can arise even in small family groups.

Dean Ing.
Pulling Through (Ace, 1983). Another post-nuke survivalist novel, particularly noted for its excellent, realistic, and precise detail on preparation and the post-disaster construction of various crucial devices. The book has sometimes been described, roughly, as, "half fiction, half survival manual", which is pretty fair; but it is also a good read.

Larry Niven and Jerry Pournelle.
Lucifer's Hammer (Del Rey, 1977). In this book, the cause of the apocalypse is a massive meteor strike. A long-time major favourite in the field by one of science fiction's best collaborative pairings; many interesting explorations of survival (and changing social) possibilities after a sudden catastrophe.

John Ringo – Council War series. A rather clever and quite entertaining twist on the post-apocalyptic, starting in a far-future world where genetic manipulation and nanotechnology give us the stuff of fantasy in a science-fiction manner. An induced breakdown throws the world back upon primitive devices; there is a good explanation for why gunpowder, etc., can't be utilized.

Progresses in some interesting ways as the series goes along; and for all its occasional flaws (metric system, Ringo, metric system! No, you can't just extract numbers from the lowest section of your GI tract when you want them!), one can't complain too hard about a series in which, eventually, "orcs in space" is actually made to work pretty well.

Ringo's thorough knowledge of military organization, psychology, theory, and practice is the "thumb" to his realist hand, even if once in a while he might make that hand work like a foot in some other ways.

There Will Be Dragons (Simon & Schuster, 2003); The Emerald Sea (including the novella "In the Time of Darkness"; 2004); Against the Tide (2005); East of the Sun, West of the Moon (2006).

Neville Shute.
On the Beach (Heinemann, 1957). A really depressing post-nuclear novel from the late '50s, when nuclear war was on everyone's mind. Again, one of the classics of the genre, though it is less survivalist and more philosophical/psychological.

George R. Stewart.

Earth Abides (Random House, 1949). An occasionally worryingly realistic post-plague novel, pointing out that there is no guarantee that random survivors will necessarily be the most capable or motivated people in the world. Yet another great post-apocalyptic classic.

S.M. Stirling –

Nantucket series. In which the whole island of Nantucket ends up back in the Bronze Age, with their only modern resources being what is present on the island at the time or what they can make themselves.

Island in the Sea of Time (Roc, 1998); Against the Tide of Years (1999); On the Oceans of Eternity (2000).

Emberverse series. In which everyone who was not on Nantucket when the island was translocated (transtemporated?) in the previous trilogy finds out that the laws of nature have changed – electricity, gunpowder, and a number of other things no longer work. Society disintegrates and gradually re-evolves in some very interesting ways indeed. Reading the Nantucket trilogy first is a good idea; there are some bits later on in the series that don't make much sense otherwise.

Dies the Fire (Roc, 2004); The Protector's War (2005); A Meeting at Corvallis (2006); The Sunrise Lands (2007); The Scourge of God (2008); Sword of the Lady (2009); High King of Montival (2010); Tears of the Sun (2011); Lord of Mountains (2012); The Given Sacrifice (2013); The Golden Princess (2014); The Desert and the Blade (2015); Prince of Outcasts (2016); The Sea People (2017); The Sky-Blue Wolves (2018).

Almost everything written by S.M. Stirling is, in my opinion, pretty wonderful; even his bottom percentile is well above the level of most other authors. These, however – especially the Nantucket series and the first three Emberverse books – are the books of most interest in a post-apocalyptic sense. His Peshawar Lancers (Roc, 2002) is also technically post-apocalyptic (massive meteor strikes); but since it is set generations after the apocalypse in question, it isn't really particularly relevant to the survival-novel context - though a brilliant read in and of itself, especially if one loves Kipling and/or harbours a sneaking fondness for Sir Harry Flashman.

Image Sources

Blue Poppy-1855 Sketch by Walter Hood Fitch [19=817-1892]
P. nudicaule-1830 Sketch by L. Curtis, Botanical Magazine, Issue 52
P. oriental-Oriental Poppy & Virginal Bluebells, 1812, The New Botanical Garden, v.1 page 42. Sketch by ST. Edwards
Red Poppy-Sketch by John Lindsey [1821-1826]
Drama Queen-http://lindacochran.blogspot.com/2012/06/papaver-drama-queen.html

Some Images/illustrations for those seeking out plants in the wild.

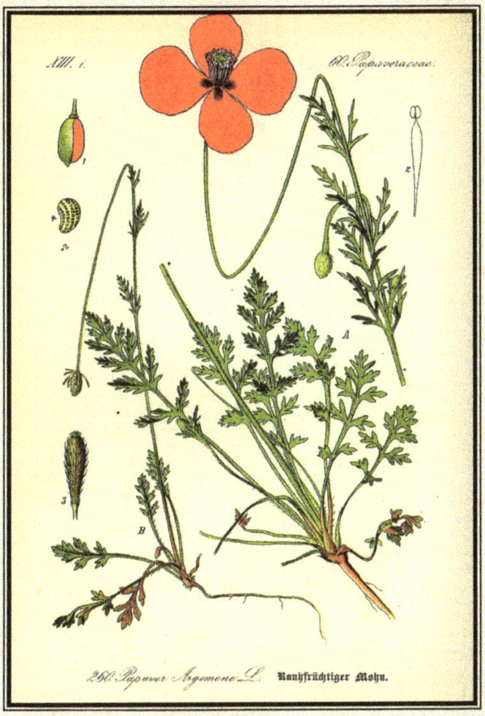

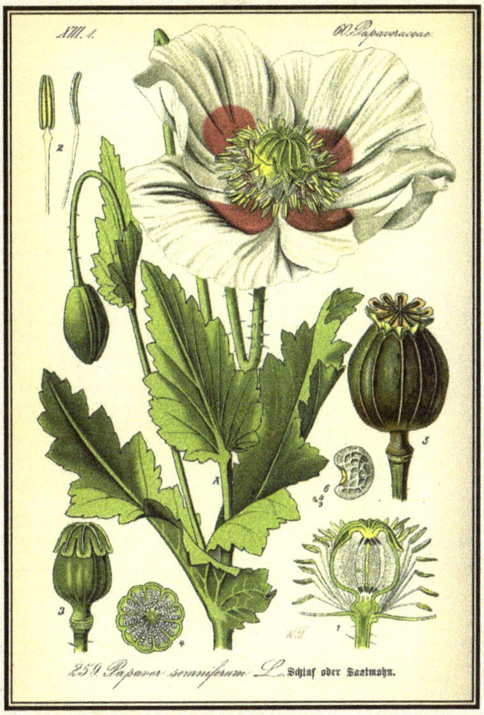

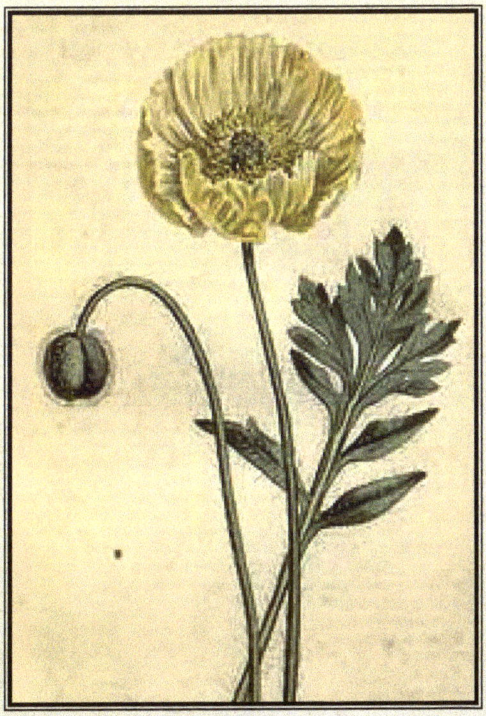

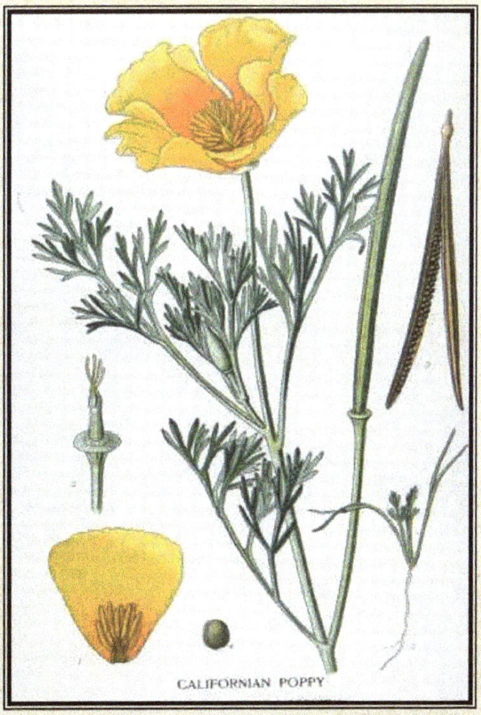

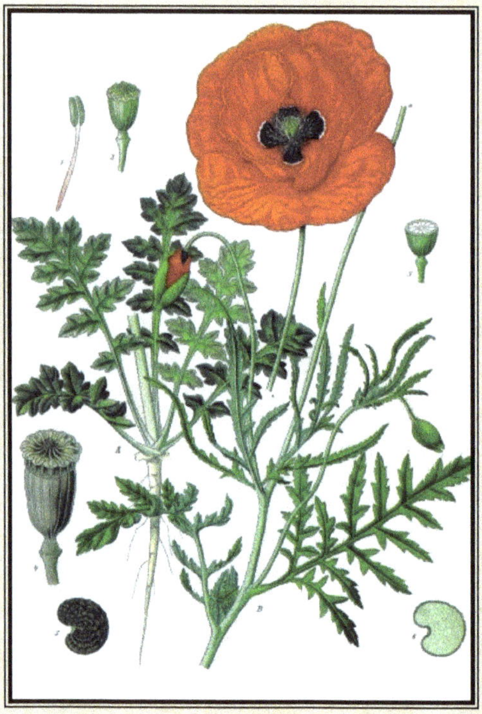
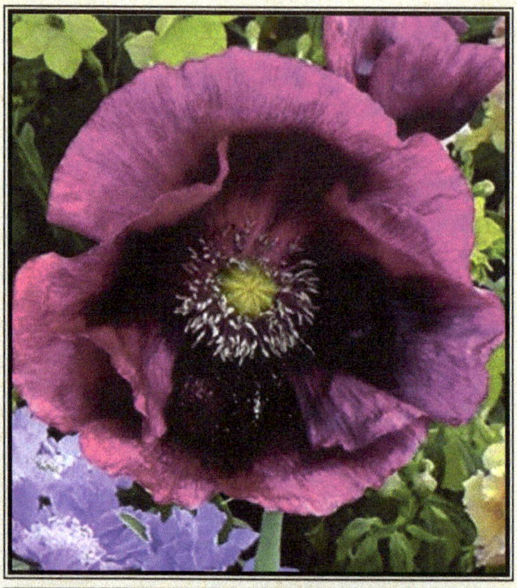
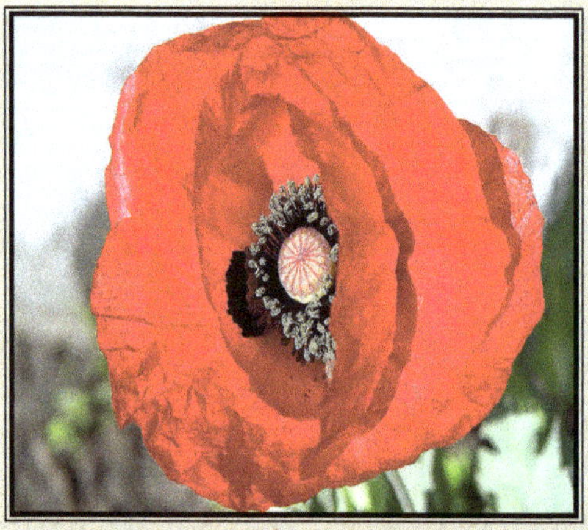
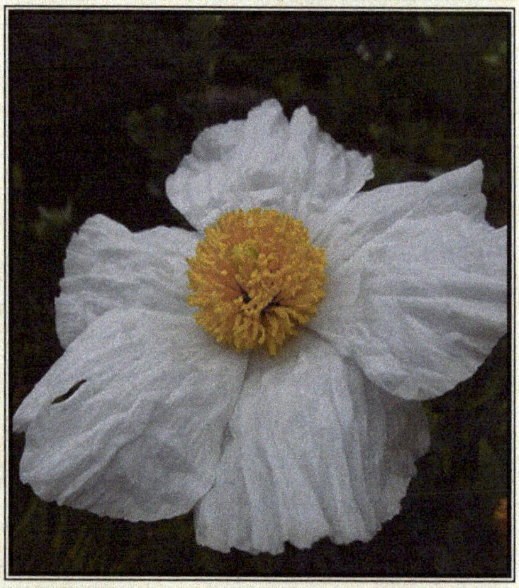
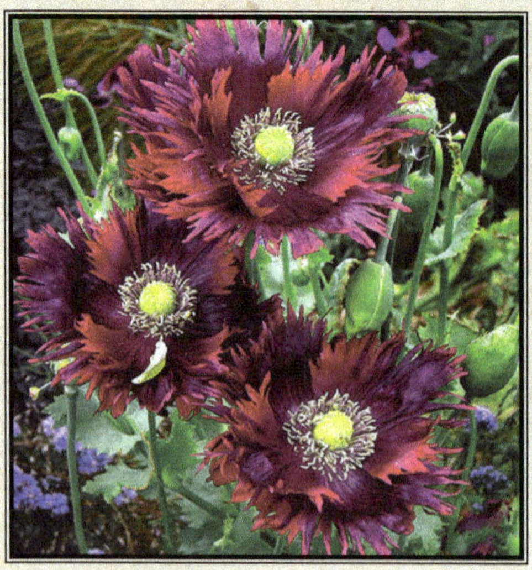
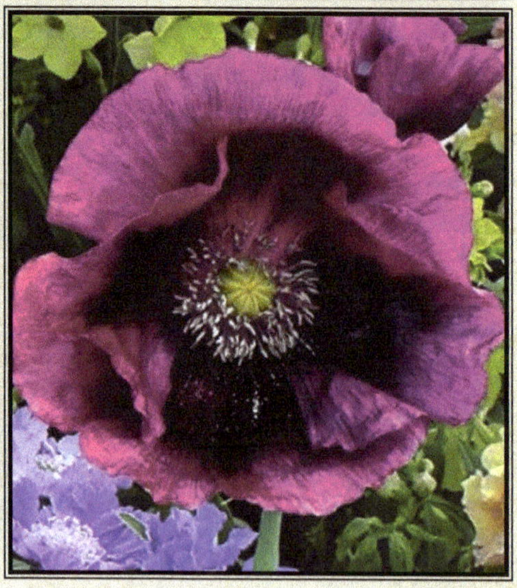

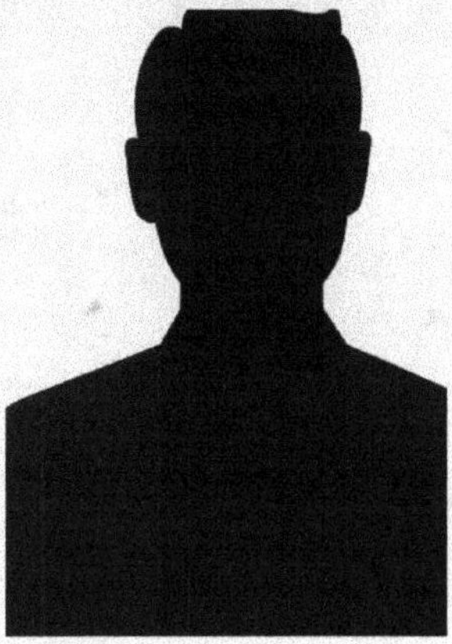

Simon Von Wolife is a survivalist and author of the Curiosity Apothocarious newsletter, in which he advocated using correct research, dosages and proper preparation in film, books and television to keep people from harm. His work was sought out by those seeking to have a better understanding of herbal medicines. Post Apocalyptic Herbology is his attempt to educate, promote and support authors in writing that involves periods of time for which pharmaceuticals may nor may not exist. His current abode is accessible to those who seek out the mysterious places of the imagination where creatures of the past still roam.

TLS

The Three Little Sisters

The Three Little Sisters is an indie publisher that puts authors first. We specalize in the strange and unusual. From titles about pagan and heathen spirituality to traditional fiction we bring books to life.

https://the3littlesisters.com

www.ingramcontent.com/pod-product-compliance
Lightning Source LLC
LaVergne TN
LVHW070849210926
848482LV00016B/896
* 9 7 8 1 9 5 9 3 5 0 0 8 8 *